Confronting the AIDS Epidemic:

Cross-Cultural Perspectives on HIV/AIDS Education

Edited by

Davidson C. Umeh

Africa World Press, Inc.

P.O. Box 1892
Trenton, NJ 08607

P.O. Box 48
Asmara, ERITREA

Africa World Press, Inc.

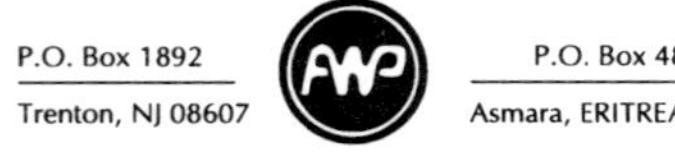

First Printing 1997

Cover and Book design: Jonathan Gullery

This book is set in Times New Roman, Helvetica and Missive

Library of Congress Cataloging-in-Publication Data

Confronting the AIDS epidemic : cross-cultural perspectives on
HIV/AIDS education / edited by Davidson C. Umeh.
p. cm.
Includes bibliographical references and index.
ISBN 0-86543-526-X (cloth). -- ISBN 0-86543-527-8 (paper : alk. paper)
1. AIDS (Disease)--Cross-cultural studies. 2. AIDS (Disease) --Prevention--Cross-cultural studies. I. Umeh, Davidson Chukwuma.
RA644.A25C634 1997
614.5'99392--dc21

97-550
CIP

PRINTED IN CANADA

To the memory of my parents
Jonah and Priscilla Umeohanu

Contents

Acknowledgements

Confronting the AIDS Epidemic could not have been completed without the support and encouragement of several people. First, I want to thank the students in my class, "Contemporary Health Problems," where the need and idea for this book was initiated. I am also grateful to Susan Larkin for her unfailing support and confidence in me which played a great role in the completion of this anthology. I am very indebted to Robert Fox for constant referral to relevant articles that were of immense help. Special thanks goes to Chikwenye Okonjo-Ogunyemi for reading and suggesting improvements to the introduction of the book. I am very indebted to my mentor and friend, Edward J. Hart, for reading the introduction to the various parts of the text, his inspiration and superb suggestions. I also thank Uchenna C. Nwosu for reading through the entire manuscript and for his invaluable suggestions.

I am especially grateful to my wife, Marie Umeh, who edited, and critiqued my work. A special debt of gratitude goes to my children, Esther, Ikechukwu, Uchenna, Chizoba and Ugochukwu for their maturity and understanding.

I thank John Taveras for transfering files from computer diskettes and making the computer environments compatible. I am most grateful to my publisher Kassahun Checole and his editorial staff for their patience and competence in managing the project.

Finally, my deepest gratitude goes to my parents Mr. and Mrs. Jonah Umeohanu, who taught me the virtues of patience, confidence and perseverance which I really needed to complete this book.

Foreword

One chapter in the story of the human struggle for survival is the epic battle against disease. In this arena, the struggle seems endless, punctuated by moments of triumph and despair, marked by an illusion of hope when a new vaccine or therapy is discovered and tempered by the specter of threat and helplessness when some new disease arises. No war, no circumstance of political oppression, no famine or natural disaster has ravaged us both physically and mentally the way disease has over the course of human history.

The great plagues that swept through Europe in the 14th and 15th centuries are a testament to the suffering and misery levied by unchecked disease. In recent years new diseases have begun to emerge that remind us of our own vulnerabilities and, in some ways, connect us with our past. HIV/AIDS is a reminder that the plagues of the past may be lying in wait, nearer than we would like to admit.

One wonders how our ancestors responded to the great plagues of yesteryear, how much of their behavior was rooted in their beliefs and perceptions of the world around them. Looking back, there is no doubt that the course of those great epidemics was, in part, sustained by human ignorance, myths and cultural imperatives that existed at the time. How far have we come since then? In one sense, a long way. Modern medicine has joined with science (rather than superstition) to produce cures unimagined four or five centuries ago; yet, in another sense, little has changed. Ignorance, myth and cultural beliefs still play important roles in our response to the modern plague:AIDS.

AIDS is a special disease. It is special because, among other things, it is tied to a topic that has almost universal conflict and myth associated with it: sexuality. One cannot discuss the issue of AIDS without considering the role of sexual attitudes as part of the problem. From an international perspective, each culture presents certain unique features but in each the burden of sexual tradition is unmistakably clear. The inability of women to negotiate condom usage with their partners because of male domination and male attitudes toward sex roles, the dependency of women on men for economic security:perpetuated by poverty and tradition, and the impact of prostitution dominate the human side of the AIDS equation. Cultures as varied as Nigeria, Kenya and Native Americans are brought to life in this collection of original essays showing how universal themes such as power inequities between the sexes serve to bridge the gap between the past and the present, as well as between these diverse cultures around the world, revealing a common thread across humanity.

The insidious epidemic continues to spread, fueled by ignorance and cultural belief systems. Special populations in the U.S. appear particularly at risk. For example, gay and lesbian individuals still labor under the yoke of "mainstream" sexual attitudes, while the reproductive mandate of the Judaeo-Christian heritage often times serves to create a climate of blame for their lifestyle rather than to promote solutions to the problem. Other groups, such as the physically or mentally challenged may lack their own resources to deal with the problem and often get little help from mainstream America. Minorities and recent immigrants may be dealing with priorities in their lives other than AIDS prevention and, even if they are concerned, the resources, educational or otherwise, may not be forthcoming.

AIDS continues to touch upon some of our most deep-seated moral dilemmas. The conflict between long-cherished values of tolerance for persons who are different or needy may clash with the irrational urge to reject and distance ourselves from those afflicted. In part, the rejection is rooted in self-preservation but one also wonders how much of it is flavored by bigotry toward those whose lifestyle is different from our own.

Dr. Umeh's collection of essays contributes much to our understanding of AIDS. The reader is immediately struck by the diversity of human responses to this complex and baffling disease but, on closer scrutiny, one is also struck by how similarly we react to the threat,no matter where we live.

Edward J. Hart, Ph. D., CHES
Bridgewater State College,
Bridgewater, Massachusetts

PREFACE

In my practice as a specialist in High Risk Obstetrics I often have occasion to watch a sexual power-play between couples. I would like to share the following typical play, bearing in mind that the names are fictitious:

> It is a Monday afternoon. Cheryl is sitting across from me in my office with her partner Bill. She has been dealing with the complications of her high risk pregnancy, and today she is requesting tubal sterilization after delivery. I inform the couple about the risk of the procedure, the failure rate, and the alternatives to tubal sterilization. I mention vasectomy as a possible alternative. Smilingly, Cheryl casts a coy glance at Bill. He shakes his head with a "don't-you-look-at-me" expression on his face and then laughingly mutters "not me,"or words to that effect. Cheryl begins to make excuses for Bill, who "does not like operations" (as if anyone does!). Still smiling, she proceeds with plans to undergo the additional operative procedure after her delivery.

If Cheryl is upset with Bill's attitude toward sexual equity she is careful to hide it by smiling throughout the negotiation that never was. For as with most sexual relationships the world over, Cheryl is a junior partner who does not enjoy sexual equity. Sexual inequity may be more extreme or subtle from one country to another, or one sub-culture to another within a given country.

This book clearly points out that sexual inequities are due to gender-determined cultural, economic and political factors in practically all societies. These factors culminate in the lack of control by women over their sexuality.

The AIDS virus is a cunning organism. Biologically it has "learned" to change its spots through frequent alterations of its immunological envelope. These changes so confound and confuse our immune system that the latter cannot produce effective antibodies to fight the virus. In terms of spread of the virus from person-to-person there is a greater ease of male-to-female transmission. In other words, the same female who is disadvantaged in sexual bargaining also acquires the virus more readily through sexual transmission.

It should be recalled that this virus was once thought to be an affliction of gay men only, but was later found to be heterosexually transmitted as well. Today, the heterosexual rate of transmission far outstrips the homosexual rate.

This book also considers some ethical issues in the control of vertical transmission of HIV, vis-à-vis the findings of the United States AIDS Clinical Trial Group (ACTG). Misconceptions in disease transmission are explored in the chapter on HIV and sports participation.

AIDS education campaigns have traditionally centered on the use of condoms, adherence to monogamous relationship, or abstinence. This book examines the cultural impediments to successful AIDS education campaigns in various countries of the world as well as in various subgroups within the United States of America.

However, as very clearly articulated in this book, we may have in some cases reached a saturation point of education as a preventive strategy for the disease. Of what use to the female is the knowledge about the preventive role of condoms if she has no power to make her partner use them, or if she must face violence by raising the issue? Of what use is her knowledge of the role of high risk sexual behavior in viral transmission if she has no power to regulate her partner's behavior in that regard, or if she could lose his material or social support by trying to do so? Or if she has no other economic opportunity other than prostitution to provide for herself or for her children? It becomes clear that the next and more fundamental chapter in AIDS prevention campaigns the world over must begin with strategies for sexual empowerment of women through economic liberation.

The other mode of transmission of the AIDS virus is through intravenous drug use. The rate of this mode has overtaken the rate of heterosexual transmission in some cultures. Interruption of intravenous mode of transmission appears closely linked to the eradication of drug addiction. Here again, while drug education plays a key role, it may also have reached its saturation point. The needle exchange program is a means of facing reality in HIV transmission. Such a program does not confer society's blessing on drug use. It simply acknowledges the fact that the HIV is a greater threat to mankind than intravenous drug use.

This book is for you if you are a heterosexual, bisexual or homosexual male or female. This book is for you if you are a business leader, an elected official, a community leader, a teacher or a sociologist. This book is for you if you wish to influence the course of human history.

Uchenna C. Nwosu, M.D.
Professor, Department of Obstetrics & Gynecology
East Tennessee State University
James H. Quillen College of Medicine
Johnson City, Tennessee

Introduction: Fact and Fiction About HIV/AIDS

One of the most complex and complicated health problems confronting the world is human immunodeficiency virus (HIV) infection and the acquired immune deficiency syndrome (AIDS) disease. The National Commission on AIDS in 1991 classified AIDS as the most deadly sexually transmitted disease ever to confront humanity. Within the past decade, scientists have achieved significant strides in identifying HIV, the modes of transmission and several drugs to reduce the proliferation of the disease. But as yet, there is no cure or vaccine for AIDS. Our knowledge of virology and the epidemiology of HIV has increased quickly, but a vaccine or cure remains elusive (Lampert, 1994).

AIDS became prominent in 1981 through reports of an unusually high incidence of illness: kaposi sarcoma and pnuemocystis carinii pneumonia found among homosexuals (CDC report, 1989). As the number of reported cases increased, scientists concentrated their investigations among gay men and initially called the disease gay-related immune deficiency (GRID). The connection of AIDS with homosexuals resulted in negative consequences for gay men and people living with AIDS. Goodwin and Roscoe (1988) reported that college students viewed AIDS as a gay disease and blamed homosexuals for its spread. The manifestation of opportunistic diseases in healthy young men eventually resulted in a new name for the disease: acquired immune deficiency syndrome (Hochhauser & Rothenberger, 1992). AIDS is the last stage of the breakdown in the immune system.

Several theories have been advanced on the origin of HIV/AIDS. Some people believe that HIV was mistakenly released from a germ warfare laboratory. Others argue that HIV developed from the African green monkey and infected those who ate the monkey's meat. Simian immunodeficiency virus (SIV) which is similar to HIV-2 does infect some African monkeys, but they do not get AIDS. This fact and the high incidence of infection of people in

Central Africa have led to the opinion that HIV originated there and mutated to become virulent for humans (Gallo, 1993). Another argument suggests that HIV/AIDS originated from the homosexual group in the United States and was spread by American tourists to Central and East Africa. Further reasoning explains that Haitians who worked in Africa contracted the disease from Africans and infected American tourists who visited Haiti. Finally, some people theorize that HIV/AIDS is a punishment from God for immorality. Latham (1993) reports that in some African societies, AIDS is blamed on bewitchment or a curse from the gods due to some moral transgression. There is no scientific evidence to support any of the claims on the origin of HIV/AIDS. The fact is that HIV/AIDS is here and the origin may be only of academic interest, since it is devastating human populations throughout the world.

HIV is the virus that causes AIDS. The virus was simultaneously discovered by Luc Montagnier at Pasteur Institute in Paris and Robert Gallo at National Institute of Health in the United States. There are two types of HIV that cause AIDS-related conditions and cancer in human beings: HIV-1 and HIV-2. HIV-1 is the most common cause of AIDS around the world. HIV-2 is more predominant in West Africa. The less virulent HIV-2, virtually confined to West Africa, is most nearly similar to a virus termed simian immunodeficiency virus (SIV). This virus is widespread and harmless in wild sooty mangabey monkeys living in the same part of West Africa where humans are affected by HIV-2. It is most similar to viruses occurring harmlessly in wild populations of various African primates, including African green monkeys, mandrills and (rarely) chimpanzees (Diamond, 1992).

It takes 8-10 years for AIDS to manifest after infection. The virus cannot survive unless it is inside living tissue. When in the body, HIV attacks the lymph cell which is responsible for protecting the body against infection. There are two types of lymph cells: the B-cells and the T-cells. The B-cells are responsible for producing chemicals as a reaction to the presence of an antigen in the body. These chemicals are called antibodies. The T-cells are responsible for fighting the micro-organisms that invade the body. The T-cells are in three categories: the Killer T-cells, Memory T-cells and the Suppressor T-cells. The Killer T-cells fight with the invading micro-organisms to prevent infection for the body. The Memory T-cells gives specific coding to the invading micro-organisms for easy identification. The Suppressor T-cells stop the activities of the Killer T-cells to prevent further fighting. HIV destroys the lymph cells and exposes the body to opportunistic diseases which attack the body due to the weakening of the immune system.

Scientific evidence shows three patterns of HIV transmission across the world (Mann et al., 1989). Pattern 1 was recognized in the United States, Western Europe, Australia and New Zealand. Transmission was mainly through homosexual intercourse and intravenous (IV) drug use. HIV infection was more prevalent in men than women. Pattern II was identified in Africa and the Caribbean. The number of HIV infected cases was equal between men and women. Transmission was mainly through heterosexual intercourse. Pattern III was traced in Asia, Eastern Europe, Middle East and North Africa. The transmission of HIV is through blood transfusion, heterosexual intercourse, IV drug use and homosexual intercourse. Proportional numbers of men, women, adolescents and children are infected by HIV. The socio-cultural and economic factors in these environments influence the epidemiology of HIV.

However, the epidemiological trend of HIV transmission has changed considerably in most parts of the world. The virus which was previously predominant among the homosexual group is now the leading cause of death for women between 20-40 years of age in the major urban areas of North America, South America, Western Europe and SubSaharan Africa (Centers for Disease Control, 1991). The data from the World Health Organization indicates that Asia is expected to have 10 million infected people by the year 2000 and will become the center of the epidemic, surpassing Africa in the number of new infections each year (Pollack, 1994).

Several drugs to reduce the proliferation of HIV have been approved by the Food and Drug Administration (FDA). In 1987, AZT (azidothymidine or zidovudine) became the first drug used for the treatment of AIDS. In 1991, DDI (Dideoinsine) and in 1992, DDC (Zalcitabine) became the second and third drugs approved for the treatment of HIV/AIDS. In 1994, D4T (Stavudine) was approved as an alternate drug for treating HIV/AIDS. All of these drugs produce toxic effects to HIV/AIDS patients, and the evidence shows that they do not have a significant impact in improving the health of HIV/AIDS patients. "All these drugs were originally developed for chemotherapy to kill human cancer cells, and they bring with them all the usual effects: hair loss, muscle degeneration, anemia, nausea and vomiting-a severe price for questionable benefits" (Duesberg, 1996). To aggravate matters, HIV mutates and becomes resistant to the drugs.

The HIV/AIDS epidemic has had a significant impact on the socioeconomic life of people around the world. The cost of drugs and hospital and medical care reduces the financial status of people. Economic activities in some countries are affected because of reduced labor force caused by illness or death. In Uganda and Tanzania, coffee and other cash crops remained unharvested in 1991 due to an agricultural labor shortage resulting from mounting AIDS deaths (Schear, 1992). In developed nations with social welfare services, the demands on these departments have increased tremendously due to an increased number of HIV/AIDS patients. Thousands of African American children are being orphaned as their parents die from AIDS. This reality has spawned concern regarding the future of these children, the burden placed on other family members (particularly grandparents), and the ability of an already overloaded foster care system to effectively care for them (National Commission on AIDS, 1993). Among the developing nations in Africa, the extended family systems have broken down because AIDS kills the economic elite, leaving their children to the care of grandparents. The responsibilities of sick relatives and their children overburden friends, family and the society in general.

Several ethical, legal, and political issues have arisen because of the HIV/AIDS epidemic. People with HIV/AIDS experience discrimination in schools, housing, employment, hospitals and other public institutions. Mandatory testing of athletes and people in other professions that involve group participation is controversial. Longman (1995) states that the admission by Greg Louganis that he had AIDS ignited a debate about whether athletes should be tested for HIV. The issue of confidentiality and disclosures of HIV status arose because of the fear, stigma and taboo associated with HIV/AIDS. The discrimination of people with AIDS is based upon poor knowledge and misconceptions about HIV/AIDS. These viewpoints may be improved through better HIV/AIDS education.

HIV/AIDS-related issues have generated several legal actions in different courts around the world. Litigations have arisen regarding discrimination in schools, patient care, employment, housing, infected blood, and a host of other aspects. AIDS has become the most litigated of diseases in the United States (Jurgens, 1994). Legislation has been enacted at State and Federal levels to protect the rights of individuals who are HIV positive or have AIDS.

Politically, many governments have responded to HIV in different ways. African governments, like most others around the world, responded lethargically to the threat, allowing the virus to gain a foothold and spread (Schear, 1992). Leaders in Africa denied that HIV/AIDS existed to prevent scaring tourists who are necessary for the maintenance of the country's economy with their input of hard currency. In the USA, politicians and people in other health care institutions refused to provide appropriate facilities to safeguard public health. The erroneous notion that AIDS was a homosexual disease influenced the unwillingness of the U.S. government to provide funding to address the HIV/AIDS program in the early stages of the disease (Shilts, 1988).

Cultural factors in the human environment influence the HIV/AIDS epidemic. The interrelationship of these factors shows in the pattern of HIV transmission around the world. Walter et al. (1994) point out that the growing awareness of the impact of cultural issues in health education prompted educators to experiment with using cultural elements in HIV education and prevention efforts. The reality is that HIV/AIDS cuts across all cultural groups and sub-groups. These groups and sub-groups which include women, men, children, adolescents, homosexuals, and athletes have different norms that influence their behavior. The HIV/AIDS education program must recognize these group cultures and integrate them into the existing education processes for each group. To ensure universal commitment, the culture of every society must be understood. Social science research on such issues as community dynamics, social relationships, youth culture and group norms (including how they are defined and influenced by factors such as sex, race, ethnicity, culture and class) is vital to developing effective strategies for preventing the spread of AIDS (Etzioni, Gamson & Levine 1994).

The success of HIV/AIDS education depends upon how effectively the cultural norms of each group are incorporated into the programs designed for them. Planned educational strategies to empower people to initiate change of behavior must factor in their cultural background. HIV/AIDS is a sensitive issue. Therefore, health educators must employ culturally sensitive methods to examine varied health behaviors in terms of positive/beneficial beliefs that must be encouraged, existential/cultural beliefs and practices that do not threaten health, and negative/harmful health practices that should be changed (Airhihenbuwa, 1995).

Singer (1991) and Stevenson and Davis (1994) have expressed the importance of culture and other environmental factors in the education about HIV/AIDS. Health educators and other allied disciplines need a volume that contains articles that discuss different perspectives of HIV/AIDS. The more reliable the information that is available, the better can be humanity's fight against this virulent disease.

References

Airhihenbuwa, C. O. (1995). *Health and Culture: Beyond the Western Paradigm.* Thousand Oaks, CA: Sage Publications.

Center for Disease Control.(1989). *Morbidity and Mortality Weekly Report. AIDS and Human Immunodeficiency Virus Infection in the United States.* 1988 Update. 38(S-4), 1-38.

Center for Disease Control. (1991). *HIV/AIDS Surveillance.* U.S. Department of Health and Human Services, 1-22.

Diamond, J. (September, 1992). The Mysterious Origin of AIDS. *Natural History*, 24-29.

Duesberg, P. (1996). *Inventing the AIDS Virus.* Washington, DC: Regency Publishing Inc.

Etzioni, A., Gamson, W. & Levine, F. (Nov. 30, 1994). Build on Knowledge from the Social Science to Fight the Spread of AIDS. *The Chronicle of Higher Education*, A56.

Gallo, R. C. (1993). *Acquired Immune Deficiency Syndrome.* Microsoft (R) Encarta; Microsoft Corporation, Funk and Wagnall's Corporation, B510.

Goodwin, M. P.and Roscoe, B. (1988). AIDS: Students' Knowledge and Attitude at a Midwestern University. *American Journal of College Health*, 36, 214-222.

Hochhauser, M. and Rothenberger, J. H. (1992). *AIDS Education.* Dubuque, IA: Wm. C. Brown Publishers.

Jurgens, R. (Feb. 16, 1994). AIDS Law Today: A New Guide to the Public (Book Review). *JAMA*, 271(7),

Lamptey, P. (August, 1994). Slowing AIDS: Lesson From a Decade of Preventive Effort. *Family Health International Journal*, 1(3), 3.

Latham, M. C. (1993). AIDS in Africa: A Perspective on the Epidemic. *Africa Today*, 3rd Quarter, 39-53.

Longman, J. (Feb. 26, 1995). Debate About HIV Tests Sparked by Diver With AIDS. *The New York Times*, E2.

Mann, J. M., Chin, J., Piot, P. and Quinn, T. (1989). The International Epidemiology of AIDS. In J. Piel (Ed.), *The science of AIDS* (pp. 51-61) New York: W. H. Freeman and Co.

National Commission on AIDS. (1993). *The Challenge of HIV/AIDS in Communities of Color*. Washington DC: U.S. Government Printing Press.

National Commission on AIDS. (1991). *America Living With AIDS*. Washington DC: U.S. Government Printing Office.

Pollack, A. (August 7, 1994). Japan May Have to Face Up To AIDS. *The New York Times*, 18L.

Schear, S. (Summer, 1992). AIDS in Africa. *Dissent*, 397-398.

Shilts, R (1987). *And the Band Played On: Politics, People and the AIDS Epidemic*. New York: St Martin's Press.

Singer, M. (1991). Confronting the AIDS Epidemic Among IV Drug Users: Does Ethnic Culture Matter? *AIDS Education and Prevention*, 3(3), 258-283.

Stevenson, H. C. & Davis, G. (1994). Impact of Culturally Sensitive AIDS Video Education on the AIDS Risk Knowledge of African-American Adolescents. *AIDS Education and Prevention*, 6(1), 258-283.

Walter, J. L., DMin, R. C. and Stein, T. (October 1994). Evaluating Multiculturai Approaches to HIV/AIDS Educational Materials. *AIDS Education and Prevention*, 6(5), 446-453.

Part One

Social and Cultural Issues

Introduction

The articles in this section examine the social and cultural factors that influence the perception of HIV infection. These articles focus on the roles that gender, language, group norms, beliefs, economy and power play in the transmission of HIV and practice of HIV preventive behaviors. The complexity of the cultural and social norms raised in these articles challenges HIV/AIDS educators to reassess their programs to be more culturally sensitive.

In "Cultural and Societal Impediments to HIV/AIDS Education in the American Indian Community," Claudia L. Windal identifies the major cultural and societal impediments to HIV/AIDS education in a Native American community. She suggests a variety of strategies for working through these impediments to promote a successful HIV/AIDS education program for Native Americans.

In "Uganda and the Challenge of AIDS," Kabahenda Nyakabwa discusses the enormous social, economic, demographic and developmental challenges posed for Uganda by the HIV/AIDS epidemic. She identifies the mortality rate which has reached such apocalyptic proportions that government, families and communities can no longer cope with the financial and emotional costs involved in caring for the sick and the dying. According to Nyakabwa, the gendered structure of social, economic and political inequalities which are unfavorable to women makes them the most adversely affected group of HIV/AIDS victims.

Charles Uwakwe investigates the "Socio-Cultural Factors that Predispose Women to HIV/AIDS in the Middle Belt of Nigeria." His study involves 164 subjects and confirmes an alignment in the opinions of the subjects' perceptions of the predisposing factors to HIV/AIDS and STDs. He stressed the need for evolvement and implementation of HIV/AIDS prevention strategies in that part of Nigeria where a high incidence of HIV and STDs has been reported.

Carolie Blair, et al. conduct a focus group discussion in a high HIV/AIDS incidence area in Kenya on barriers to behavior change. Their results indicate that there was no significant change in behavior and people continue to practice unsafe sex. The respondents identified malaria as a more problematic illness than AIDS. The results show that many traditional and cultural practices prevented the adoption of positive sexual health behaviors. The authors suggested that to improve the effectiveness of HIV/AIDS preventive programs, the message should address the fears and beliefs of the audience.

Ralph DiClemente and Gina Wingood, in "Prevention of Human Immunodeficiency Virus Infection Among African-American Adolescents...," indicate that there is a growing threat of HIV infection among adolescents. In fact, African-American adolescents are disproportionally represented among AIDS cases and have higher seroprevalence rates relative to other ethnic groups. In designing HIV/AIDS education programs for African-American adolescents, it is important to understand not only the broad context in which adolescence takes place, but also the cultural and psychosocial factors that exert considerable influence on behavior. A number of contextual barriers were identified as affecting African-American adolescents' willingness to modify high-risk behavior. These include: suspicion and mistrust, economic constraints, perceived risk of HIV infection, perception of peer norms as supporting high-risk behavior and sexual communication. To develop maximally effective programs for African-American adolescents, they must be designed within the context of the African-American community.

Cultural and Societal Impediments to HIV/AIDS Education in the American Indian Community: Mitakuye Oyasin[1]

Claudia L. Windal

The early days of the HIV/AIDS pandemic were filled with myth: heterosexual women and men believed themselves to be safe because this was a "gay disease," and women believed themselves safe because, "only men get AIDS," and children were believed to be safe from HIV infection because "only adults became infected," and persons of color believed themselves to be safe because, "AIDS is a white man's disease." Within a short time, these beliefs began to dissolve as heterosexual women and men, children as well as adults, and persons of color along with Caucasians, became infected with the virus known as HIV. Despite this reality, HIV/AIDS education continues to be met by great resistance in the American Indian community. This essay will identify and explore several of the undergirding reasons for this resistance.

In 1992, the Health Resources and Service Administration Bureau of Health Resources Development, brought together twenty one Native Americans and Alaskan natives as well as a group of federal representatives, to discuss providing HIV/AIDS services to these two groups of native persons. This group then, identified several societal and cultural issues[2] that impact and act as impediments to HIV/AIDS education and services. Some of these issues are: 1. Native American societies are culturally distinctive, diverse, and complex, 2. HIV/AIDS is only one of many problems in most Native American communities, 3. A Native American spokesperson has not been identified to make HIV/AIDS real for Native American communities, 4. AIDS hysteria is high, in part because Native Americans, like many others, do not understand how it (HIV) is transmitted, 5. Racism is an important complicating factor, and 6. Confidentiality is an important underlying issue in dealing with HIV among Native American populations.

This list of concerns and issues was expanded during a conversation with Chani Phillips (Cheyenne River Lakota), a colleague from the Indian Health Board, who identified the following additional impediments to HIV/AIDS education in the Native American community: 1. Variations in religious beliefs; "Tunkashila"[3] (grandfather) is responsible for what happens to us as opposed to those who believe that we are responsible for our own destinies, 2. The need for involvement of elders and spiritual leaders in HIV/AIDS education, 3. A similar need for tribal chairpersons and council members to speak about concerns regarding HIV/AIDS, and 4. Most HIV/AIDS education has been approached as working for native persons rather than doing education with native persons.

One final impediment to HIV/AIDS education identified by a client in our case management program is: a mistrust of White people and White bureaucracy. He stated specifically, "You must remember that it's only been a hundred years since Wounded Knee." Admittedly, this is not a comprehensive list of societal and cultural impediments to HIV/AIDS education in the Native American community. It is, I believe, a well-informed beginning to understanding the resistance of many Native American people to discussing and learning more about HIV and AIDS.

The remainder of the chapter will discuss in detail, each of the impediments to HIV/AIDS education that have been previously identified.

American Indian Societies Are Culturally Distinctive, Diverse, and Complex

In early April, 1995, nearly one thousand Native American women from the United States and Canada, gathered in Portland, Oregon for the Women and Wellness VI Conference.[4] The cultural diversity within the group was both evident and celebrated. The social pow wow, especially, demonstrated this diversity in the variation of dance attire, music, dance style, and languages used in singing; diversity that is all too frequently amalgamated and defined simply as "Indian."

That which constitutes a wonderful diversity among Native American tribes and people, creates a dilemma in HIV and AIDS education. As a workshop presenter for this conference, I frequently heard statements such as, "On my reservation... no one will talk about HIV/AIDS," and "My people don't talk about sex... there's no way you could come in and begin to mention condoms." Others continued, "The elders of my tribe become upset if anyone even mentions Two Spirits[5] as okay." Each of these statements brought home to me the reality that is obvious to Native Americans and not so obvious to others, which is that we must be aware and respectful of Native American tribal and cultural diversity, as we attempt to present HIV/AIDS education especially on various reservations.

An additional consideration is the influence of the dominant culture on the reservation. One must ask whether there are small groups of non-natives who live on the reservation. How much interaction do they have with the natives and how much do the natives have with them? Do the non-natives attend school with the native children? Who are the teachers: Native Americans or Euro-Americans? If the schools are mixed, what lessons are taught about Native Americans? How dependent is the reservation on the dominant culture in meeting basic needs such as food, clothing, shelter?

Traditional values have been greatly influenced by the dominant culture. An example of this was clearly articulated by a woman who attended the Portland conference who said that traditionally, Two Spirits (lesbian and gay) held a place of honor in her tribe and often became medicine men and women. They were considered wise and their counsel was often sought. Now, Two Spirits are often ridiculed and many say that they brought AIDS to Indian country. Many don't want them to live on the reservation. She continued by saying that all of this is the influence of white people. She, in fact, has a cousin who is Two Spirited and he is kept from seeing his family because he is treated so poorly when he comes home. Another example of this occurred last year when I was invited to present an HIV/AIDS in-service workshop for a tribal health clinic. While driving to the clinic the morning of the presentation, the health educator warned me that there are horrible attitudes on this reservation toward homosexuals and he further cautioned me to not reveal my sexual orientation lest everyone leave the presentation.

The dominant culture has influenced those on the reservation also by the presence of Christian churches and schools. Thomas (1993), addresses the influence of boarding schools:

> ... since remaking the Indians meant converting them to Christianity, it was natural for (President) Grant to replace the corrupt civilian agents on reservations with men picked from various church groups. The denominations divided up their potential flocks;

> Episcopalians taking the Lakota tribes, Presbyterians assigned to the Navajos, and Quakers working with the southern Plaines tribes that were willing to relocate to reservations in Indian Territory.
>
> Children,... presented a much better opportunity for genuine reform—provided they could be cut off for a prolonged period from their "savage" environment. Thus has developed the notion of government boarding schools for Indians in which native children could be safely ensconced during their formative years.... Quite aside from the terror any child feels at being torn from family and familiar surroundings, these children suffered personal humiliation when their long hair was hacked off and their bodies were physically abused; and certainly there was irreparable harm done when their Indian heritage and languages were suppressed.

Consequently, entire generations of Native American people grew up believing their traditional ways, their spiritual practices, their language, dress, music, and dance, were all bad and somehow wrong. Replacing the familiar words, "the elders have spoken," were "Sister said" or "Father said." Guilt replaced tradition and shame replaced pride. The grandfathers, grandmothers, mothers and fathers, aunties and uncles who are the teachers of the youth to whom we must reach out with HIV and AIDS education, are the former boarding school students and those who are too frequently guided by what the church or the government says rather than by Tunkasila.

In contrast to the vast cultural diversity experienced by those living on reservations, is that of urban Native Americans. One of my saddest experiences is asking a new client to which tribe she or he belongs and hearing that they don't know: "I think Sioux... maybe. I was adopted by whites and no one really ever talked to me about my real parents... whether they're both Indian... what tribe or tribes they came from..." Many of the women with whom I visited during the Women and Wellness Conference reported that they did not have a clear understanding of their tribal affiliation until they were young adults. A growing number of these women reported that they are finally beginning to learn their Native language and dance and are also passing on these traditions to their children and grandchildren.

Some of our case management clients have not visited their reservations since they were small children. They have no sense of recollection of either home or school experiences, and there are no pleasant memories that inspire attachment to their reservations. Several other clients do not know to which reservation they would belong if they desired enrollment. These same persons neither speak nor understand their native language nor do they recognize the beadwork common to their tribe; they rarely attend pow wows and none of them dance. Although most do identify themselves as Native American, they identify more closely with the dominant culture than with their native traditions and culture.

HIV/AIDS Is Only One of the Many Problems In Most American Indian Communities

For many Native Americans, struggling to meet the basic human needs of shelter, food and clothing takes precedence over HIV/AIDS information and education. Where unemployment is greater than the national average on most reservations,[6] (high as 80%) it is impossible to consider issues that are believed to be someone else's problem. In reviewing conversations with twenty two Native American clients, the following was noted: nine of them report that they have been homeless at least once in the past two years;[7] four of them have been homeless two or more times during that same period of time. Nineteen clients report that they get food regularly from at least one food pantry. An additional fourteen clients regularly visit up to three food pantries a month for food assistance. Twenty clients received county or federal financial assistance; only four of those twenty are considered disabled by their HIV or AIDS. Twelve clients reported that they were raised in homes where their parent(s) did not work and that their only income was what they received from the county.

It seems that only on occasion, are my clients and I able to only discuss issues and concerns regarding HIV/AIDS. During a typical 40 hour work week, approximately eight hours are devoted to HIV/AIDS concerns. Another 20 hours are spent in securing housing, food, and financial assistance. Bereavement work (letters, phone calls, and visits) averages about 4 hours a week, while the final 8 hours are spent in general office management (reports, professional reading, meetings, and so on) and community projects (high school HIV/AIDS education, HIV/AIDS consultation with other agencies). The urban environment in which the Indian Health Board is located, has not obliterated the struggle to meet basic needs that is common to the Native American community.

Beginning the second month of my employment with the Indian Health Board, I sent a monthly form letter to each client, containing regular HIV/AIDS educational information, community news regarding HIV/AIDS, and recreational/social opportunities for those interested. This letter has grown to a full four page (double-sided) monthly newsletter with a circulation of 70-80 people. Information contained in this monthly mailing has expanded to address AIDS clinical trials, basics of HIV/AIDS, sex and sexuality, nutrition, and a variety of current topics. The response from clients and others alike, has been most positive. The newsletter is seen as both a non-threatening way to receive this information and something that can be read when there is time and energy to do so.

HIV/AIDS is only one of several health concerns in the Native American community. Diabetes and alcoholism top HIV/AIDS as two of the leading health problems. It is estimated that over 47,000 of the more than 2 million Native Americans in the United States have diabetes (Diabetes Fact Sheet,

1993). This same resource indicates that the Pima Indians of Arizona have the highest rate of diabetes in the world and that serious complications of diabetes are increasing in frequency among Native Americans. With this increase come the rise of kidney failure, amputations, and blindness.

Between 1989 and 1991, the age-adjusted alcoholism mortality rate for the Indian Health Service area population8 was 37.6%. When the three IHS areas with apparent problems in under-reporting of Indian race on death certificates are excluded, that rate is 51.8% (630% higher than the United States All Races rate of 7.1% for 1990). These health concerns are of far greater importance to most Native Americans than HIV, simply because many of them have had either their lives or the lives of family members and loved ones, touched by diabetes or alcoholism. Neither carry with them the prejudice and the misunderstanding of HIV and AIDS. Perhaps Maslow (1954) explains that domination by one's need is enough to totally change one's outlook and attitude. An example of this from experience with homeless clients is that the greatest happiness and peace of mind for most of these clients is in finding shelter. They believe that this then, is all that is needed to have a good life. All other considerations such as disease prevention and personal feelings are considered unimportant since they have nothing to do with resolving their homelessness.

A Native American Has Not Yet Been Identified to Make HIV/AIDS Real for the American Indian Community

Certainly there is no identified Magic Johnson, Ryan White, or Arthur Ashe speaking as a Native American who is living with HIV/AIDS. There are however, an increasing number of Native American people who are HIV positive and who are willing to speak publicly about their infection and the need for others to be cautious and learn means of prevention.

Here in Minneapolis, we are fortunate to have C.L.F., an Ojibwa woman who was diagnosed HIV positive in 1986 and who has shared her story throughout Indian country. Another outspoken native woman is L.T. who has traveled across the United States to tell the story of her infection through unprotected sexual intercourse with an HIV-infected male, to countless numbers of Indian youth. Just this week, three of my clients agreed to give a panel presentation to several large audiences of ninth grade students at a local high school. One of the panel members is a Native American mother and grandmother who shared the painful story of shared needle use and subsequent HIV infection. Another Native American client, however, who has been open and honest about his HIV status and AIDS-related declining health, was recently contacted by someone on a reservation regarding his availability to present HIV/AIDS educational information at a community meeting. Before he was formally asked if he would be willing to speak, he was asked about his sexual orientation. He was honest about being a Two Spirit, and said that he would be honored to visit the reservation and participate in the planned educational event. Despite this person's willingness, he has not yet received the invitation that he believed was initially being extended to him. Imagine the lost opportunity for members of the reservation community if he is not invited to participate in their AIDS education! This is the reservation to which he belongs as an enrolled member. At last, there would be one additional identified spokesperson for one more reservation, willing to join the handful of others who will publicly discuss their HIV status and speak about protection, education, and compassion.

Conversely, when I speak in the Minneapolis Public Schools, I often meet large numbers of African-American students and I generally ask who they can think of who has lived or is living with HIV or AIDS. It takes no time at all for someone to respond with the names of either Magic Johnson or Arthur Ashe. The need for this cultural identification was further illustrated several years ago when I was privileged to attend a large gathering of students to hear Pedro Zamora, an 18 year old Hispanic, tell of his journey with HIV and AIDS. Although the Hispanic students who were present had received as many hours of HIV/AIDS education as every other student present, this was the first time that they engaged in open dialogue, asked questions, and sought further information from someone with whom they could so closely identify.

There is an effort among HIV/AIDS educators, prevention specialists, and case managers who work in the Native American community, to utilize culturally specific materials such as pamphlets, brochures, posters, and the like, and to use phrases and language that are easily recognizable and frequently used by Native Americans. Nothing can replace interpersonal interaction with someone of the same race, culture, and tradition as the audience.

AIDS Hysteria Is High, in Part, Because Native Americans, Like Many Others, Do Not Understand How It (HIV) Is Transmitted

This is, it seems to me, the essence of our dilemma in bringing HIV/AIDS education to the Native American Indian community: AIDS hysteria is high, in part, because Native Americans, like many others, do not understand how HIV is transmitted. This is partly because their AIDS hysteria and "Two Spirit-phobia" keep them from developing a willingness to concentrate on behavioral means of transmission and instead they dwell on other means of transmission that don't trigger the same hysterical responses or that keep HIV/AIDS as their problem and not ours.

Native Americans show an obvious resistance to discussion around behaviors that lend themselves to HIV transmission. This was especially evident to me when I gave an HIV/AIDS in-service presentation to a large group of tribal clinic workers and members of the local reservation community. I began by acknowledging that the things we needed to focus on that day:

> ... are traditionally not discussed by Native American people. I

> apologize if anyone finds this information or the terms that I must use, offensive. HIV/AIDS education is essential to the preservation of Native American lives and I believe the grandfathers would want everything possible to be done so that entire tribes of people will not vanish because of a preventable illness. We are individually called to wellness, and Native American people comprising tribes are also called to wellness. The Wellness Circle consists of four directions or dimensions which are: physical, emotional, mental, and spiritual. Today, we must concentrate on the mental dimension, using our minds to begin to understand HIV and how the virus is transmitted and how it is not transmitted; how we can protect ourselves from infection and what behaviors and actions put us at risk for infection with HIV...

When I finished this introduction, I asked if anyone could tell us where HIV is found in the body so that it can be transmitted to another person. The clinic health educator had pre-warned me that this group would probably not be especially verbally responsive and to not be disappointed if this was the case during the day. Rather than silence, nearly a dozen hands went up and we were told that HIV is transmitted by blood and body fluids. Elated by their response, I pushed on to define specific body fluids, and again many hands were raised and members of the local community poured forth the correct response. Before I could become too overjoyed at what appeared to be a transcending of expected resistance to HIV/AIDS education, one of the clinic staff members raised her hand and asked about the safety of the blood supply. I responded that blood is now very safe for transfusion and then continued that great caution is taken through testing and other precautions with all donated blood. Despite my best efforts, this woman tried to monopolize our time with her concerns and questions until I wondered if we would have time to discuss behavioral means of transmission. Finally, I acknowledged that she and I would apparently not come to an agreement during the time of the presentation and I suggested that we continue our discussion over lunch. From this, I attempted to move on and define how HIV is transmitted, only to have another hand raised. This time, the questioner was an older clinic worker who said that he couldn't understand why he needed to wear gloves anytime he might come into contact with blood. "You can tell who they are," he told us. I perceived the "they" to be Two Spirits and I asked him to define who he believed "them" to be. With much coaxing, he said that he could tell Two Spirited clients and that he was always especially careful to not even get near them, let alone their blood.

As we took a break, it became apparent to me that this dwelling both on the safety of the blood supply and on knowing who is living with HIV by identifying the Two Spirits, went much deeper than the personal convictions of those who had spoken. Although I could not substantiate my belief, I surmised that these questions were a means of re-focusing HIV transmission away from behavior and rather, to others or to substances that put HIV into an "us and them/it" modality. When the in-service resumed, two of the non-native nurses assisted in re-focusing our attention on behaviors that permit HIV to be transmitted to another. Although the dialogue continued to be animated and informational, the verbal participation of the Native American staff members greatly diminished.

I believe that given the ideal circumstance of on-going HIV/AIDS education in the Native American community, AIDS hysteria would lessen and the facts of transmission would be more easily heard. This dovetails directly into the point previously made regarding no identified Native American HIV/AIDS spokesperson. When enough HIV positive, heterosexual Native Americans, who were infected through unprotected sexual intercourse, are identified and are willing to step forward and share their stories in the Native American community, the "we/they" barriers will begin to crumble and Native Americans will hear the facts and understand that they are at risk of becoming HIV/AIDS statistics if they engage in risky behaviors. Native American traditions are rich in story telling. In order to dispel the myths and misunderstandings regarding HIV/AIDS, perhaps educational information would be best conveyed by story-telling. Who is better to do this in the Native American community than a sister or brother who is living with the virus? We can begin to encourage this story telling in safe places such as the small group setting of the Indian Health Promotion Conferences. Although no one has identified him or herself as HIV positive during the conferences I have attended, there have been participants who have identified as family members of someone living with HIV /AIDS. Each of them shared that this was the first time that they had told their story. As more and more Native Americans living with HIV/AIDS share their stories in supportive and caring environments with other Native Americans, the more they will be encouraged to take the risk of telling those stories to larger groups within the Native American community to help others avoid HIV infection.

Racism is an Important Complicating Factor

> What was it I so avidly wrapped with rags,
> And hidden, dragged through dark months and years?
> In these concealing rags, I hid my heart,
> When found, it was sorely bruised
> Shrivelled red from stigma I sought to lose.
> (Song, 1987).

Racism is an important complicating factor in HIV/AIDS education in the Native American community. Native Americans have been "marked" by several labels and by many generations. Among these labels are: lazy, uncooperative, un-American, alcoholic, and troublemaker. If those who are responsible for HIV/AIDS education believe these labels, what is the motivation to bring their educational materials into the American Indian community? Their thinking is undoubtedly like the following: "If Indians are alcoholic, they're not going to be in any shape to change their sexual or needle-sharing behaviors and reduce the risk of HIV infection, so why bother?" "Since they're irresponsible, nothing that anyone says will make them change their risky behaviors." "Lazy as they are, they're not about to come out for a community awareness forum or educational meeting so why waste the energy?" "All they would probably do is cause some big free-for-all if we were to try to present AIDS education." No, these are not statements that I have ever heard; they don't come from the Bureau of Indian Affairs (BIA) or the Center for Disease Control (CDC) or from any other government agency of which I am aware. It doesn't however, take much imagination to understand how these thoughts might be even covertly formulated in the minds of non-Indian HIV/AIDS educators given the racism, the "mark," that has been placed upon Native American people.

"In these concealing rags, I hid my heart. When found, it was sorely bruised, shrivelled red from stigma I sought to lose." What "sorely bruised heart" would be open to hearing yet another message bringing with it shame, disgrace, and death to the one infected with this virus? I believe that there is an internalized racism for many Native Americans, just as there is an internalized homophobia for many Two Spirits, that perpetuates the negative messages that are repeatedly given to them: "I am an alcoholic and when I drink I go to jail for something pretty awful. I am a bad and undeserving person." "I never did listen to my teachers or to my parents or to the elders; if I had, I wouldn't be in this mess. I am a bad and undeserving person." "I'm 25 years old, have three kids; I didn't finish school and can't read more than the label on a beer bottle and most of that I've memorized. I am a bad and undeserving person."

Another aspect of racism is the belief that "I'm not like them." "I'm an Indian; AIDS is a White man's disease and has nothing to do with Indians." This is where "Mitakaye Oyasin" (all my relations) begins to disintegrate and conditions are put upon just who are all my relations. "I'm Lakota and the only Indians I know with HIV/AIDS are Navajo." "I'm heterosexual and only Two Spirits get AIDS." "We don't have enough money to deal and use drugs, so... AIDS is a rich white man's disease." "I believe what the grandfathers taught us, and the white man's words don't fit." The entire thought process begins to sound like the childish "Ha, ha, ha, ha, ha... I've got the truth and you don't... you've got AIDS, and we don't." The more dis-similarities that can be imagined, the less likely one is to become infected with "Someone else's problem."

Although great harm has occurred due to racism, the greatest harm is in it's subtle and covert manner of operation. The phrases used to illustrate this phenomenon rarely surface as spoken word or even conscious thought. In the darkness of the unconscious, they take control and send the messages of "I'm a bad person and I am undeserving of good," or "I'm not like you, I'm an Indian and AIDS is a white man's disease." The reality is that the more messages and the stronger the messages of racism, the less likely that HIV/AIDS education will become an integral part of the Native American community.

Confidentiality Is an Important Underlying Issue in Dealing With HIV/AIDS Among Native Americans

Our afternoon workshops were nearly ready to begin on the second day of the Women and Wellness VI Conference. I arrived at my room early so that I could list several important points on the board. This was to be the "Grief: Women Infected and Affected by HIV/AIDS" workshop and I had anticipated that with about 1000 participants, there would be 25-30 people in each of two sessions. As our start time drew near, there were only nine women sitting in the room; all looking nervous and none speaking to any others. Many had stopped by the room, looked at and read the workshop title, and then quickly moved on to other rooms. I shared my surprise with the assembled group. One woman said that she was amazed that there were nine people present. "You know, it's risky sitting here where anyone can see us. Some of them probably think that we're here because we have AIDS, and now who knows who they'll tell."

Several months ago, I realized that the monthly client newsletter could be sent at a much more reasonable cost if I simply folded and stapled it and didn't place it in an envelope. Within days of this change in mailing, I received a call from a client who said that I had made him extremely angry by not using an envelope for his newsletter. His most recent newsletter had been placed in his mailbox, opened and unfolded as if it had been read. "Now I suppose everybody in my building will know that I have AIDS."

During the Christmas holiday season, a local HIV/AIDS organization fills Christmas baskets for several hundred people living with HIV or AIDS. It is my responsibility to deliver the baskets to my clients. While bringing in the "goodies" to one client, she pulled me aside and asked, "What's this doing in my stuff?" She was holding up a can of ADVERA, a nutritional supplement especially for those with AIDS. The product literature that had been included in the basket, had AIDS boldly written all over it. "Get it out of here without anyone seeing it... I haven't told any of these people that I have AIDS and I'm not going to tell them today because of this!"

Early in my employment at the Indian Health Board, I mentioned to someone in the clinic that I needed to call one of our clients to remind him of an upcoming appointment. "Don't bother," she replied, "He's my mother's girlfriend's auntie's uncle. I'll just tell my mother who can let—know and she'll tell—when they go to BINGO tomorrow.

The Native American community is one of the most tightly knit groups within which I've ever worked. Our clinic staff is filled with relatives, and if not relatives, with people who know one another so well that they seem like family. What one person hears or sees, ten or twelve or more people could learn before the end of day. This makes HIV testing and, for some, HIV care, difficult. Chances are great that a Native American who comes in for testing will either receive pre-test counseling or his HIV blood drawn by someone they know. When the result come back, it is possible that the person who receives the result will know to whom it belongs. In each case, the opportunity exists for confidential information to not remain confidential even if it goes no further than one clinic employee who is known by or who knows the client. I might add that we are all extremely aware of this potential and go to great lengths to keep information to ourselves and to those providers who must absolutely know.

So great are issues of confidentiality, that most of our case management clients do not know one another. Although clients frequently speak of establishing a support group, they fail to follow through because this would put them at risk for having their diagnosis revealed by other clients who might either be related to or know some of their friends or family members. They fear meeting other clients from their reservations for risk of exposure of their HIV status at home. One client, the mother of a large family, shared her concerns with me when she explained, "If they find out at home that I have AIDS, not only will I not be accepted, but my kids will have nowhere to go when I die. No one will want the kids to come home to live with my parents. I know someone else at home who has AIDS. She doesn't even know this, but they burn her dishes and silverware when she leaves. They're scared to death of her... that by using her same plate, even after it's washed, that they'll catch HIV."

Given the stigma of HIV/AIDS in much of the American Indian community, confidentiality is an important consideration in both HIV education and care. No one wants it gossiped about or told to others that they are HIV positive or have AIDS before they make the decision to reveal that information themselves. Certainly, no one wants others to believe that they are HIV positive or have AIDS based upon their presence at an educational seminar or conference workshop, or by their expression of interest in knowing more about HIV. This was, in part, what motivated my workshop title: "Grief: Women Infected and Affected by HIV." With this title, I believed that it could as easily be surmised that those in attendance were health care professionals who work with those living with HIV. Despite my best efforts to lessen possible labeling and stigma, many were fearful of attending lest the worst be assumed by others; that those in attendance were infected by HIV or living with AIDS. Even if no one acted differently toward them during the remainder of the conference, maybe someone would mention to an employer, a family member, a co-worker, a spiritual leader, an elder, or a spouse, that they were seen at this workshop and that they might have AIDS! How does one go about undoing the damage of a breach of confidentiality? Obviously, this is a difficult enough task that many were not willing to take the risk and attend the workshop.

As my first summer as the Indian Health Board AIDS Case Manager, came to an end, I proposed an end of summer picnic for all of our clients that would be held at my home. I was astounded when a colleague from another clinic, suggested that I should not be too disappointed if the turnout was very small. She said she would be surprised if many clients would have enough trust to come together with other Native Americans living with HIV/AIDS, "for fear that news of their HIV status would travel... " I was thrilled to welcome nine clients and their families to our home. Initially, there was little conversation between this group of strangers, beyond the beautiful weather. As the afternoon drew on and supper was finished, I noticed that several small clusters of people had gathered around the yard, back porch, and house. One group was comparing their medications. Each had a handful of medication and several were commenting that they didn't take anything that looked like what they saw! Another group was engaged in prayer, burning sage and singing, and a third group had gathered in the dining room where they were discussing and comparing their central lines.[9] All three of these men had their lines surgically placed in their chests and they had lifted their shirts to compare dressings. Although I could not have been happier at the wonderful interaction of the group of Native Americans living with AIDS, my heart ached for those who could not trust enough to join us. Among those present, much was gained in better understanding of medications, various symptoms of HIV and AIDS, spiritual means of coping with a positive diagnosis and knowledge that others had similar equipment, experiences, and feelings. It is to this end that we must strive as we work to eliminate breaches of and the potential for breaches of confidentiality in our Native American communities.

Variations in Religious Belief Have an Impact on How HIV/AIDS Education is Received

This particular point is made in the opening comments of this chapter regarding the many variations in Native American cultures and traditions. True and traditional Lakota people understand Tunkashila as grandfathers who possess the power to impact their destiny. They turn their concerns over to Tunkashila while continuing to take responsibility for the outcome. Both traditional Ojebwa and Lakota medicine people emphasize self-determination as an essential aspect of Native American spirituality. Groups of Indian people have developed however, the belief that Tunkashila is responsible for their destiny and take no responsibility in shaping the outcome. This, emphasized the Indian Health Board of Minneapolis Executive Director, is contrary to native tradition and the victimization that results from this attitude is something that is being fought constantly in the native community.

Those Native Americans who believe that Tunkashila, the Great Spirit,

Creator, God, or whatever term is theirs for the divine, is responsible for what happens to them, are likely to be numerous in the group who oppose HIV/AIDS education as unnecessary. If it is to be that their people do not become ill with HIV, the Creator will take care of it without help from mere mortals. In addition, the discussion of sexuality, sexual practices, and human reproductive organs, did not take place among the grandfathers. Discussion of this type was considered inappropriate and wrong; therefore the same remains true today. Unable to discuss sexuality, sexual practices, and/or human reproductive organs precludes a discussion necessary to the very essence of HIV/AIDS education. Rather than work within these beliefs, many educators find the restrictions insurmountable and either do not attempt to educate those who hold them, or make an attempt to change the beliefs and then introduce

HIV/AIDS Education

Those of course, who believe that we are each responsible for our own destinies, tend to be much more receptive to HIV/AIDS education. This does not mean that the traditions of the grandfathers are ignored or disrespected. Rather, the wise educator will begin a class or forum by burning sage and offering prayer to the Tunkashila recognizing that this might seem contrary and apologizing for any perception of disrespect.

"It is not the way of the grandfathers," can easily become a phrase behind which those who have fears and concerns regarding HIV/AIDS or who are fearful someone will suspect them of being Two Spirits or of being HIV positive themselves, might easily hide. Some educators have reminded these same persons that wearing shoes and Euro-American clothing; using washing machines, and buying pre-packaged buffalo is also not the way of the grandfathers, yet many of these things have become a part of the daily routine and life of a large number of Native Americans.

I believe in my heart-of-hearts that HIV/AIDS education is as possible with those who consider Tunkashila responsible for their destiny as it is for those who follow the traditional belief that they are responsible for their own destiny. The answer to what appears to be an almost insurmountable dilemma is in the educator's approach to those he/she hopes to bring information to. Sincerity, honesty, and respect can and, in most cases, will bring with them the blessings of Tunkashila for the education that is essential to the well-being of Indian nations.

There Is a Need for Involvement of Elders and Spiritual Leaders in HIV/AIDS Education

Most parents who have had their children in parochial schools will always remember hearing, "Sister said," or "Father said." What Sister or Father said might be the very messages that mothers and fathers had given their children day after day. These words were heard in an entirely new light when spoken by Sister or Father. Much the same is experienced in the Native American community: messages spoken by the elders and spiritual leaders carry a great deal more weight than do the same messages spoken by any member of the tribe, and certainly are taken more seriously than when spoken by someone from outside the tribe.

As I spoke about HIV/AIDS during several workshops of a Wellness and Spirituality Conference, I made many references to the importance of receiving these messages being received by elders and spiritual leaders. During the next few days, several people asked to see me. Two of these people were sweat lodge leaders. They had attended the HIV/AIDS workshop and had questions. They had encountered concerns about someone with AIDS coming to a sweat and infecting others. There were elders who also had attended the workshop and they acknowledged their responsibility to talk about HIV/AIDS, yet they felt inadequately prepared to do so. Some who asked to speak with me were medicine men who were concerned about having persons with HIV or AIDS participate in ceremonies. In the case of the sweat lodge leaders and medicine men, I asked what they knew of HIV transmission. Some of them had at least partial knowledge of transmission while others were uncertain and hesitant to speak. I asked further if they would be interested in taking time before the end of the conference to increase their knowledge of HIV and transmission so that they would feel more fully prepared to respond to questions asked of them. All of those leaders returned during a long break one day, to discuss what they knew and what they believed they knew about HIV and its transmission. We burned sage, prayed, and talked together while they gained a great amount of knowledge to share on their reservations in a small amount of time.

With the elders, I acknowledged my respect for their dilemma in wanting to bring HIV/AIDS education to their people and I asked what they thought would be the greatest help to them now, during the conference. They had questions about things that they had heard or read about HIV/AIDS and wondered if I might answer some of the questions and add to their knowledge and understanding. Once again, I met with these elders and we burned sage, prayed and discussed their concerns. With their questions answered, I then suggested that it might not be as necessary for them to take on the entire responsibility of providing the AIDS education as it would be for them to endorse this education. I further suggested that there are many people, both native and non-native who are familiar with HIV/AIDS education and work in the Native American community, who could actually provide this education and I offered to provide them with the names and addresses of several people.

Native American communities are blessed with the wisdom of elders and spiritual leaders. I have found these persons more than willing to participate in HIV/AIDS education when approached with respect and when their wisdom and insight are acknowledged. Because HIV/AIDS is a topic which only a few are comfortable in presenting, it is important that we offer resource persons with whom they might work: the elders and spiritual leaders as endorsers and the others as the actual instructors.

There Is a Need for Tribal Chairpersons and Council Members to Speak to the Need for HIV/AIDS Education

In many ways, this point is not dissimilar to that of the preceding point regarding elders and spiritual leaders. Not infrequently, if the tribal chairperson doesn't think that something is important enough to recommend, then it is not going to occur. I can easily translate this into the operation of many Christian congregations. If the pastor never addresses specific issues from the pulpit, in the newsletter, or during the adult forum, they must not be important enough to be considered by or acted upon by members of the parish. Members of a congregation then, whose pastor never addresses lesbian and gay concerns, will tend to believe that it is not important that they know anything about these issues, let alone the people most deeply affected by them. They might also perceive by the pastor's silence that it is somehow wrong to be gay or lesbian. If the pastor doesn't include a need for outreach to the poor in an occasional sermon, members of the congregation might well believe that the poor are "the problem of some other congregation and pastor" and so on.

Although my experience working with tribal politics is quite limited, I did encounter some of this when presenting HIV/AIDS education in a tribal clinic. Following the presentation, the health educator and I visited at length. She was initially enthusiastic and energetic in planning additional programs and activity, yet she sounded much less enthusiastic toward the end of the day. "I really would like to do further HIV education here and then do some in the schools, but I only have six months left for all of that." I inquired about the time frame. She continued by telling me that in six months there would be tribal elections. If the same chairman is elected, there is a good chance that further AIDS education would be encouraged, but if someone else is elected, they might not see this as a priority and might even ban it from the clinic. "Programs here at the clinic," she said, "are pretty much controlled by the chairman who is the chair of the board, and has all of the control. If he thinks Fetal Alcohol Syndrome (FAS) is where our focus should be, then FAS it is and AIDS education simply won't happen."

Tribal chairpersons and council members are elected. And although I don't doubt their concern for the welfare of the tribe, their priorities are set on keeping happy those whose votes won the election for them. Both realities must be understood and acknowledged by anyone suggesting that HIV/AIDS education be presented in a tribal setting.

It Is Essential That HIV/AIDS Education Be Approached as Working With Native Americans Rather Than Doing for Them

The BIA does FOR Native Americans: "See all of the things we can do for you if you will live on reservations: housing, roads, schools... you name it." if the Pine Ridge Reservation is representative of what the BIA does for Native Americans, their comments can only fuel mistrust and ill feelings toward Euro-Americans. As I drove through the reservation recently, I experienced these broken promises first hand: pot holes so large that I feared the car would be engulfed and irreparably damaged, homes that were merely shacks, broken and missing windows in most of these dwellings, mud holes nearly as deep as swimming pools, and abandoned automobiles everywhere with tires, mirrors, doors, and other parts missing. These are the images that I expect many of our Native American sisters and brothers have when they hear that someone will do for them.

Not only does the BIA fail in doing for Native Americans, but so do many other large, bureaucratic institutions: medical assistance, Social Security, Aid to Families of Dependent Children (AFDC), and others. My clients have shared that the paper work required of them is itself oppressive; especially when the vocabulary used is not familiar. They immediately feel intimidated and inadequate. In many instances, these same people further report that their workers are Euro-American women and men who "just don't understand Indians." They report feeling that they can't seem to express their needs in the ways workers understand and because of this, they often don't get the full benefits that they deserve.

Much of this eventually translates to health care and finally to HIV/AIDS education. The AIDS "experts" that Native Americans see and hear on the nightly news are not indigenous people; they are for the most part, Euro-Americans who look much like people from the BIA and the Social Security office; people that Native Americans have learned to distrust. Their message is: "Listen to this information and be safe; do what we say and you won't become infected with HIV." The message sounds vaguely similar to, "Live on reservations and see what we'll do for you." I can imagine that a message heard in that context will not be heard or heeded.

On the other hand, if the message is, "Please listen to the information about HIV/AIDS so that we can discuss it and think about what we can do together to stop the spread of the virus," there is a far greater chance that at least some of the message will be heard and received. When speaking to groups of Native Americans about HIV/AIDS, I frequently acknowledge being "washichu"[10] (Euro-American person) and how it can affect their level of trust. I make my message brief and factual, using commonly understood terms rather than medical vocabulary and explaining the terms that are not easily simplified. When mistrust of the CDC arises, as it most often does, I acknowledge once again, that it must be difficult to trust large, bureaucratic institutions that are made up mostly of washichu doctors. Most importantly, the educator must not present him/herself as doing for, but rather, uphold the ability of those assembled to find solutions for these difficult problems. "This is simply one more difficult problem that needs your attention if complications from HIV infection are not to destroy your tribe." A member of the Women and Wellness Conference planning committee told us how she dislikes the phrase "to empower." She feels that this implies that someone or some group of people, are without power until another person or group gives them the power. Native Americans do not need to be empowered to fight HIV and AIDS; they do need to be able to work side by side with people who are knowledgeable about the virus, it's transmission, and testing, until they are secure in their own knowledge and understanding. This is very different from doing for or empowering them to do. This in fact, reaches to the very heart of the chapter subtitle, "Mitakuye Oyasin," "All my relations." We as HIV/AIDS educators must stand side by side with our Native brothers and sisters as "All my relations" and work with them in bringing HIV/AIDS education to the people.

It's Only Been a Hundred Years Since Wounded Knee

By the 1870's, prayers for release from the oppression and the violence of White settlers were common among Native Americans. Perhaps the Ghost Dance best exemplifies this, where dancers gathered and swayed in dance while entering into a trance-like-state where they were able to visualize promises of a brighter future. As the Ghost Dance grew in practice, a great deal of it's violent message was lost and what non-Indians understood was that the dancers dreamed and prayed for a life where there were no white settlers. This was perceived as a threat to the settlers who then notified the army and troops were dispatched to detain several hundred Indian men, women, and children who had gathered for the Ghost Dance at Wounded Knee. From somewhere, a shot was fired and in the ensuing gunfire, over two hundred Native Americans were critically wounded or killed. Many of the women were able to briefly escape. These women were captured and killed only a few miles away and the rest eventually froze to death in the harsh elements of the surrounding hills.

While visiting the Pine Ridge Reservation for the first time, a newly made Oglala friend told me that he hoped I would make time during my brief stay to visit Wounded Knee. Several hours later, he and another friend offered to drive out to Wounded Knee with me. We parked the car some distance away and walked to the small burial place of those savagely murdered only one hundred years ago. After several minutes of reading the names of the dead, my young friend spoke. Although I don't remember his words verbatim, I do remember the essence of his message.

> I'm never certain what people expect to see here. I've been out here when an occasional group of white tourists comes by. Most of the time they stay just a few minutes and then head back to their cars. As they leave, I've heard many of them say, "Is this all that there is?"
>
> I want to scream. This is where hundreds of innocent women, children, and men were slaughtered! What did you expect: Tepees? Native men in feathered head-dresses with their faces painted? Women all decked out in buckskin? If you want that, head up the Black Hills to Mount Rushmore.
>
> This huge loss of life is the result of white expectations and the fear that was generated by those expectations.

Before any of us (even the best-intentioned) Euro-Americans charge into the Native American community, hell-bent on providing HIV/AIDS education, let us remember that it has been only a hundred years since Wounded Knee and that a hundred years is only time enough to begin the process of healing and trust rebuilding. Throughout those hundred years, Native Americans have not lived in a void, but have been keenly aware of the systematic annihilation of European Jews and others during World War II, and the slaughter of hundreds of thousands on the African and European Continents. How does one with such a history trust that the messages regarding HIV/AIDS are not really some means of masked genocide; after all, AIDS did begin by taking the lives of thousands of "sinful" Two Spirits.

It is easy to think, "But, we're not our ancestors; we mean no harm." Only time will prove that to those so severely wounded by our ancestors for many generations. Perhaps we must learn to think less globally and concentrate first on working with individual Native Americans who are living with HIV and AIDS who can, in turn, take the message of prevention and education to the larger Native American community. I believe that we Euro-Americans do have a place in HIV/AIDS education and work with our Native American sisters and brothers, walking, teaching, learning all alongside of and with them. As we walk the path together, we gain not only understanding and knowledge, but trust and mutual respect. This is the spirit of Mitakuye Oyasin.

Epilogue

Since beginning the writing of this chapter in February, 1995, three of our HIV/AIDS case managed clients have died; two of them Native American with strong ties to their reservations. Both of these young men exemplified the need to pursue HIV/AIDS education in the Native American community in an attempt to not only bring a message of prevention, but also of compassion and acceptance in the spirit of Mitakuye Oyasin.

Because he was a Two Spirit, and fearful of rejection, one young man never revealed his HIV status or his AIDS diagnosis to his family. So great was his fear of discovery that he was constantly on the move and only on the reservation for brief visits. He called me one evening from the reservation to ask what he would be experiencing if he had anemia. I described the symptoms to him and asked if this seemed to be the problem. He said that he was certain that he was experiencing what I described and asked what he should do. I suggested a trip to the PHS hospital for laboratory work that would confirm our suspicion and if positive, a change in medication. A trip to the local hospital was impossible, because someone there would know why he was experiencing anemia—and would then know about his HIV status. This young man then asked about the possibility of wiring money to him so he could make a two hour bus trip to a large city hospital and have the laboratory work done there. I could not honor his request, but learned from him several days later, that he hitch hiked the entire way to the large city, had blood drawn and was indeed, experiencing anemia—as we suspected.

As he became increasingly ill, this young man remained in the large city and was eventually admitted to the hospital there. When his family was notified of his admission and subsequent death, they were told that he died of a non-AIDS related problem. His body was returned home and he was buried in the tradition of his tribe. AIDS was not spoken of at the wake or funeral and to this day, his true cause of death is not known by the family.

In the second instance, a young male client living in Greater Minnesota, was open and honest about his HIV status and his AIDS diagnosis. Not only was this shared with his family and former wife, but he revealed it openly during his NA/AA meetings in an attempt to educate others. After months of saving, he was finally able to have a telephone installed in his home. Finally, we were able to have regular personal contact other than by letter and Newsletter. I called one day, to find that the number he had given me had been discontinued. Alarmed that this young man might be ill and hospitalized, I called his parents. His mother shared with me that because of his honesty during meetings and other gatherings, her son had begun to receive death threats by phone and eventually had no choice but to have the phone discontinued. Although this client did not live on the reservation, his community was comprised of a large number of Native Americans and they were located in close proximity to the reservation. Would HIV/AIDS education have prevented the death threats? Would this young man have been warmly welcomed and accepted by a circle larger than his immediate family? I expect that both would have occurred. As I began these closing thoughts and comments this morning, I received word that this client died several days ago.

The number of Native Americans who have tested positive for HIV infection is small in comparison to Euro-Americans, Afro-Americans and others. The fear of HIV/AIDS educators is that many Native Americans who are positive have yet to be tested, and while not knowing their diagnosis, are continuing to transmit the virus to others. One more Native American infected with HIV is one too many. It is our obligation to walk alongside of our Native American sisters and brothers, as colleagues, friends, companions, health care professionals, and educators, as in-roads are made in bringing HIV/AIDS education to the Native American community. Mitakuye Oyasin.

Notes

1. Lakota meaning all my relations.
2. These issues are identified throughout the document, "HIV/AIDS Work Group on Health Care Access Issued for American Indians and Alaska Natives" produced by the U.S. Department of Health and Human Services, 1992.
3. Lakota meaning the grandfathers.
4. Sponsored and developed by the Indian Health Promotion Program of the University of Oklahoma.
5. Used by many tribes to describe those who are lesbians or gay
6. As high as 80% on the Pine Ridge Reservation of South Dakota
7. 1993-1995
8. Indian Health Services which is comprised of eleven regional area offices: Aberdeen, Alaska, Albuquerque, Bemidji, Billings, California, Nashville, Navajoland, Oklahoma, Phoenix, Portland and Tucson. In the fiscal year 1992, the IHS user population was approximately 1.150,000. The population is younger, less educated, and poorer than the U.S. all races population.
9. Intravenous catheters placed in large veins for the purpose of administering medications, fluids, and/or nutrition.
10. Lakota word meaning white or Euro-American person.

References

American Diabetes Association. (1993). *Diabetes Fact Sheet.* Washington, DC: Government Printing Press.

Maslow, A. H. (1954). *Motivation and Personality*. New York: Harper and Row.

Song, C. S. (1987). *Tell Us Our Names*. New York: Orbis Books.

Thomas, D. H. (1993). *The Native American: An Illustrated History*. Atlanta: Tumer Publishing Inc.

Uganda and the Challenge of Aids

by Kabahenda Nyakabwa

In the 1980s when Acquired Immune Deficiency Syndrome (AIDS) first appeared in Uganda, Ugandans mused at its emaciating effect and gave it the euphemistic name of "slim." Uganda was the first African country to openly acknowledge the existence of this disease and to conduct an aggressive campaign towards its prevention. In spite of a phenomenal effort to fight the AIDS epidemic, Uganda is currently one of the countries worst-hit by AIDS in Africa. Reportedly 1.7 million Ugandans are infected with the HIV virus (*Africa Report*, May/June 1994). The total Ugandan population of 17 million is directly and indirectly affected: mortality and morbidity rates have reached ominous proportions, whole communities may be decimated, and the country is threatened with destitution, economic devastation and social disruption.

Many factors can account for the explosive AIDS situation in Africa and Uganda but none as dramatically as economic misery, patriarchy, culture, religion and inadequate health care resources (Barnett and Blaikie, 1992; Latham, 1993; Turshen, 1991).

The purpose of this paper is to illustrate the reality of the AIDS epidemic in Uganda as a medical and social disease that poses enormous economic, social, and developmental challenges for Uganda in general, and for women in particular. The implications of the AIDS epidemic for the country are discussed and policy strategies proposed.

AIDS has become Uganda's number one killer disease and the following statistics illustrate the magnitude of the problem:

• 1.7 million Ugandans are allegedly infected with the HIV virus but the epidemic has not yet peaked (*Africa Report*, May/June 1994, 28).

• AIDS in Uganda is a plague that cuts across age, gender, sexual orientation, class, religion, tribe, social and economic status, rural and urban boundaries. Young, affluent, urban professionals, prostitutes, school children above the age of 15, as well as people in the rural areas are equally affected (*Africa Report*, May/June 1994; Barnett and Blaikie, 1992;).

• A joint study conducted by UNICEF and Makerere University in 1990 reported that 83% of all reported AIDS cases were among individuals between 15-40 years of age.

• According to the latest World Bank report on Uganda's social indicators, AIDS will lower the population growth rate from the 3.7% it would have been without AIDS, to 3.1% during 1995-2000. "Because of the long latency period, even if effective AIDS control practices were adopted today, the annual number of AIDS deaths would continue to increase for the remainder of this decade" (The World Bank, 1993, 9).

• The mortality rate has reached such crisis proportions that the government, families and communities are beginning to feel the strain.

• The financial and emotional burdens involved in caring for HIV/AIDS patients and the millions of orphaned children are beyond the capabilities of the government and families.

• People with AIDS are survived by their elderly parents and their orphans who are financially and emotionally incapable of looking after themselves (*Christian Science Monitor*, 16 Mar. 1994; *Toronto Star*, 24 Mar. 1994).

The following case studies depict the situation of many women in Uganda today.

Ms. Namukasa is a 45 year-old single parent of six children. Her oldest daughter, Margaret, who has just died of AIDS, left her three children in Namukasa's care. Ms. Namukasa's elder brother and his wife died in the war of liberation in 1985, leaving their five children in the care of Namukasa. Margaret was a petty-trader in Kampala, the capital city. Two of Ms. Namukasa's other daughters are HIV positive and keep falling sick. Each has two very young children. Ms. Namukasa has never worked outside the home and can barely read and write. She grows all her food and was depending on her oldest daughter for money. She now has to care for her five daughters, her seven grand-children, her brother's five children (two nieces and three nephews) and does not have time to grow as much food as she used to. The death of her oldest child, the sickness of the two daughters and their impending death have had an emotional toll on her. She was recently diagnosed with high blood pressure and has been advised to take bed-rest. Her three younger daughters have had to quit school because she cannot afford to pay their school fees. Moreover, they have to help her take care of their sisters, nephews, nieces, and cousins.

Mrs. Bagonza, Mrs. Kintu, and Mrs. Okello are sisters in their thirties. Mr. Bagonza, a prominent lawyer and Mr. Kintu, an accountant with the Central Bank, were both young men under 45 years of age who died of AIDS. Mr. Kintu, in a desperate search for a cure, visited private doctors in Zaire and West Germany and the Kintu family has been left virtually penniless. Mr. Okello, a university professor, and his wife have full-blown AIDS and are on their death-beds. Mrs. Bagonza and Mrs. Kintu have persistently tested seronegative. There are twelve children involved in this case study, ranging from 6 years of age to 14. Mrs. Bagonza and Mrs. Kintu both have high school education but they have never worked outside the home. Since the deaths of their husbands, they have withdrawn from society and all they do is sit in their homes and cry. Mrs. Bagonza is a relatively well-off widow but her in-laws have already expropriated some of her property and she fears they may take it all. Mr. and Mrs. Okello do not have much money and their healthcare is costing their extended family a lot of money. Relations between the Okellos and their extended families are visibly strained. The three sisters claim they are victims of their marriages but are powerless against this disease. They have elderly and sickly parents.

The impact of HIV/AIDS on women in Uganda demonstrates that it is women who bear the brunt of the continent's misfortunes such as wars, famine and disease, patriarchy, gender-based oppression, lack of rights and poverty (Paulme, 1963; James, 1992). Although men and women are both infected with the HIV virus, the latter are more adversely affected because of their specific economic, social, health and biological situations (Barnett and Blaikie, 1992; Caldwell, Orubuloye & Caldwell, 1992).

Extreme economic deprivation and lack of social status, and a patriarchal system which encourages polygamy have predisposed women to high rates of HIV infection and AIDS. It is poverty that forces poor women and young girls into prostitution, thus placing them at high risk for unwanted pregnancies, HIV infection and AIDS. The "sugar daddy" phenomenon means that young school girls render sexual favors to urban middle class and affluent men known as "sugar daddies" in exchange for money and other material goods. The men and the girls both become carriers and they in turn spread the virus (*Africa Report*, 1994; Barnett and Blaikie, 1992; *New York Times*, 22 June 1992).

Monogamous relationships are not shields against infection because of a double sexual standard whereby women are expected to remain faithful to their husbands and boyfriends while turning a blind eye to their infidelities. Even when a woman knows or suspects that her husband or partner has been unfaithful to her, the notion of "negotiating safer sex practice" is out of the question because of cultural reasons, her economic dependence on the man and her lack of assertive skills (Unlin, 1992). A study done in Uganda in 1990 reported that 30% of the women surveyed believed themselves at risk because they could not stop their partners from having sex with other women for reasons stipulated above (Mariasy & Radlett, 1990).

In Uganda as in the rest of Africa, development has taken place on the backs of women because they perform most of the hard labor. However, in a male-dominated society, it is the men who own the property. Traditional female roles are centered around domestic chores and reproductive responsibilities including raising children and care-giving (UNICEF, 1989). This means that women delay seeking care for themselves because they are busy caring for children and ill family members. In addition to the burden of family care, food production also falls on their shoulders. Notwithstanding, women have limited decision-making powers within the family and within society, including power to control their own sexuality, and therefore their own bodies, to challenge men's behavior, and to negotiate the conditions under which they have sexual intercourse (Hunter, 1990; Unlin, 1990). But when their husbands or partners die they are deprived of property and inheritance rights and left virtually destitute (Barnett and Blaikie, 1992). Their predicament is further complicated by officials of the office of the Administrator General who reportedly defraud vast amounts of money from the estates of widows and children that fall under their jurisdiction (*Uganda Confidential*, 29 Nov.-6 Dec. 1993). AIDS, therefore, does not create new contexts for women; it only aggravates the problems of their existing conditions in society.

Surprisingly, for unknown reasons, seropositive women are reported to live longer than men (Barnett and Blaikie, 1992). As caregivers, the role of women in the fight against AIDS in Ugandan society should not be overlooked. As survivors they cannot effectively participate in the country's development without an amelioration in their social conditions. By implication, therefore, women form a special category that requires special attention in terms of health delivery services and AIDS prevention programs. Apart from maternity and ante-natal clinics, medical clinics that cater exclusively to women are scarce. Yet, AIDS symptomatology is different in women than in men and consequently, many women are misdiagnosed. The need for female-centered clinics to respond to the specific needs of all women and particularly seropositive women is urgent in Africa and Uganda.

The economic and moral challenges posed by the AIDS epidemic for Uganda are frightening. In most cases, people with AIDS (PWAs) particularly in urban centers, are young, educated professionals and their death implies direct and indirect deprivation of human and financial resources necessary for Uganda's present and future development. The economic and developmental impact is harsh. First, the country loses directly because civil servants, taxpayers, potential investors, consumers and young parents, who, at the peak of their earning and reproductive capacity, are dying in great numbers. Second, the disease may make governments and companies dysfunctional through increased deaths among the managerial, professional and skilled labour supply. These losses "can be expected to slow the growth of the modern sector of the Ugandan economy, over the medium to long term" (The World Bank, 1993, 10). Third, increased deaths in the rural areas could lead to a drop in coffee production which accounts for 90% of Uganda's foreign exchange earnings. Time spent caring for the sick and dying means that less time is devoted to food production and in the long term this may cause famine. Fourth, the country also loses indirectly because governments and companies accord sick-leave to those dying of AIDS, death benefits to surviving family members, time off for co-workers to attend funeral services and burial and grief-leave, all of which affect production and efficiency. In the long run, therefore, capital that could be used for developmental and investment purposes is being diverted to AIDS education and prevention programs thereby slowing down progress. AIDS is an incurable and expensive disease. The cost of medical care is clearly above the means of a debt-burdened Third World nation like Uganda. Palliative drugs such as the controversial AZT, DDI (Dideoxyinosine) and DDC (Dideoxycytidine) which are prolonging the lives of PWAs in the western countries are not accessible to nor affordable by Third World countries. The implication is that in less-developed countries PWAs have virtually no chance of survival. For example PWAs in western countries can lead healthy lives for 12 to 15 years after diagnosis while the longevity of an ordinary PWA in Uganda varies from six months to three years following diagnosis. According to a Canadian doctor, "the cost of drug therapy for the direct and indirect treatment of HIV and AIDS can range from about two thousand dollars upwards to tens of thousands of dollars annually per person. These costs usually increase as a person progresses from HIV infection to full-blown AIDS" (Kilby, Mar. 1993, 31). As the number of PWAs increases treatment costs will soar; the government has to choose between PWAs who are going to die in the long run and development projects. The moral dilemma posed by this epidemic becomes obvious. Hard-pressed families have to devote all their resources to doctors and medicines and by the time the PWA finally dies, their financial and emotional resources are severely depleted. The total effect on the country will be increased poverty at both the macro and micro levels.

As more people die, increasing numbers of the elderly, spouses and children are left without adequate financial and emotional support. One of the most visible social impacts of the AIDS epidemic on Uganda is the increasing number of orphans and their elderly grandparents (*The Christian Science*

Monitor, 16 March 1994; Toronto Star, 24 Mar. 1994). By the end of 1991, it was estimated that the total number of children orphaned by AIDS ranged between 620,000 and 1,200,000 (Hunter 1990). Forty per cent were under the care of guardians who are over 50 years of age while 25% were under the care of individuals above the age of 60 (Uganda/UNICEF Report October 1991). Caring for PWAs and the orphans left by them places an enormous burden on surviving families and societies.

Depending on the age of a child, the death of a parent can be the most catastrophic event in his or her life. The younger the child the more he or she is dependent on his or her parents. Loss of a parent in early childhood means loss of a central figure of attachment in the child's emotional life (Osterweis, et al. 1984). Some children may have witnessed their parents dying of AIDS and are psychologically traumatized by the manner in which their parents died. Due to their tender ages, the psychological effects may not manifest themselves until late adulthood.

In cases where both parents die, the parental role is assumed by grandparents, uncles, aunts, or close family friends. Change of homes and guardians, especially in early childhood, creates chaos and disorganization in the lives of children and has deleterious effects on their emotional, social, psychological and intellectual development (Osterweis, et al. 1984).

Generally speaking, Uganda is a very poor country and many families already experience severe economic hardships. In African culture adoption is relatively unknown and a practice that is not easily acceptable. The cultural expectation is that surviving immediate and extended family members will take care of the orphans of their deceased/dying relatives. But the size of Ugandan families and the sheer numbers of children involved makes it practically impossible for Ugandans to provide adequate care for these children. Grandparents and the extended family are the only social support networks and welfare system available to orphans. With increasing deaths, inflation and rising costs of living, the economic effects on the families become apparent. A study done in Uganda in 1990 found that both guardians and children were experiencing stress.

> Guardians report psychological stress from dividing already scarce resources among natural and orphaned children. Orphans leave home at young ages because they are continually disadvantaged in the distribution of material resources and psychological support. They may be overworked by relatives or other guardians who consciously or unconsciously view them as a burden. Lack of supervision, proper caretaking and school or vocational activities lead to poor socialization, alienation from guardians and the community and possible delinquency (Hunter, 1990, 686).

This has serious implications for the country's development. Essentially, these children may be emotionally, socially, and financially incapacitated to the extent that they may become unproductive members of society. Therefore, their participation in Uganda's development process will be ineffective.

Governmental, non-governmental and community groups have organized locally, and the international community has responded with financial and material generosity towards HIV/AIDS prevention educational programs.

AIDS support organizations (ASO) have mushroomed in Uganda. The first and internationally recognized one is The AIDS Support Organization (TASO). Although TASO provides counselling, practical support and training for people with AIDS (Barnett and Blaikie 1992, 108), it does not have branches in all parts of the country. Other local initiatives include The Uganda Women's Efforts to Save Orphans (UWESO) which helps orphans with clothing and scholarships; Orphans Community Based Organization (OCBO) is run by the National Resistance Councils to register orphans (Barnett and Blaikie, 1992, 108); the National Council for Children (NRC) under the Ministry of Labor and Social Affairs was recently established reportedly "to coordinate a national program of action for children." The NRC entrusts Resistance Councils' (RCs) vice-chairpersons and members with the children's "protection and welfare." (*The New Vision*, 23 May, 1994).

AIDS in Uganda should be addressed in a developmental context. Such a proposition would take into consideration the definition of the United Nations Declaration on the Right to Development which states that development is a comprehensive economic, social, cultural and political process that aims at the attainment of a better life for the entire population on the basis of their active, free and meaningful participation in development and in the fair distribution of benefits resulting therefrom (*Encyclopedia of Human Rights*, 1991, 384).

Ugandans do not participate equally in the development process. The unequal status of women and the marked regional differences in terms of wealth distribution and healthcare infrastructure mean that AIDS affects Ugandans disproportionately (World Bank, 1993). Without a revision of some of the aspects of existing health, political and social institutions and a total change in individuals' world views, the fight against AIDS will be futile. In spite of alarming death rates in the whole country, health services are not equitably distributed and the seriousness of the epidemic is not readily apparent to the people at risk. For example, "AIDS control is still confined largely to health ministries; health infrastructures are grossly inadequate; churches continue to campaign against condom use; soldiers rape with impunity" (*Africa Report*, May/June 1994, 29).

On the basis of the above considerations, the following policy strategies at the national, regional and international levels are proposed:

1. Health must take precedence over other government priorities because without a healthy society, other developmental efforts will be fruitless. The World Bank reports that "Uganda's aggregate health indicators are among the world's worst" (1993, 52).

2. Health services and blood screening centers must be equally distributed throughout the country and available to all Ugandans.

3. In the absence of a miracle cure, Uganda's salvation in terms of future development lies with its children. The care of orphans in African societies was always assumed by the extended family based on the assumption that the extended family was itself intact. Given the present circumstances in Uganda, extended families are also dealing with their own deaths, bereavement and orphans. Therefore, their financial and emotional resources are depleted and they are no longer in a position to cope with the situation. Institutional care is not a viable alternative for Uganda for the following reasons: (a) because it is an alien concept in African culture; (b) because it would isolate children from their kin and familiar surroundings, marginalize them and expose them to the stigma of being known as "AIDS orphans" (*The Christian Science Monitor*, 16 March, 1994); (c) because it raises issues of child sexual molestation which are becoming public concerns in Uganda today (*The New Vision*, 12 Jan., 1994); and (d) because the country does not have the necessary infrastructure and human resources for institutional care. Hence, a foster care/parenting program that helps orphaned children to cope with their deprivation while simultaneously offering them an opportunity for self-development should be implemented.

4. There should be strong and effective legislation to protect women and children from seropositive men. Those who rape women and children are a menace to society and should be prosecuted, and if found guilty, incarcerated.

5. Regardless of their social, economic or political status, the justice system must serve all Ugandans fairly.

6. Legal education on the rights of women and children to property and inheritance, and freedom from violence must become an integral part of all programs offered by AIDS support organizations.

7. An effective surveillance system would contribute to better and adequate data collection methods on mortality from AIDS. Without accurate statistics it is difficult to fathom the reality and magnitude of the epidemic. For example, the war in eastern and northern Uganda renders the area inaccessible to researchers and government officials. Consequently, the reality of the AIDS situation in these parts remains obscure (Barnett and Blaikie, 1992, 23).

8. Research has tended to concentrate in the central region of Buganda particularly Rakai district and the surrounding districts of Kigezi and Hoima. More research should be undertaken in remote parts and other regions of the country such as Toro in the western province and Mbale and Tororo in the eastern province. This could provide Uganda with a useful comparative framework in terms of rates of infection, morbidity and mortality, community responses, coping mechanisms and population decimation. The last point is very important, especially for smaller tribes of less than one million, and should not be underestimated.

9. There should be more female-centered research geared to exploring women's knowledge, attitudes and practices, support systems and coping resources particularly of long surviving seropositive women.

10. AIDS programs must give particular emphasis to women and children as target groups and should incorporate women in the development of AIDS prevention strategies at the national, district and county levels in recognition of the role they play in society, that they are more adversely affected than men and that they tend to survive longer (Barnett and Blaikie, 1992).

11. In order for AIDS support organizations to function effectively, they must be democratic, and accountable to the communities that they serve. Representatives from these communities must be included at the planning and implementation levels of AIDS prevention education programs. There must be coordination and evaluation at the national and community levels to avoid duplication of efforts.

12. AIDS support organizations should act as media for raising individuals' consciousness about issues such as sexuality, rape and violence against women, their effects on women's lives and implications for society, and the risk of HIV infection and AIDS.

13. "Peer Counselling Models" like those developed in Canada and the United States for PWAs should be introduced in Ugandan colleges and universities. These may prove to be more effective than counselling offered by existing organizations. This point is significant for African countries where seropositive young people may deliberately avoid such organizations because of the cultural reverence and fear of those older than themselves. As a result, this impedes open communication about sexuality, sex and use of condoms.

14. A system whereby community elders would identify some responsible members of their communities to volunteer to provide homes for orphans should be explored. A family support allowance would be provided to such families. Social workers or community development officers would visit the homes regularly to evaluate the care the children are receiving and to help foster families deal with behavioral problems.

15. Mortality rates directly affect labor and food production. Agricultural policies to ensure continued food production to mitigate against famine due to loss of productive labor power should be implemented.

1. Research done in Third World countries by western academics and medical personnel has tended to enhance the careers and fame of the same while obscuring the efforts and contributions of local professionals; research findings should be shared equally.

2. The availability of vaccines or any other therapeutic drug to affected countries should be mandatory.

3. More funding should be channeled towards social science research and should focus on the effect of multiple bereavement on the elderly, children, families and communities. How are children, families and communities coping? What are the effects, if any, of multiple bereavement? How does the nation plan to cope with the psychological effects of this epidemic?

4. Fighting AIDS and its effects in Uganda requires a concerted effort of the government, local and international NGOs and the international community.

International donor agencies can play a key role in providing additional resources—physical, financial and technical—to enable the government to meet the shelter, educational, nutritional, clothing, and health needs of the orphans.

Summary

This paper has illustrated that AIDS poses enormous social, economic, demographic and developmental challenges for Uganda. Mortality rates have reached such apocalyptic proportions that the government, families and communities can no longer cope with the financial and emotional costs involved in caring for the sick and the dying. Because of the gendered structures of social, economic and political inequalities, women, who are society's most vulnerable group, are most adversely affected. Thus, massive financial assistance from the international community is necessary if the country is to deal effectively with the short term and long term challenges of the AIDS epidemic.

Conclusion

In conclusion, the AIDS situation in Uganda begs the following question: Why is it that despite an open and aggressive AIDS campaign, and in spite of the knowledge acquired about this epidemic through the traumatic experience of high death rates in families and communities, the AIDS situation in Uganda has not abated?

Dr. Mann, acknowledged specialist in the fight against AIDS, recently admitted that "AIDS prevention programs are losing strength and credibility and can do little to prevent the epidemic from spreading to vulnerable countries" (*Ottawa Citizen*, 10 August, 1994). The evidence leads the author to conclude that increased knowledge is a necessary but insufficient mechanism to fight AIDS; prevention programs provide only a partial solution and therefore new strategies must be explored.

The selective nature of AIDS and its direct and indirect economic and social costs portend destitution and social and economic devastation at macro and micro levels. In order to halt the ravages of this disease in Africa, AIDS prevention education must be combined with a change in the pre-existing conditions that predispose people to HIV and AIDS. Such conditions include economic, social and gender inequalities such as women's lack of control over their own sexuality, lack of property and inheritance rights, lack of legal and political rights, unequal access to healthcare, and cultural practices such as polygamy which relegate an inferior and powerless position to women in families and society. This calls for a developmental model which emphasizes the provision of basic human needs with a human rights component. One of the most important aspects of such a model would be the involvement of women in all phases of AIDS-related planning, program development, implementation and monitoring. The other would be the recognition of the worth of every Ugandan, and women not only as agents of reproduction, but as productive members of society with equal political, social and economic rights as preconditions for a healthy society.

References

Africa Takes Small Steps to Help AIDS Orphans. (March 16,1994). *Christian Science Monitor*, Boston: Robert M. Press.

Blaikie, P. (1992). *AIDS in Africa: Present and Future Impact*. New York: Guildford Press.

Caldwell, J.C., Orubuloye, I.O. & Caldwell, P. (1992). Underreaction to AIDS in Sub-Saharan Africa. *Social Science and Medicine*, 34 (11), 1169-1182.

Cheeye, S. (November 29, 1993). Women: The Death Industry. *Uganda Confidential*, Kampala, 13.

Flint, J. (May/June, 1994). AIDS: The Plague Years. *Africa Report*, 27–29.

Government of Uganda & UNICEF Programme of Cooperation (October 1991). Expanded Programme of Communication for Control of AIDS in Uganda. Plan of Action 1991-1992.

Hunter, S. (1990). Orphans As a Window on the AIDS Epidemic in Sub-Saharan Africa: Initial Results and Implications of Study in Uganda. *Social Science and Medicine*, 31(6), 681-690.

James, S.N. (1992). Transgressing Fundamental Boundaries: The Struggle for Women's Human Rights. *Africa Today*, 39(4), 34-45.

Kilby, D. (March 2, 1993). Playing Catch-Up With Reality: The Future Challenges Are Already Here. *In AIDS: The Challenge*. Proceedings of the Conference on AIDS at the Westin Hotel. Ottawa, Canada.

Lawson, E. (1991). The Declaration On the Right to Development. In *Encyclopedia of Human Rights*, (1986). New York: Taylor and Francis Inc.

Latham, M.C. (1993). AIDS in Africa: A Perspective on the Epidemic. *Africa Today*. 40(3), 39-53.

Mariasy, J. & Radlett, M. (1990). Women the Vulnerable Sex. *AIDS Watch*, 10 (23).

Our Children: Our Future. (May 23, 1994). *The Kampala New Vision*, 12.

Osterweis, M., Solomon, F., & Green, M. (1984). *Bereavement: Reactions, and Care*. Washington, DC: National Academy Press.

Parlez, J. (June 22, 1992). Briton Sees AIDS Halting African Population Rise. *New York Times International*, 21.

Paulme, D.(Ed.) (1979). *Women of Tropical Africa*. Berkley, CA: University of California Press.

Samuels, L. (March 24, 1994). A Land of the Orphaned and Old. *Toronto Star*, 6.

Saunders, J. & Valente, S. (1987). Bereavement in Survivors of AIDS. In M.A. Morgan (Eds.), *Proceedings of the 1987 King's College Conference*, (pp. 203-208). London: Ontario.

Schoepf, B.G. et al. (1991). Gender, Power and Risk of AIDS in Zaire. In M. Turshen (Ed.). *Women and Health in Africa*. Trenton, NJ: Africa World Press.

Turshen, M.(Ed.) (1991). *Women and Health in Africa*. Trenton, NJ: Africa World Press.

The World Bank. (1993). *Uganda Social Sectors: A World Bank Country Study*. Washington, DC: The International Bank for Reconstruction/World Bank.

Ulin, P.R. (1992). African Women and AIDS: Negotiating Behavioral Change. *Social*

Science and Medicine, 34(1), 63-73.
UNICEF. (1989). *Children and Women in Uganda: A Situational Analysis*. Kampala, United Nations Children's Fund.
We Are Worried About Our Kids. (January 12, 1994). *The Kampala New Vision*, 8.

Socio-Cultural Factors That Predispose Women to HIV/AIDS in the Middle Belt of Nigeria

Charles B. U. Uwakwe

Introduction

Contemporary discussion on the Acquired Immunodeficiency Syndrome (AIDS), and its causative pathogen, the human immunodeficiency virus (HIV), often focus on the frightening power and magnitude of the disease. The World Health Organization estimates that 13 million people worldwide are infected with HIV, the majority of whom are in sub-Saharan Africa (Merson, 1993; Asindi et al., 1994). In parts of this sub-region, HIV... the deadly virus which erodes the body's ability to fight off infection..., has been detected in over 25% of some communities (Merson, 1993). Nigeria which has erstwhile been categorized as a low seroprevalence country is suddenly awakening to the rude shock of an imminent epidemic with recent epidemiological data showing that as many as 500,000 persons are HIV-infected (Asagba, 1992; Gashau et al., 1993; Harry et al., 1994). Thus Nigeria with a population of 85 million has the highest pool of susceptible people with HIV in Africa. Furthermore, recent sentinel survey reports indicate that the prevalence rate of HIV infection has increased from approximately zero percent in 1986 to about 1.7% in 1992. With an annual increase of HIV prevalence of 1%, the number of infections is projected at four million in 1996, and 7.2 million in the year 2000.

Surveys in Nigeria (Makinwa-Adebusoye, 1993; Uwakwe et al., 1995), however show that a high proportion of young urban Nigerians are currently sexually active—as many as 78% of males and 86% of females aged 20-24. According to the survey of more than 5,500 males and females aged 12-24, sexual intercourse appears sporadic and unstable; many of these young people of both sexes have had more than one sexual partner. Similar findings were made among female university students by a more recent study (Uwakwe, Mansaray and Onwu, 1993). Findings such as these are only the tip of the iceberg and reinforce the extremely urgent need for measures to address HIV/AIDS risk among young people.

In general, the upper socio-economic strata has a lower rate of AIDS/STDS than the lower socio-economic strata. Studies in other cultures, the United States of America for example, indicate that two out of every three persons under poverty line are women who have the highest rate of illiteracy, lowest educational levels and may not even have access to radio and television (Panos Institute, 1990). This makes it difficult for them to receive information about AIDS/STDs. Hernandez (1993) stated that poor women everywhere have difficulty with the consequences of this lack of information. This perhaps has been one of the major reasons for the rapid spread of AIDS in Nigeria and other African countries. Many women in the lower economic strata lack information and so may be ignorant of AIDS. Even when they are aware of HIV risk, they lack the power to change the sexual behavior of their partners on whom they depend economically. They are usually afraid of being abandoned or of physical violence should they attempt to increase their bargaining power in heterosexual relationships (Shayne and Kaplan, 1991).

The growing urbanization in Nigeria and other African countries make cities attractive to men and women. Most men leave their families behind in rural areas to go to the cities, where they form relationships with other women only to go back to the rural areas to infect their wives (Bassett and Mhyloyi, 1991). Some women migrate to the cities in search of social mobility through acceptance of money, gifts and favors in exchange for sex.

The socio-economic factors that contribute to the high risk of HIV infection in Africa are culturally determined attitudes to increasing exposure to sexual activity. In the past, religion and traditional societal strictures served to limit the incidence of venereal disease in Africa. However, the modern and more permissive sexual attitudes are being adapted not only by the younger but also by the older generation (Hardy, 1987). There is increased tolerance for heterosexual and homosexual activity, more frequent pre-marital and extra-marital intercourse and multiple sexual contacts. These practices increase the chances of HIV infection in the continent. Certain cultural belief systems in Africa are perhaps potent forces for the promotion of the risk of HIV infection. In Mozambique, it is believed that a sick person can be cured by passing the disease to another, which could encourage the raping of young women by men with STDs. Other studies (Alausa and Osaba, 1980; Bello and Dada, 1983) have also corroborated these findings that the Yorubas and Hausas of Nigeria believe that having sexual intercourse with a virgin will cure a man of any form of STDs.

With this background, the present study investigated the socio-cultural factors that predispose and possibly expose women in the Middle Belt of Nigeria to HIV/AIDS.

The following three hypotheses were tested at the 0.05 level of significance:

-There will be no significant difference between male and female subjects' knowledge about HIV/AIDS in the Middle Belt of Nigeria.

-There will be no significant difference between male and female subjects perception on the socio-cultural factors predisposing women to AIDS/STDS in the Middle Belt of Nigeria.

-There will be no significant difference between health and non-health workers' opinions on socio-cultural practices predisposing women to AIDS/STDS in the Middle Belt of Nigeria.

Design and Procedure:

Design of the study:

The simple descriptive survey was utilized to investigate the socio-cultural factors that predispose women to AIDS/STDS in the Middle Belt of Nigeria.

Subjects:

The subjects consist of 164 people (87 males and 77 females) drawn from the general population in the Middle Belt area of Nigeria. Of this sample, 75 were health workers, the remaining 69 were non-health workers. The subjects' ages also ranged between 25 and 34 years. The lowest educational qualification of the respondents was the West African School Certificate. Of the 20 subjects taken from the illiterate segment of the populace, six were males, and 14 were females.

Instrument:

The AIDS/STDs and Cultural Practices Scale for men and women was utilized for the study. The scale has three sections covering subjects' demographic data, knowledge about HIV/STDs, and the socio-cultural dimensions that predispose women to AIDS and STDS infections. The scoring was based on three points: true, false and don't know paradigm; while the section 'C' was evaluated on a five point Likert-type scale of Strongly Agree, Agree, Undecided, Disagree and Strongly Disagree.

The study also used the Focus Group Discussion (FGD) method for data collection. The FGD consist of seven items with the first three items tapping information on subjects' knowledge on AIDS/STDS while the last four items elicited the subjects' opinions on socio-cultural practices predisposing women to AIDS/STDS.

The split-half statistical method was employed to determine the reliability of the study. The computation was done using the Pearson Product Correlation coefficient.

Data Analysis:

A simple Student's t-test was used to test the hypotheses at the 0.05 level of significance. The findings are as summarised in the tables below showing a pairwise comparison.

Results and Findings

There follows a pairwise comparison table reflecting the t-values at the 0.05 level of significance.

Discussion:

The three tested hypotheses in the study were confirmed. This finding seems to contradict the common notion that women do not have as much access to information as men, (Shayne, and Kaplan, 1991), and may therefore not be as knowledgeable on such matters when compared to their male counterparts. That the hypothesis states that no significant difference exists between male and female subjects in terms of their knowledge of AIDS/STDS was further explained by the fact that most of the respondents were educated. Thus the level of education is probably associated with different enlightenment and awareness programs embarked upon throughout the country (Adamolekun and Boyibobe, 1987). Wilson et al., 1989, corroborate the present finding by confirming that better education among the upper socio-economic strata may increase awareness of AIDS/STDS.

The results emanating from the study have been summarised as indicated below.

Differential Groups	N	X	SD	't'observed	't' critical	Df
Knowledge of male subjects on AIDS/STDS	63	22.7	3.4	1.47	1.96	142
Knowledge of female subjects on AIDS/STDS	81	23.1	2.8			
Opinion of male subjects on socio-cultural factors	63	107	13.2	0.84	1.96	142
Female subjects response on socio-cultural factors	81	109	14.5			
Health workers on socio-cultural factors	75	110	11.8	1.73	1.96	142
Non-health workers on socio-cultural factors	69	106	15.5			

*$p < 0.05$

The second hypothesis was confirmed by the study. The analogy drawn here is that both the male and female subjects tested were aligned in their opinions on the socio-cultural factors that predispose women to AIDS/STDS in the Middle Belt of Nigeria. Such socio-cultural factors included prostitution, multiple sexual partners and the subservient status of most women among others. In corroborating this finding, Cameron et al. (1989) posited that sexual behaviors such as prostitution, multiple sex partners and promiscuity constitute a high risk of contracting HIV/STDS infections. The findings also lend support to the views of Campbell (1990) and Mahmoud (1991) who stated that the subordinate status of women in the family and society restricts their ability to protect themselves from HIV infection and other health-compromising behaviors. In the words of Hernandez (1993) "poor women everywhere have difficulty in preventing AIDS/STDS." It is implied from this study therefore that a wide spectrum of social, economic and cultural factors, which women have very little control over, actually contribute to their vulnerability to AIDS/STDS in the Middle Belt of Nigeria. The consensus of opinion among the respondents in the present survey is that such socio-cultural norms and practices as prostitution, submissiveness and poor bargaining power of the female folks, poverty, promiscuity and the use of circumcision instruments among others are implicated in this epidemic in the Middle Belt of Nigeria. No efforts should be spared in stemming the tide of the threat of the HIV/AIDS pandemic, which is presently acknowledged as one of immense proportions. Considering the dynamics of these cultural, social and economic factors, responsibility for this task should be shared by both men and women. In other words, since these socio-cultural factors have been implicated as high risk factors predisposing to HIV/AIDS infection, such practices should either be outrightly abrogated, discouraged, or modified to reduce the risk factors associated with them. Furthermore, the systematic community-based sensitization drive should be intensified to increase awareness about the inherent risks associated with such behaviors and practices.

References

Adamolekun, A. and Boyibobe, B. (Oct. 1987). Prospects of Effective Sex Education in Nigeria Secondary School. *Journal of Moral Education,* 15.

Alausa, K.O., Osaba, A.O. (1980). Epidemiology of Gonococcal Valvo-Vaginith's Among Children in the Tropics. *British Journal of Ven. Disease,* 56, 239-242.

Asagba, A.O.(Ed.). (1992). Focus on AIDS in Nigeria. *Nigerian Bulletin of Epidemiology,* 2(2), 1-24.

Asindi,A.A., Ibia,E.O., & Young, M.U. (1992). Acquired Immunodeficiency Syndrome: Education Exposure, Knowledge and Attitude of Nigerian Adolescents in Calabar. *Annual Tropical Pediatrics,* 12, 397-402.

Bassett, M. T. and Mliyoli, M. (1991). Women and AIDS in Zimbabwe. *International Journal of Health Services,* 21(1), 143-156.

Bello, C.S.S. and Dada, J.D. (1983). Sexually Transmitted Disease in Northern Nigeria. *British Journal of Venerology Diseases,* 59, 202-205.

Cameron, C. (1989). Female to Male Transmission of Human Immunodeficiency Lions Type 1 Risk Factors for Sero-Conversion in Men. *Lancet,* 2, 403- 407.

Campbell, A.C. (1990). Women and AIDS. *Social Science and Med.* 30(4), 407- 415.

Gashau, W., Harry,T.O.,Ekenna,O., & Mohammed,I. (1993). *HIV Infection in Spouses of Maiduguri, Nigeria.* Paper presented at the IXth International/Conference, Berlin, Germany.

Hardy, B. D. (1987). Cultural Practices Contributing to the Transmission of Human Immunodeficiency Virus in Africa. *Review of Infectious Diseases* 9(6), 1109-1119.

Harry,T.O., Bukbuk,D.N.,Idrisa,A., & Akoma,M.B. (1994). HIV Infection Among Pregnant Women: A Worsening Situation in Maiduguri, Nigeria. *Tropical Geographic Medicine,* 46, 46-50.

Hernandez, M. (1993). Research Approach to HIV/AIDS and Women's Reproductive Health. *National Institute of Public Health,* Mexico.

Mahmoud, F. (1991). Addressing AIDS From a Women's Perspective: Interview. *The Carrier,* No 126, 75.

Makinwa-Adebusoye, P.K. (1991). Adolescent Reproductive Behaviour in Nigeria: A Study of Five Cities, *NISER Mimeograph Series,* No. 3, NISER, Ibadan.

Merson, M. (1993). Slowing the Spread of HIV: Agenda for the 1990s. *Science,* 260(5112), 1266-1268.

Panos Institute. (1990). *Triple Jeopardy: Women and AIDS,* London: The Panos Institute.

Shayne, V.T. and Kaplan, B.J. (1991). Double Victims: Poor Women and AIDS. *Women Health,* 17 (1), 21-37.

Uwakwe, C.B.U., Onwu, G. & Mansaray, (1993). *A Psychoeducational Program to Motivate and Foster AIDS Preventive Behaviours among Female Nigerian University Students.* A Technical Report to the Women and AIDS Program, International Center for Research on Women, Washington DC, USA.

Uwakwe,C.B.U., Adeniyi,E.O., Imoh, G. & Egunjobi, O. (1995). *An Evaluative Survey of the Impact of the STD/AIDS Control Intervention Programs in Nigeria.* A Technical Paper for a Project Jointly Sponsored by The Federal Ministry of Health and Human Services, Lagos, and The World Health Organisation (WHO), Geneva, Switzerland.

Wilson, D., Greenspan, C. Sibanda, R. & Msimanga, P.(1989). Towards an AIDS Information Strategy for Zimbabwe. *AIDS Education and Prevention,* 1, 96-104.

Barriers to Behavior Change: Results of Focus Group Discussions Conducted in a High HIV/AIDS Incidence Area of Kenya

Caroline Blair, David Ojakaa, S.A. Ochola, and Dishon Gogi

The Homa Bay District of Kenya is among those worst affected by the AIDS epidemic. The district, before the creation of Migori as a separate administrative district, accounted for 11.2% of all reported AIDS cases in the country. This makes the two districts combined the leader in reported cases among all 52 districts in Kenya (Kenya National AIDS Control Programme, 1995).

In 1993, the district, situated on the shores of Lake Victoria had a total labor force of 315,640 people. Agriculture employs most of the labor force. Other activities in which the labor force is engaged include fishing, rural self-employment, and commercial enterprises. Homa Bay town offers most of the wage employment in the district, but this is very limited. The district generally experiences seasonal employment in agriculture and fishing, mainly during the rainy peak harvesting and fishing seasons. Most employees are paid very low wages and live in poor housing in small towns. Wage earnings in the district range between $ U.S. 25 and 117 per month among rural households. Poverty is a major problem in the district. It is estimated that over 100,000 people are dependent on the fishing industry in some way (Republic of Kenya, 1993).

While sentinel surveillance and other quantitative studies (such as the 1993 Kenya Demographic and Health Survey- KDHS) provide useful information for the planning and implementation of AIDS prevention activities in Homa Bay district and beyond, they leave some major questions unanswered. For example, compared to a national average of 40%, in Nyanza Province (the province in which Homa Bay is situated), over 50% of women and over 60% of men know someone who has AIDS or has died of it. When asked about perception of personal risk in the same survey, 65.6% and 46.2% of men and women respectively said that they could possibly become infected (National Council for Population and Development (NCPD), Central Bureau of Statistics (CBS), Office of the Vice-President and Ministry of Planning and National Development (Kenya), and Macro International Inc. (MI), 1994).

One would expect that on the basis of these figures, people would be changing their behavior to lower their potential risk of infection. This does not, however, appear to be the case, except among a limited numbers of persons in selected sub-groups of the Kenyan population. (NCPD et al., 1993; Plummer, F.A., Ngugi, E.N., and Moses, S, 1994; and Moses et al., 1994)

Another curious finding of the KDHS is that in spite of all of the public education which has taken place, asked about ways to prevent HIV/AIDS, only 32.6% of Kenyan men and 16.6% of Kenyan women cited the use of condoms, with usage figures being even lower at 20% and 6%, respectively for men and women. The United Nations Children's Fund (UNICEF) has been implementing AIDS prevention programs in partnership with the Ministry of Health in Homa Bay District since the late 1980's.

This UNICEF-supported study sought to gather, through qualitative research, information which would help to answer some of the questions unanswered by quantitative research. It was also intended to use focus group discussions to help identify barriers to behavior change as perceived by the residents of a geographic area which has been particularly hard hit by HIV and AIDS. These findings would then be used to improve program design and delivery as well as to provide a basis for strengthened message development.

Method

Focus group discussions were held with a total of 34 groups in November of 1994. These groups were comprised of school youth, traditional healers, clan elders, members of women's groups, widows, widowers, community health workers, traditional birth attendants, church elders, teachers, fish mongers, fishermen, and bar attendants.[1] See Table 1 for details on the groups interviewed.

This study was developed based upon a draft research proposal submitted to the UNICEF office in Nairobi by the Ministry of Health in Homa Bay and by using techniques suggested by Scrimshaw and Hurtado (1987), and by reviewing the results of a similar study undertaken earlier in Zimbabwe (Ministry of Education and Culture, Zimbabwe, 1993).

The discussion guide had two parts. The first covered background issues related to the participants. The second part dealt exclusively with the subjects of HIV infection and AIDS. The guide went through several pre-testing sessions before it was finally translated from the English into Dholuo, the local language of the Homa Bay area where the discussions were conducted.

The pre-selected target groups were identified and invited to participate through local Community Health Workers (CHW's). A letter inviting each of the participants to attend the discussion was sent out by the CHWs. The letter also specified the venue and time of the discussion. The selection was carried out in such a way that all the ten divisions in the district were covered. The discussions took exactly twelve days. On average, three discussions, each lasting between one and one and one half hours were held on each of the twelve days.

A total of two hundred and four respondents were thus interviewed. Of these, 69 were male, while 135 were female. The ratio of about two to one for women over men came about without a deliberate attempt being made. However, in light of the fact that it is well documented that women are disproportionately burdened with the care of the sick in Africa, that they have little control over their sexuality and of the sexual behavior of their partners (McGrath et al., 1993; Moses et al., 1994; Ulin, 1992) and that, unlike in the West, they make up 50% of persons with AIDS, this imbalance was not regarded to be problematic.

Attempts were made to have members of each discussion group be of the same sex. In most cases, this was achieved. An exception is bar attendants: one of the groups had two male bar workers; in one group of widows two widowers were present. Similarly, the following target groups had a combination of men and women in at least one of their sessions: traditional healers, church elders, CHWs, TBAs, and teachers.

TABLE 1: FOCUS GROUP DISCUSSIONS HELD

GROUP INTERVIEWED	NUMBER OF GROUPS
WIDOWS	3
BAR ATTENDANTS	3
TRADITIONAL BIRTH ATTENDANTS	3
COMMUNITY HEALTH WORKERS	3
CLAN ELDERS	3
CHURCH ELDERS	3
FISH MONGERS	3
TRADITIONAL HEALERS	3
BEACH WORKERS	1
WIDOWERS	2
TEACHERS	3
OUT OF SCHOOL YOUTH	2
WOMEN'S GROUP MEMBERS	3

RESULTS

Sexuality

Although some groups reported that they perceived at least marginal changes in behavior, for the most part, respondents felt that life was continuing as usual and people continued to practice unsafe sexual behavior. The general feeling that seems to have been expressed is that people are very busy and that as such while there is a considerable degree of fear of AIDS and that it is frequently discussed, they are more concerned with day to day survival than with something that might happen to them in five to ten years. In addition, while AIDS is a serious health problem, other illnesses, most notably malaria, continue to be major worries to residents of Homa Bay and have a more obvious cause and effect pattern. Sexually transmitted diseases (mainly gonorrhea) were mentioned by young people as another recurrent problem.

Of the persons interviewed, all the participants had heard about AIDS, first in whispered tones in the 1980s, then in more frequent and open discussions in the 1990s. Funerals of persons suspected to have died of AIDS were mentioned repeatedly as a place were AIDS was commonly the topic of conversation.

While all groups mentioned sexual intercourse as the main mode by which HIV/AIDS is spread, many misconceptions about routes of transmission persist. Among these, mosquito bites, public toilets, and kissing were mentioned. Men still also seem to believe that women are more resistant to HIV, making them more dangerous than men.

While most participants could correctly identify HIV prevention methods, many of them were not convinced that condoms were very effective, and although remaining faithful to one's partner was frequently cited as a method of prevention, it came out very clearly in the study that both premarital and extramarital sex are very common and that it was extremely unlikely that this would change anytime in the foreseeable future. Table 2 lists some of the statements made by participants regarding sexuality which illustrate the strong feelings which exist on this subject.[2]

TABLE 2: STATEMENTS ON SEXUALITY

"God gave Adam a partner and for that reason, sex is natural."
"The sexual urge is strong—at times uncontrolable."
"The sexual urge is natural and incessant in man. It is like a thief going to steal in the place where another thief was killed."
(The sexual appetite)..."is insatiable."
"Human beings are human beings who forget easily and go back straight into the ditch."
"One cannot resist the sexual urge acquired from the Garden of Eden."
"Even God's people still have women friends."

Mistrust between partners and spouses also seemed prevalent, with men and women blaming each other for affairs outside the relationship. Sexual relations among in-laws were also said to take place frequently. Reasons given for these relations included boredom with one (or in the case of polygamous unions, more than one) partner ("you should not eat vegetables only every day - you should change your diet"), and feelings of neglect on the part of women in polygamous unions. Experiencing long separations (a common occurrence in Kenya as men migrate to urban areas for employment) from spouses was also cited as a reason why people engaged in extra-marital relations, as was financial need, particularly in women's cases, and the desire to seek revenge for hurt feelings.

Of particular interest was that in spite of the commonly expressed views that sexual desire was almost uncontrollable, the discussions nonetheless exposed a great deal of ambivalent and conflicting feelings and opinions about sexuality in general and about AIDS prevention and condom use in particular. Moreover, when asked whether they could contract AIDS, most respondents answered that it was possible (this tallies with the KDHS findings referred to earlier), but their discussions quite clearly indicated that they did not think that it was at all likely that they themselves would become infected. Thus when discussing behavior change, respondents almost always talked about other people's behavior and not their own, thus indirectly implying that they themselves were not at risk.

The very frequent use by members of all groups (although this was less pronounced among the bar attendants, community health workers and traditional birth attendants) of words like promiscuous, promiscuity, immorality, and prostitute was very much in conflict with the almost universally expressed view that sexual desire is so strong that no one can truly expect to control it. One could perhaps assume that there is a high level of discomfort when dealing with one's personal sexual life and that this discomfort leads to denial of risk. This denial of risk in turn reduces an individual's personal responsibility to almost nothing, as the problem is one which only afflicts the "promiscuous." Although engaging in unsafe sexual practices with multiple partners would result in labelling the person practicing this behavior as "immoral" in the case of other people, it seems that individuals are more lenient when judging themselves, justifying their behavior by citing loneliness, need for money, or some other reason.

The opinion that persons with HIV should be isolated was quite frequently expressed. It was perceived by the respondents that this would make persons with HIV "stop spreading the virus." Related to this perception was the one that there were numerous HIV-infected individuals who willingly and knowingly infected others on a regular basis. These opinions/perceptions further demonstrate the general tendency to blame others for the spread of HIV infection rather than to take responsibility for one's own actions. Rather than make an objective and difficult examination of one's own behavior patterns and thus face the conflict between actual behavior and the desire to avoid one of the pejorative labels (immoral, promiscuous, etc.) given to persons who engage in extra-marital sexual behavior, the choice which is often made is to put the blame on others. This very human tendency makes it very difficult to change behavior, as individuals come to the conclusion that their behavior is not directly related to their potential for infection.

Traditional Practices

The Luo community traditionally has required that widows are married by one of the surviving brothers or another close male relative of the deceased husband. The original purpose of this tradition was to provide a home, protection, and comfort to the widow and to her children. The act of sexual intercourse between the widow and the new husband sealed the bond between the widow and her new family.

According to a number of the respondents, this tradition has continued but in many cases has lost its intended meaning. Rather than being a custom through which widows were protected, it is now often practiced mainly to get access to the wealth or property left by the deceased. Many widows complained of neglect by their inheritor and in some cases expressed that they might have been better off if left alone.

In spite of these expressed feelings, it was quite clear that the desire to adhere to the practice of inheritance remains very strong, as women and men both fear social sanctions and the curse that is believed to fall upon people who shun these practices (see discussion of "Chira" below).

This fear is such that many groups told stories of women who rather than not go through the rites, hire outsiders ("drunkards or mad people or people desperate for money") to perform the sexual rites. This use of outsiders to perform a ritual rather than expose the true inheritor to potential HIV infection from a woman whose husband is suspected to have died of AIDS was mentioned by several groups, and in only one case was it reported that the ethicality of this practice was questioned ("what if it was your son?").

Some suggestions were made as to possible alternatives to the sexual intercourse normally engaged in between the widow and the inheritor. Two of those mentioned, which apparently were performed in the past, was the man placing his leg on the woman's thigh, or hanging his coat in the house.

There nonetheless appears to be a small but growing group of persons who feel that the practice should be abolished. In our study, clan elders and church leaders were largely against the continuation of the practice, as were a number of individuals in several other groups. Until quite recently, the issue of this practice needing to be changed or abolished would not even have arisen.

Condom Use

Condom use has been growing rapidly in Kenya (NCPD, 1993). Verbal communication with USAID and the World Bank (who together with the United States Agency for International Development (USAID) have been the major suppliers of condoms to Kenya) have confirmed that the distribution figure for 1994 was close to 90 million, up from 6 million in 1988. In the case of the Homa Bay district, while specific figures are not available, usage rates remain relatively low. This may be due to lack of access, negative attitudes toward their use, lack of knowledge on proper use and continuing misconceptions. Most likely it is a combination of all of these factors. It should perhaps be noted at this point that the Homa Bay District (and Nyanza Province as a whole) continue to lag behind the national average on other related indicators such as contraceptive use (NCPD et al., 1993).

It appears that while virtually all respondents have heard of condoms, few people are actually fully equipped to use them. They either are uncomfortable or shy about using them, about negotiating their use, or do not have access to them. The conflict between the reality that sexual activity is common, frequent and natural, and that one who thinks about and plans for sex is "immoral" was made evident in the discussions on condoms. A notable number of respondents were willing to state that should counselling fail, condoms should be made available, although a strong opposition to this view was apparent. Fear exists that promoting condoms will promote "immoral behaviors." The out of school youths interviewed seemed more willing to accept condom use than did most other groups, although some of them also voiced opposition on "moral" grounds. Overall, however, this group stated that sex existed before condoms did and that people would engage in sex even if condoms had never been invented, so claiming that condoms increase the frequency of sex is an invalid argument.

Also of note on the subject of condoms is that many respondents indicated that commercial sex workers did demand condom use, and the bar attendants also mentioned that they saw an increase in condom use in bar and lodging settings while simultaneously seeing a decline in the number of clients.

A frequently offered reason for non-use is that condoms are not 100% effective. While this is true, using this reason is not consistent with other prevention measures used in the same community. As mentioned earlier, malaria continues to plague Homa Bay, and chloroquine-resistant strains are very common. Furthermore, it is commonly accepted that the use of impregnated bed nets is not an absolute guaranty that one will not contract malaria. Yet the demand for these nets remains very high as they are seen as "much better than nothing." Thus fatalism cannot be said to be a general characteristic of the community in question. Thus we are led to believe that the problem is with the messages and promotion strategies which have so far been used to promote the condom.

Chira (Curse)

No discussion of HIV/AIDS in Nyanza Province would be complete without reference to the belief in the concept of "chira" which continues to thrive there. Chira can be roughly explained as a curse which befalls persons and the families of persons who go against an established taboo or who fail to perform the expected traditional rites. Unfortunately, the symptoms of chira resemble those associated with full blown AIDS (loss of weight, rashes, diarrhea). Attempts have been made in the campaign of the last few years to disassociate the two. Community Health Workers now teach about the differences between the two, such as the fact that chira can be cured by correcting the "mistake" which had been committed (for example, practicing the rite which had not been performed), but that AIDS cannot be cured. Also, AIDS tends to affect young people while chira was normally believed to affect older people for transgressions they had made earlier in life. AIDS also afflicts persons who have observed customary laws as well as those who have not observed them.

The concept of chira originally served the purpose of being a method of social control. It was meant to create fear and to entice people into observing sexual or other behavioral taboos. According to many of the respondents, the existence of chira (or of AIDS for that matter) no longer seems to have any impact on sexual behavior patterns, but that in many cases it is used as a convenient explanation of death which does not carry the stigma that admitting a family member died of AIDS does. In spite of this realization, the concept is perceived by the respondents as one that will continue to exist and which has the potential to reduce the effectiveness of any AIDS prevention campaign, at least in the foreseeable future.

Discussion

The most significant finding of these discussions is that program planners and implementers have so far failed to find ways to effectively deal with the conflicting feelings and ambivalence which exist in Homa Bay between the recognized very strong sexual desires and the continued practice of condemning persons who appear to behave in such a way as to satisfy these desires.

While respondents overwhelmingly expressed skepticism about people's ability to remain celibate or monogamous due to jealousy, the wish to adhere to cultural practices, the need for money, the physical separation of spouses, desire for revenge, or just plain sexual desire; at the same time, people who are seen to have sex outside of marriage are persecuted for following their urges and for not following customary law.

Related to this finding was the persistence of the practice of placing blame on other individuals or groups rather than genuinely recognizing personal risk and taking responsibility for one's own actions. The persistence of this practice may be due to a lack of feelings of control over HIV/AIDS and sexual behavior and a feeling that the options which exist to protect people are inadequate.

Some encouragement may be found in the fact that the community health workers and traditional birth attendants who have been trained through the UNICEF/Government of Kenya program were much less judgmental in their views on sexuality and condom use. Additional training on communications skills could prove useful and effective.

In addition, the authors regularly get requests for condoms from community members, most notably from young men roughly under the age of 35 during their ongoing field work. The profile of current condom users will be the subject of a separate study in which we wish to establish ways to better target condom promotion campaigns in rural areas.

In order to improve the effectiveness of HIV prevention programs, it is imperative that better-targeted messages, ones that address the fears and beliefs of the population of Homa Bay be developed and that the reliance on standardized generic messages must be discontinued. These messages should emphasize risk, responsibility and control factors. These messages must be conveyed through credible sources, such as the CHW's and in the case of youth, through peers.

It was apparent from the discussions that parents felt that their children wouldn't listen to their advice, even if they could bring themselves to discuss the sensitive subjects of AIDS and sexuality. A fear was also expressed by parents that, since in the absence of a social security system they expected to in the future be fully dependent on their children for survival, they did not wish to risk angering them by implying that their behavior was perhaps inappropriate. The young people interviewed claimed that their parents were not good role models: preaching one thing and practicing another.

Regarding condoms, it was very clear from this study that a concerted effort must be made to popularize the condom and to make it a more attractive and acceptable method of HIV prevention. The promotion of condoms is likely to be much more effective if targeted to younger men. This and previous studies, as well as observations in the field, indicate that they are much more open to the use of condoms but need to be made to feel more confident about their use and effectiveness. The success of the promotion campaign could possibly be enhanced by placing as much emphasis on their role in preventing sexually transmitted diseases (STD's) as in preventing AIDS. The young people interviewed indicated that STD's were very common and many respondents had had first hand experience with gonorrhea. Young people could perhaps be encouraged to use condoms to prevent recurrences of such known illnesses which have more meaning for them than does a disease which may or may not afflict them some time in the future.

As stated earlier in this article, women in Africa are in most cases more affected by AIDS than are men. When women fall sick, they are often banished from the home, while when men fall sick women almost always tend to their needs. Women's lack of power to negotiate for safer sexual practices is limited. Although the empowerment of women is one of the keys to the prevention and control of AIDS in the long run and should be addressed in a broader context—as is being done through a number of UNICEF/Government of Kenya programs—in the short to medium, successfully encouraging young men to practice safer sex (and particularly to use condoms) is likely to have a greater impact than focusing on the general public. If a man is made to protect himself, he will also indirectly protect his sexual partners. This does not mean, however, that services should not be extended to women who want them.

The practice of wife inheritance and the belief in chira are likely to continue for some time to come. It may be more effective, as suggested by a number of respondents, not to make attempts to abolish the practice or the belief, but to modify the former to a less dangerous form and to emphasize the differences between AIDS and chira. Suggestions provided were allowing inheritance to continue but not performing the sexual rites.

In spite of the above possible alternatives to ritual sex, if as described by so many of the respondents, widows thus inherited continued to engage in sexual intercourse with other men, and if the cause of her husband's death was AIDS, while this might prevent transmission to her new husband, it would not prevent the spread to her other partner(s). Therefore encouraging alternatives to sexual intercourse at inheritance or faithfulness in marriage are unlikely to have much impact.

Finally, the AIDS prevention program should make its information and services more accessible to the community by redoubling its attempts to provide existing community health workers with additional training, information, and teaching materials. These workers should then be encouraged to focus their outreach activities on the places and groups whose behavior they are most likely to impact through counselling and condom distribution. In the case of Homa Bay, this may well be young men, persons employed near the beaches (they spend up to 18 hours per day there and are believed to engage in high risk sexual behaviors) and persons who work at or frequent bars and lodgings both of which are known to be places where high risk behaviors are practiced or initiated.

Notes

1. In Kenya, bar attendants are often providers of commercial sex to bar patrons.
2. In some cases these are translations from the Dholuo language.

References

Kenya National AIDS Control Programme. (1995). Verbal Communication of June 1994 Sentinel Surveillance Data.

McGrath, J.W., Rwabukwali, C.B., Schumann, D.A., Pearson-Marks, J., Nakayiwa, S., Namande, B., Nakyobe, L., Mukasa, R. (1993). Anthropology and AIDS: The Cultural Context of Sexual Risk Behaviour Among Urban Baganda Women in Kampala, Uganda. *Social Science and Medicine,* 36, 429-439.

Ministry of Education and Culture, Zimbabwe. (1993). *A report on focus group discussions with out of school youth on perceptions and strategies for communicating about AIDS.*

Moses, S., Muia, E., Bradley, J.E., Nagelkerke N.J.D., Ngugi, E., Njeru, E.K., Eldridge, G., Olenja, J., Wotton, K., Plummer, F.A., Brunham, R.C. (1994). Sexual Behaviour in Kenya: Implications for Sexually Transmitted Disease Transmission and Control. *Social Science and Medicine,* 39, 1649-1656.

National Council for Population and Development, Central Bureau of Statistics, Office of the Vice-President and Ministry of Planning and National Development (Kenya), and Macro International Inc. (1994). *Demographic and Health Survey:*(1993).

Republic of Kenya.(1993). *Homa Bay District Development Plan 1994-1996.* Office of the Vice-President and Ministry of Planning and National Development, Kenya.

Scrimshaw, S.C.M. & Hurtado, E. (1987). *Rapid Assessment Procedures for Nutrition and Primary Health Care.* Los Angeles, CA: The United Nations University, Tokyo Japan, and UCLA Latin American Center Publications.

Ulin, P.R. (1992). African Women and AIDS: Negotiating Behaviour Change. *Social Science and Medicine,* 34, 63-73.

Prevention of Human Immunodeficiency Virus Infection Among African-American Adolescents: The Importance of Understanding Cultural and Psychosocial Influences in the Development of HIV Prevention Programs

Ralph J. DiClemente and Gina M. Wingood

Introduction

There is a growing awareness of the threat HIV infection and AIDS pose for adolescents (DiClemente, 1990; 1993; Hein, 1992; 1991). While the number of diagnosed cases of AIDS among adolescents remains relatively small compared with older age groups there is ample cause for concern. There is substantial epidemiological data describing the prevalence of HIV-related risk behaviors among adolescents that increase the probability of infection (DiClemente, 1990). Behaviors such as inconsistent condom use among sexually active adolescents, multiple sex partners, injection drug use and the use of alcohol and other drugs that result in sexual disinhibition are associated with greater likelihood of exposure to HIV (Vermund et al., 1989). While each behavior singularly increases the probability for HIV infection, they are more often reported in combination, further elevating an adolescent's risk for infection.

Adolescents are not a homogeneous population. However, adolescents are a mosaic of subgroups defined by subcultural norms, values and mores. Importantly, the risk of HIV infection is not uniform across these subgroups. One understudied and underserved subgroup at increased risk of HIV infection is African-American adolescents.

Risk for AIDS Among African-American Adolescents

African-American adolescents are disproportionately represented among AIDS cases (Bowler et al., 1992). African-American adolescents are five times more likely to be diagnosed with AIDS than their white peers. Gender-specific analyses reveal a greater differential. Among males, for instance, African-Americans have a prevalence approximately five times greater than whites, while African-American women have a prevalence 11 times higher than whites (DiClemente, 1992).

While AIDS data is informative, it represents a clinical endpoint in a disease process with a long and variable latency period. More informative for gauging the impact of HIV on African-American adolescents is HIV seroprevalence data. HIV seroprevalence data also identify African-American adolescents as being at substantially higher risk of infection relative to other ethnic groups. Seroprevalence among African-American applicants for military service was 1.00 per 1000 compared with white (0.17) and Latino (0.29) applicants. Separate analyses by gender and race/ethnicity show that, for males, prevalence for African-Americans, whites and Latinos was 1.06, 0.18 and 0.31, respectively. Corresponding rates for African-American, white and Latino females were 0.77, 0.12 and 0.16 (Burke et al., 1990). Similarly, a recent study of U.S. army active-duty personnel has identified substantial variation in HIV seropositivity by ethnicity, with African-Americans 4.0 times more likely to be seropositive compared to white soldiers (Kelley et al., 1990).

Seroprevalence studies in a non-military population, entrants to the Job Corps, confirms previous findings (St. Louis et al., 1991). African-American males had the highest seroprevalence rate of all ethnic-gender groups. African-American males had a seroprevalence of 0.55% relative to a rate of 0.30% and 0.14% for Latino and white males, respectively. Similarly, African-American females had the highest seroprevalence (0.48%) compared with Latino and white females (0.18% and 0.08%, respectively). More recent findings from the Job Corps surveillance data indicate that there have been considerable changes in HIV prevalence over time. In 1988, for instance, African-American males had the highest rate of seropositivity of any applicant group. By 1992, while African-American males still had the highest prevalence rate among ethnic groups for males, the rate had declined significantly. Unfortunately, the HIV seroprevalence for African-American women had increased markedly, surpassing that of same-age African-American males (Conway et al., 1993).

While seroprevalence data is informative with respect to identifying the existing number of HIV-infected individuals, it is also important to obtain incidence data, that is, the number of persons who are uninfected at one timepoint, then, on subsequent HIV testing, are identified as seropositive. Direct measurement of the incidence of new HIV infections greatly enhances the ability to track the evolving epidemic and substantially improves the accuracy of epidemic forecasts. Given the widespread dissemination of information about HIV and AIDS, incidence data also provide some insight into the differential effectiveness of prevention efforts for various subpopulations.

HIV Incidence Among African-American Adolescents

Since 1985, soldiers on active duty in the U.S. Army have been routinely tested for the presence of HIV antibodies and are required to undergo repeated serologic evaluation every two years. While the actual number of adolescents (less than 20 years of age) who seroconverted (went from being seronegative on initial antibody evaluation to being seropositive on repeated testing) was not great, the incidence was markedly different for white and African-American, being 0.22 and 0.76 per 1000 person-years, respectively (McNeil et al., 1991). When the data was divided into period-specific incidence rates to identify changes in the incidence of HIV infection over time, African-Americans had higher period-specific incidence rates for 1987, 1988 and 1989. Further, period-specific incidence rates declined significantly among white adolescents from 1987 to 1989. However, this decrease was not evident among African-American adolescents. African-Americans had sharply higher seroconversion rates in 1989 than in 1987. This is particularly alarming given that this was a period when HIV prevention education programs and media campaign information were rapidly being disseminated. Clearly, the prevention message was not affecting this population as HIV-related risk behaviors among African-American soldiers were increasing. This sharp rise in HIV incidence indicates a need for more intensive HIV education tailored for African-American adolescents.

Although clinically overt disease remains uncommon relative to older age groups, results of the screening of civilian applicants for military service, seroprevalence studies of select adolescent populations and seroconversion (incidence) studies conducted with U.S. active-duty military personnel indicate that subclinical HIV infections are not uncommon among African-American adolescents. While adolescents presenting for military service and the Job Corps may not be representative of the U.S. population in general, nonetheless, the data are alarming and warrant considerable attention from health educators, policy analysts, school officials and, most importantly, the African-American community.

Psychosocial and Cultural Influences on Behavior

The epidemiological data indicate that African-American adolescents have been disproportionately affected by the HIV epidemic. Moreover, future projections suggest that the forecast for African-American adolescents is bleak: increased HIV-related morbidity and mortality. While epidemiological data are informative with respect to quantifying the differential risk for AIDS/HIV infection, they provide little insight into the influence of pervasive cultural and psychosocial factors that are the determinants of HIV-associated risk behavior.

In examining the threat of HIV for African-American adolescents, it is important to understand not only the broad context in which adolescence takes place, but also the cultural and psychosocial factors that exert considerable influence on behavior. Understanding the influences that shape behavior is critical in developing and implementing targeted and more efficacious programs designed to reinforce the adoption and maintenance of HIV-preventive behaviors (Auerbach, Wypijewska, & Brodie, 1994; DiClemente, 1993).

HIV as a Cultural and Psychosocial Phenomenon

As HIV prevention programs, for the foreseeable future, represent the only practical strategy for preventing the spread of infection (DiClemente & Peterson, 1994), it is noteworthy to underscore that HIV disease is as much a psychosocial and cultural phenomenon as it is a biological phenomenon. While HIV is the etiologic virus associated with AIDS and, while it is a necessary factor in disease pathogenesis, it is not sufficient to drive the epidemic. HIV causes disease, but behavior, more specifically, the lack of appropriate preventive behavior, propels the epidemic. And precisely because HIV disease links sexuality with disease, it is inextricably a psychosocial and cultural phenomenon. To understand the HIV epidemic and the behaviors which result in infection, then, we must ultimately confront it as much in sociocultural as in biomedical terms (Yankauer, 1986; Coates, Temoshok, Mandel, 1984; Auerbach, Wypijewska, & Brodie, 1994; DiClemente & Peterson, 1994).

HIV-associated sexual risk behavior is not random, uncontrollable, or inevitable. Many factors, both individual (intrapersonal) and social (interpersonal) contribute to an adolescents' propensity to engage in HIV-related sexual risk-taking. Risk behavior is, therefore, not a simple behavioral response, but rather the culmination of a complex social and interpersonal interaction, reflecting a multifactorial decision-making process in which many factors—biological, developmental, social, and psychological—underlie the decision-making process (Irga & Irwin, in press; DiClemente, 1992). Most important, from an intervention perspective, many of these factors are modifiable. Historically, most HIV prevention programs for African-American adolescents have been developed without sufficient empirical information about the strategies that would be most effective in motivating health-promoting behavior change. Consequently, behavior change interventions which have attempted to modify HIV-related risk behaviors have not, unfortunately, demonstrated sufficient and stable health-protective behavior change over time. To a large extent, this is attributable to the use of broad-based concepts and generalized theoretical models of behavior change not directly applicable to African-Americans (Cochran & Mays, 1993). As culturally inappropriate programmatic frameworks account for the failure of many social and behavioral programs (Airhihenbuwa, 1989), contextualizing adolescents' behavior within a psychosocial and cultural matrix, e.g., the beliefs, mores, social roles and values that may contribute to the maintenance or reluctance to modify high-risk behaviors, can further the development of culturally-specific explanatory models of behaviors, e.g., models developed from empirical data derived from studies of African-American adolescents. These models may be more appropriately suited to explain behavior and, thus, can be of substantial value in the design of more targeted and, potentially, more effective HIV risk-reduction interventions (Wingood & DiClemente, 1992).

A number of contextual barriers have been identified as affecting African-American adolescents' willingness to modify high-risk behaviors. These include: suspicion and mistrust, economic constraints, perceived risk of HIV infection, perception of peer norms as supporting high-risk behavior and sexual communication. Each of these influential contextual factors is described in turn below.

Suspicion and Mistrust

One cultural barrier which has hampered the effective development and implementation of HIV prevention activities among African-American adolescents has been the feelings of suspicion and mistrust (Dalton, 1988; Thomas & Quinn, 1991). The perception that HIV education is being imposed on the African-American community by the white majority further fuels this suspicion (Mays & Cochran, 1988; Dalton, 1988). Much of this suspicion is rooted in a longstanding neglect of African-American problems; neglect of the decaying living environment, jobs and job training for inner city youth, neglect of meaningful social programs to combat high unemployment among adults, teen pregnancy, the influx of drugs and the prevalence of violence in African-American communities. While it is clear that many of these social ills are prevalent in the African-American community, it is less clear that society in general has attempted to address these problems in a concerted and systematic manner that could produce meaningful changes in the standard of living for many African-Americans.

HIV prevention programs targeted towards African-American adolescents must foster trust and respect in order to gain the acceptance and legitimacy of these programs. They must also take into account the needs of their culture, especially as it reflects the adolescents' experiences within the context of the broader American culture. Overcoming these perceived and real barriers will not be quick nor easy. Given a history of neglect and lack of health care services in the African-American community, adolescents will be less likely to acknowledge and be receptive to overtures of expressed concern about their well-being. Eroding this longstanding distrust will take time and, most importantly, a palpable demonstration of good will; not "bandaid" approaches but comprehensive health care and economic reform within the African-American community which will allay fears and enhance the likelihood of a more trusting relationship.

The Role of Economic Constraints

The daily choices of many African-Americans are highly influenced by their economic situation (Mays & Cochran, 1990). Unemployed and underemployed out-of-school African-American adolescents who may be coping with the inequalities of society while seeking a sense of belonging, creativity or achievement may find sexuality a ready means to demonstrate manhood or womanhood through having children and being sexually active (Fullilove, Fullilove, Haynes & Gross, 1990). HIV prevention efforts targeted towards African-American adolescents therefore need to enhance economic opportunities and stability in the African-American community. This may be one of the most promising hopes for the establishment and maintenance of protective sexuality (Fullilove, Weinstein, Fullilove, Crayton, Goodjoin, Bowser, & Gross 1990) since the promise of economic rewards leads to the delay of sexuality and family formation (Bowser, 1986).

Perceived Risk of HIV Infection

African-American adolescents, relative to their white counterparts, appear less knowledgeable about the protective value of condoms to inhibit transmission of HIV (DiClemente, Zorn & Temoshok, 1986; DiClemente et al., 1987; DiClemente et al., 1988). Compounding this lack of crucial information, African-American adolescents tend to perceive themselves as less at-risk for HIV infection (Mays & Cochran, 1988) and are less likely to increase self-protective behaviors, such as condom use during sexual intercourse. One factor influencing African-American adolescents' appraisal of personal risk may be their belief that AIDS is exclusively a disease of white, homosexual men (Evans, 1988). Substantial ethnic/racial differences in the proportion of adolescents endorsing statements about the prevalence of AIDS among homosexual men and lesbian women have been reported, with African-American adolescents, relative to similar age white peers, being 2-3 times more likely to believe that AIDS is overwhelmingly a disease of homosexual men or women (DiClemente, Boyer & Morales, 1988).

Without accurate appraisal of their personal risk, African-American adolescents may be less motivated to attend to prevention messages and to modify risk behavior. In addition to imparting basic information about HIV, the overriding theme of the prevention message should be that African-American adolescents are at equal, or greater risk, for contracting HIV infection depending on the extent of their HIV-associated risk behaviors. A cautionary note; communicating personal vulnerability should avoid using fear-arousal messages which may be counterproductive (Jobs, 1988), but rather, should strive to provide an unambiguous linking of personal behavior and epidemiologic data on HIV prevalence. Such a message linkage is designed to reduce misplaced complacency and indifference, enhance receptivity to strategies for changing personal behaviors and increase motivation to adopt and maintain behavior changes.

Perceived Referent Group Normative Behavior

Perceived referent group norms are those behaviors that adolescents view as being socially sanctioned by their peers. Findings from studies with inner-city youth indicate that adolescents' perceptions of high-risk and low-risk behavior is directly related to their own behavior. For example, a recent study of adolescents in public housing projects found that the influence of perceived peer norms was a significant factor associated with adolescents' self-reported sexual behavior (Romer et al., 1994). Other studies with high-risk inner-city, predominantly African-American youth, have substantiated the influence of perceived peer norms on adolescents' own sexual behavior (Walter et al., 1992; DiClemente & Fisher, under review; DiClemente, 1992). One limitation of these studies has been their reliance on cross-sectional research designs. Cross-sectional designs limit the determination of the direction of causality between hypothesized predictors of behavior and actual behavior. However, one study did use a prospective research design.

In the most recent study, DiClemente and his colleagues (in press) in an effort to understand the influences on condom use, conducted a prospective study of African-American adolescents between 12-21 years of age residing in two public housing developments in San Francisco. Adolescents were recruited through street outreach and asked to complete a theoretically-derived research interview assessing HIV-related knowledge, attitudes and behaviors. After a six month time period, adolescents completed a follow-up interview similar to the baseline measure. Among adolescents reporting sexual activity in the six months prior to completing the baseline interview (N=116), logistic regression analysis evaluated the influence of demographic, psychosocial and behavioral factors on frequency of condom use. Adolescents who perceived peer norms as supporting condom use were 4.2 times more likely to report consistent condom use. Prospective analyses identified the baseline level of condom use as the best predictor of condom use at six-months follow-up. Adolescents who were consistent condom users at baseline were 7.4 times as likely to be consistent condom users during the follow-up period. A key finding from this study is that inner-city African-American youth do report using condoms consistently during sexual intercourse. Approximately 41% of sexually active adolescents reported using condoms every time they engaged in sexual intercourse in the six months prior to completing their personal interview. Thus, even in the midst of a decaying social environment, high unemployment and pervasive drug use, adolescents adopt and, in many cases, maintain consistent condom use for extended periods of time.

Adolescents are more likely than adults to be influenced by referent group normative values (DiClemente & Houston-Hamilton, 1989). Pressure, either through the perception of peer norms as supporting risky behavior or through actual peer pressure to engage in high-risk sexual and drug-related behaviors, may be more prominent in inner-city neighborhoods increasing the difficulty of promoting HIV-preventive behaviors (Morales, 1987). The image of black males has also been exaggerated to produce a stereotypical notion of their sexuality (Davis & Cross, 1979; Wyatt, Strayer, & Lobitz, 1976), and is supported by the referent group. Appearing to be concerned about AIDS or using condoms during sexual intercourse may be inconsistent with this cultural norm. In fact, sanctions may be directed at those who attempt to engage in health-promoting behaviors (Fisher, 1988). Confronting these social pressures is a challenge that must be accepted, engaged in and overcome. While the prevalence of social pressures may be pervasive and influential, findings from our previous research in public housing projects (DiClemente et al., in press) are both promising and instructive.

A theoretical framework which may be useful for designing African-American adolescent interventions may be the Social Influence Model of behavior change. Based in Cognitive Social Learning Theory, this model emphasizes and integrates cognitive, affective, behavioral and environmental factors and social skills and competency training so that adolescents can learn a set of social strategies and resistance techniques for countering social and peer pressures to participate in high-risk behaviors. Participants are first helped to identify various sources of pressures to engage in risk behaviors and are then provided with the skills needed to resist these influences. Most programs based on this model also target perceived norms to correct the perception that the target risk behavior is socially acceptable and sanctioned.

Fisher (1992) and others (Wulfert & Wan, 1993; DiClemente, 1993) suggest that this model may have direct implications for HIV prevention research. HIV preventive behaviors are often seen as inconsistent with adolescent group norms, making it difficult to achieve individual-level behavior change without initially targeting group-level social processes. Empirical findings suggest that adolescents who perceive the referent-group norm as supporting condom use are significantly more likely to report using condoms during sexual intercourse (DiClemente et al., in press; DiClemente, 1991; DiClemente & Fisher, under review). Fisher further emphasizes the importance of reframing the preventive behaviors so they appear consistent with current peer group values (e.g., being "cool", macho) in order to change norms. Interventions based on social influence models using peer leaders have been used successfully to deter the onset of the use of alcohol and other drugs among adolescents (Telch et al., 1990; Robinson et al., 1987; Hansen & Graham, 1991; Perry & Grant, 1988; Klepp, Halper & Perry, 1986; Botvin, 1986). Peer-based models, while a promising intervention (DiClemente, 1993), remain untested with African-American adolescents.

Social Competency Skills — Sexual Communication

For HIV prevention efforts to successfully modify risk behaviors requires more than accurate dissemination of information (Becker & Joseph, 1988; DiClemente & Peterson, 1994). Adolescents need to acquire the social and practical skills necessary to avoid risk-taking situations and behaviors. Perhaps the most prominent social competency skill needed by adolescents is the ability to effectively communicate with sex partners about the need for condom use. A number of studies with African-American youth identify communication as a key determinant of either condom use or unprotected sexual intercourse (DiClemente, 1991; DiClemente & Fisher, under review; Walter et al., 1992). For example, in the previously cited prospective study (DiClemente et al., in press), African-American adolescents who were able to assertively demand condom use were 11 times more likely to report consistent condom use. Moreover, findings from other high-risk adolescent populations, such as incarcerated adolescents, not only identify communication skills as a key factor associated with condom use, but observe a stronger statistical association between communication and condom use than usually reported for other adolescent populations (DiClemente, 1991).

While the findings indicate that communication skills, and the confidence to use these skills, is of paramount importance in promoting the use of HIV-preventive sexual behaviors, all too often interventions neglect social skills training. The inclusion of social skills training is a critically important component for behavior change, one which cannot be overlooked (Chesney & Coates, 1990; DiClemente, 1993). Methodologies including media campaigns, political action and group education combined with values clarification (Leviton et al, 1990) have resulted in behavioral changes in HIV risk behavior.

There is ample evidence that communication between sex partners is strongly associated with increased use of condoms during sexual intercourse (Rickman, Lodico, DiClemente, et al., 1994; DiClemente et al., in press; DiClemente, 1991; DiClemente & Fisher, under review; DiClemente, 1992). However, providing training in communication skills to adolescents whose communicative ability may not be substantial poses a challenge to prevention scientists.

Adolescents do not learn equally well, at a uniform rate or in the same manner. Communication skills training, clearly important for reducing high-risk behavior, must access the full spectrum of dissemination and education strategies. Utilizing more pro-active educational strategies, such as cognitive rehearsal of self-protective behaviors, assertiveness training, group discussions, use of video tapes and perhaps even mini-plays and skits, are more likely to yield greater skills acquisition and perceived self-efficacy to initiate communication with sex partners, change risk behavior and adopt HIV-preventive behaviors. The goals of these approaches are to resist social influence to engage in risk-taking behavior, increase perceptions of the capability to perform self-protective behaviors and enhance participation by creating an atmosphere conducive to frank and candid discussion of sensitive topics (Evans, 1988; Melton, 1988; Flora & Thoresen, 1988; Brooks-Gunn, Boyer & Hein, 1988; DiClemente, Boyer & Mills, 1987).

State of the Science of HIV Prevention Among African-American Adolescents

Although epidemiological data highlights the disproportionate impact of the HIV epidemic on African-American adolescents, these young people remain an understudied and underserved population. Few studies have focused exclusively on designing culturally-relevant HIV prevention programs for African-American youth. The more successful programs (Jemmott, Jemmott, Fong, 1992; Jemmott & Jemmott, 1994; St. Lawrence et al., 1995) have been developed within a community framework. These programs emphasized skills training in correct condom use, sexual assertion, refusal, self-management, problem-solving strategies and risk recognition. Given the importance of the social milieu and the cultural context of behavior, both high-risk and health-promoting behavior, one theoretically-based intervention approach, that has remained largely untested with African-American adolescents, is the use of peer-based models of behavior change.

Peer-Involvement: An Implementation Strategy Which May Enhance Program Efficacy

Peer-based interventions represent an under-utilized implementation strategy which may be particularly effective for promoting African-American adolescents' adoption of safer sex behaviors. Theoretically, peer-involvement offers a number of advantages over traditional, didactic, STD/ HIV prevention programs. Derived from Social Cognitive Theory (Bandura, 1992; 1994), and based in developmental theory, peer-facilitated interventions recruit and train peers indigenous to a large target population to serve as leaders, educators and counselors. Peer-involvement targets two theoretically important psychosocial constructs related to condom use: communication between sex partners and peer norms (DiClemente, 1992b; Joffe, 1993, Wight, 1992). For instance, research findings indicate that even high-risk incarcerated adolescents are influenced by these factors. In a study of incarcerated adolescents in San Francisco, adolescents who report discussing HIV with their sex partners and those who perceived peer norms to be supportive of condom use were approximately 15 and 7 times, respectively, more likely to be consistent condom users (DiClemente, 1991).

Peer-facilitated interventions have been used with adolescents to address a variety of health behavior problems. Peer interventions with adolescents have successfully delayed the onset of smoking, decreased alcohol use, and reduced initiation and prevalence rates of marijuana use (Botvin, 1986; Perry & Grant, 1988; Robinson et al., 1987; Telch et al., 1990; Hansen & Graham, 1991; Klepp, Halper, & Perry, 1986). Overall, the data suggest that peer-assisted programs are more effective than didactic programs without peer involvement in modifying health-risk behaviors.

Peer interventions offer a number of advantages over adult-led programs when working with adolescents. Peers may be more effective teachers of social skills, more influential models of health-promoting behavior, and can serve as credible role models because they are members of the adolescents' social milieu. Peers can also help to change normative expectations about the frequency of the targeted behavior in the peer group. Finally, peers can offer social support for performance of desired behaviors and for avoidance of health-damaging behaviors. These advantages are particularly important when educating adolescents in inner-city environments where social networks are limited and social norms may encourage and support risk- taking behavior (DiClemente & Houston-Hamilton, 1989). Clearly, peer involvement in the implementation of HIV-prevention interventions for African-American adolescents warrants further consideration as one strategy for enhancing programmatic efficacy.

Accessing African-American Adolescents

Though often neglected in the design and implementation of HIV prevention programs, a key factor limiting programmatic efficacy is the ability to access African-American youth. Community-based agencies have not been as aggressive as they might have been in serving as health advocates or providing information and services to African-American adolescents (Bowser & Wingood, 1992). One notable exception, however, is the Youth Environment Study (YES) conducted in San Francisco. YES uses Community Health Outreach Workers or CHOWs as part of an active, aggressive, one-on-one, street education and outreach effort which has proven successful with hard-to-reach populations especially intravenous drug users. CHOWs are typically indigenous to the target areas and familiar with the culture of the target population. Experience alone, however, is not sufficient. An essential difference between CHOWs and outreach staff in other settings is the extensive training they undergo that teaches them how to establish rapport with the target audience, thorough understanding of lifestyles and values, appropriate educational responses to interactions, and a range of empowerment techniques including practical skill-building and self-help strategies. Thus far CHOWs have concentrated on and been much more effective in modifying intravenous drug use than sexual behaviors (Jang, Moore, Houston-Hamilton, et al., 1988). However, parallel implementation with African-American adolescents is a promising strategy.

Limitations

This chapter is limited by the dearth of research attempting to identify the influence of cultural and psychosocial forces as they shape and motivate African-American adolescents' behavior. More precise information regarding these factors and their contribution to the initiation and continuance of HIV-related risk-taking and, more importantly, to the adoption and maintenance of preventive behavior is critical for the development of maximally effective intervention programs. Without such information, attempts at program development, by necessity, will lack the cultural and contextual cohesiveness that often determines whether or not programs are accepted, adopted and effective.

Conclusion

Programs designed to increase self-protective behaviors are urgently needed to avert a further increase in HIV infection among African-American adolescents. In general, programs that are theory-based and emphasize changing adolescents' perceptions of normative behavior and imparting social competency skills are more effective at motivating behavior change (Kirby & DiClemente, 1994; Schinke et al., 1990). However, HIV interventions that are not developed within the cultural context of the African-American community may have limited potential for positively impacting adolescents' risk behaviors. To develop maximally effective programs for African-American adolescents, intervention scientists and health educators need a greater understanding of the cultural and social factors within the African-American community. HIV educators also have a responsibility to consider how interventions can be culturally sensitive, as well as developmentally and gender-appropriate (De La Cancela, 1989). Cultural patterns that facilitate the spread of HIV must be identified in terms of their roots in historical tradition and/or as a symptom of socioeconomic conditions. Since differences exist along racial and ethnic lines regarding modes of transmission of HIV infection, HIV education and prevention must begin with an exploration of cultural values that may help to explain individual, family and community predisposition to engaging in risk activities. Understanding, modifying and harnessing these forces can serve as powerful change agents to reduce the risk of HIV infection among African-American adolescents.

References

Airhihenbuwa, C. (1992). Strategies for Health Interventions in the African-American Community. In R. Braithwaith & S. Taylor (Eds.), *Contemporary Health Issues: Perspectives on the African-American Community* (pp.267-280). San Francisco, CA: Jossey-Bass.

Airhihenbuwa, C.O., DiClemente, R.J., Wingood, G.M., & Lowe, A. (1992). HIV/AIDS Education and Prevention Among African-Americans: A Focus on Culture. *Journal of AIDS Education & Prevention,* 4, 251-260.

Airhihenbuwa, C.O. (1989). Perspectives on AIDS in Africa: Strategies for Prevention and Control. *AIDS Education and Prevention,* 1, 57-69.

Auerbach, J.D., Wypijewska, C., & Brodie, H.K. (1994). *AIDS and Behavior.* Washington, DC: National Academy Press.

Bandura, A. (1992). A Social Cognitive Approach to the Exercise of Control over AIDS Infection. In R. J. DiClemente, (Ed.), *Adolescents and AIDS: A Generation in Jeopardy* (pp. 89-116). Newbury Park, CA: Sage Publishing Company.

Bandura, A. (1994). Social Cognitive Theory and Exercise of Control Over HIV Infection. In R. J. DiClemente & J. Peterson (Eds.), *Preventing AIDS:Theories and Methods of Behavioral Interventions* (pp. 25-59). New York, NY: Plenum Publishing Corp.

Becker, M.H. & Joseph, J.G. (1988). AIDS and Behavioral Change to Reduce Risk: A Review. *American Journal of Public Health,* 78, 394-410.

Botvin, G. (1986). Substance Abuse Prevention Research: Recent Developments and Future Directions. *Journal of School Health,* 56, 369-373.

Bowler, S., Sheon, A.R., D'Angelo, L.J., & Vermund, S.H. (1992). HIV and AIDS Among Adolescents in the United States: Increasing Risk in the 1990s. *Journal of Adolescence,* 15, 345-371.

Bowser, B.P., & Wingood, G.M. (1992). Community-Based HIV Prevention Programs for Adolescents. In R. J. DiClemente (Ed.), *Adolescents and AIDS: A Generation in Jeopardy* (pp.194-211). Newbury Park, CA: Sage Publications.

Bowser, B.P. (1986). Community and Economic Context of Black Families: A Critical Review of the Literature 1909-1985. *American Journal of Social Psychiatry,* 6, 17-26.

Brooks-Gunn, J., Boyer, C.B., & Hein, K. (1988). Preventing HIV Infection in Children and Adolescents. *American Psychologist,* 43, 958-964.

Burke, D.S., Brundage, J.F., Goldenbaum, M., Gardner, L.I., Peterson, M., Visintine, R., & Redfield, R.R. (1990). Human Immunodeficiency Virus Infections in Teenagers. *Journal of the American Medical Association,* 263, 2074-2077.

Chesney, M.A. & Coates, T.J. (1990). AIDS: Putting the Models to the Test. In S. Petrow, P. Franks & T. R. Wolford (Eds.), *Ending the HIV Epidemic: Community Strategies in Disease and Health Promotion.* Santa Cruz, CA: Network Publications.

Coates, T.J., Temoshok, L., & Mandel, J. (1984). Psychosocial Research is Essential to Understanding and Treating AIDS. *American Psychologist, 39,* 1309-1314.

Cochran, S.D., & Mays, V.M. (1993). Applying Social Psychological Models to Predicting HIV-Related Sexual Risk Behaviors Among African Americans. *Journal of Black Psychology, 19*, 142-154.

Conway, G.A., Epstein, M.R., Hayman, C.R., Miller, C.A., Wendell, D.A., Gwinn, M., Karon, J.M., & Peterson, L.R. (1993). Trends in HIV Prevalence Among Disadvantaged Youth. *Journal of the American Medical Association, 269*, 2887-2889.

Dalton, H.L. (1988). AIDS in Blackface. *Daedulus, Spring,* 205-227.

Davis, G.L. & Cross, H.J. (1979). Sexual Stereotyping of Black Males in Inter-racial Sex. *Archives of Sexual Behavior, 8,* 269-279.

De La Cancela, V. (1989). Minority AIDS Prevention: Moving Beyond Cultural Perspectives Towards Sociopolitical empowerment. *AIDS Education & Prevention, 1,* 141-153.

DiClemente, R.J., Ponton, L. and Hansen, W., (1996). New Directions for Adolescent Risk Prevention and Health Promotion Research and Interventions (pp. 413–420) In R.J. DiClemente, W. Hansen & L. Ponton (Eds.), *Handbook of Adolescent Risk Behavior.* New York, NY: Plenum Publishing Corporation.

D'Angelo, L., & DiClemente, R.J. (1996). Sexually Transmitted Diseases and Human Immunodeficiency Virus Infection Among Adolescents. In R. J. DiClemente, W. Hansen & L. Ponton (Eds.), *Handbook of Adolescent Risk Behavior.* (pp. 333–368). New York, NY: Plenum Publishing Corporation.

DiClemente, R.J., Lodico, M., Grinstead, O.A., Harper, G., Rickman, R.L., Evans, P.E., & Coates, T.J. (1996). African-American Adolescents Residing in High-Risk Urban Environments Do Use Condoms: Correlates and Predictors of Condom Use Among Adolescents in Public Housing Developments. *Pediatrics.* 98: 269-278.

DiClemente, R.J. (1994). African-American Adolescents At Risk for HIV: Understanding Cultural and Psychological Influences on Behavior. In *HIV and Alcohol Impairment: Reducing Risks* (pp. 58-64). San Diego, CA: University of California.

DiClemente, R.J., & Peterson, J. (1994). Changing HIV/AIDS Risk Behaviors: The Role of Behavioral Interventions. In R. J. DiClemente, & J. Peterson(Eds.). *Preventing AIDS: Theories and Methods of Behavioral Interventions* (pp.1-4). New York, NY: Plenum Publishing Corporation.

DiClemente, R.J. (1993). Confronting the Challenge of AIDS Among Adolescents: Directions for Future Research. *Journal of Adolescent Research, 8,* 156-166.

DiClemente, R.J. (1993). Preventing HIV/AIDS Among Adolescents: Schools As Agents of Change. *Journal of the American Medical Association, 270,* 760-762.

DiClemente, R.J. (1992). Confronting the Challenge of AIDS in the African-American Community. *Ethnicity & Disease,* 2, 358-360.

DiClemente, R.J., Durbin, M., Siegel, D., Krasnovsky, F., Lazarus, N., & Comacho, T. (1992). Determinants of Condom Use Among Junior High School Students in a Minority, Inner-City School District. *Pediatrics, 89,* 197-202.

DiClemente, R.J. (1992). Psychosocial Determinants of Condom Use Among Adolescents. In R. J. DiClemente (Ed.), *Adolescents and AIDS: A Generation in Jeopardy* (pp. 34-51). Newbury Park, CA: Sage Publications.

DiClemente, R.J. (1992). Epidemiology of AIDS, HIV Seroprevalence and HIV Incidence Among Adolescents. *Journal of School Health, 62*, 325-330.

DiClemente, R.J., & Fisher, J.D. (under review). Predictors of HIV-Preventive Sexual Behavior Among Adolescents In An HIV Epicenter. The Effect of Social Influence Factors.

DiClemente, R.J. (1991). Predictors of HIV-Preventive Sexual Behavior in a High-Risk Adolescent Population: The Influence of Perceived Peer Norms and Sexual Communication on Incarcerated Adolescents' Consistent Use of Condoms. *Journal of Adolescent Health, 12,*385-390.

DiClemente, R.J. (1990). The Emergence of Adolescents as a Risk Group for Human Immunodeficiency Virus Infection. *Journal of Adolescent Research, 5,* 7-17.

DiClemente, R.J., & Houston-Hamilton, A. (1989). Strategies for Prevention of Human Immunodeficiency Virus Infection Among Minority Adolescents. *Health Education, 20,* 39-43.

DiClemente, R.J., Boyer, C.B., & Morales, E. (1988). Minorities and AIDS: Knowledge, Attitudes and Misconceptions Among African-American and Latino Adolescents. *American Journal of Public Health, 1,* 55-57.

DiClemente, R.J., Boyer, C.B., & Mills, S. (1987). Prevention of AIDS Among Adolescents:Strategies for the Development of Comprehensive Risk-Reduction Health Education Programs. *Health Education Research, 2,* 287-291.

DiClemente, R.J., Zorn, J., & Temoshok, L. (1987). The Association of Gender, Ethnicity, and Length of Residence in the Bay Area to Adolescents' Knowledge and Attitudes About the Acquired Immune Deficiency Syndrome. *Journal of Applied Social Psychology, 17,* 216-230.

DiClemente, R.J., Zorn, J., & Temoshok, L. (1986). Adolescents and AIDS: A Survey of Knowledge, Beliefs and Attitudes about AIDS in San Francisco. *American Journal of Public Health, 76, 1443-1445.*

Evans, P. *(1988).* Minorities and AIDS. *Health Education Research,* 3, 113-115.

Fisher, J.D., Misovich, S.J., & Fisher, W.A. (1992). Impact of Perceived Social Norms on Adolescents' AIDS-Risk Behavior and Prevention. In R. J. DiClemente (Ed.), *Adolescents and AIDS: A Generation in Jeopardy* (pp. 117-136). Newbury Park, CA: Sage Publications.

Fisher, J.D. (1988). Possible Effects of Reference Group-Based Social Influence on AIDS-Risk Behavior and AIDS Prevention. *American Psychologist, 43,* 914-920.

Flora, J.A. & Thoresen, C.E. (1988). Reducing the Risk of AIDS in Adolescents. *American Psychologist, 43,* 965-970.

Fullilove, M.T., Fullilove, R.E., Haynes, K., & Gross, S. (1990). African-American Women and AIDS Prevention: A View Towards Understanding the Gender Rules. *Journal of Sex Research, 27,* 47-64.

Fullilove, M.T., Weinstein, M., Fullilove, R.E., Crayton, E.J., Goodjoin, R.B., Bowser, B.P., Gross, S.A. (1990). Race/Gender in the Sexual Transmission of AIDS. In P. Volberding & M. A. Jacobson (Eds.), AIDS *Clinical Review.* New York: Marcel Dekker Inc.

Hansen, W.B., & Graham, J.W. (1991). Preventing Alcohol, Marijuana and Cigarette Use Among Adolescents: Peer Pressure Resistance Training Versus Establishing Conservative Norms. *Preventive Medicine,* 20, 414-430.

Hein, K. (1992). Adolescents at Risk for HIV Infection. In R. J. DiClemente, (Ed). *Adolescents and AIDS: A Generation in Jeopardy* (pp. 3-16). Newbury Park, CA: Sage Publications.

Hein, K. (1991). Risky Business: Adolescents and Human Immunodeficiency Virus. *Pediatrics, 88,*1052-1054.

Irwin, C. E., & Igra, V. (In Press). Theories of Adolescent Risk-Taking Behavior. In R. J. DiClemente, W. Hansen & L. Ponton (Eds.), *Handbook of Adolescent Health Risk Behavior.* New York, NY: Plenum Publishing Corporation.

Jang, M., Moore, M., Houston-Hamilton, A., et al. (1988). Second Year Evaluation of California's AIDS Community Education Program. San Francisco, CA: URSA Institute.

Jemmott, J.B., & Jemmott, L.S. (1994). Interventions for Adolescents in Community Settings. In R. J. DiClemente & J. Peterson (Eds.), *Preventing AIDS: Theories and Methods of Behavioral Interventions* (pp. 141-174). New York, NY: Plenum Publishing Corporation.

Jemmott, J.B., Jemmott, L.S., & Fong, G.T. (1992). Reductions in HIV Risk-Associated Sexual Behaviors Among Black Male Adolescents: Effects of an AIDS Prevention Intervention. *American Journal of Public Health, 82,* 372-377.

Jobs, R.F.S. (1988). Effective and Ineffective Use of Fear in Health Promotion Campaigns. *American Journal of Public Health, 78,* 163-167.

Joffe, A. (1993). Adolescents and Condom Use. *American Journal Diseases of Children,* 147, 746-754.

Kelley, P.W., Miller, R.N., Pomerantz, R., Wann, F., Brundage, J.F., & Burke, D.S. (1990). Human Immunodeficiency Virus Seropositivity Among Members of the Active Duty US Army 85-89. *American Journal of Public Health, 80,* 405-410.

Kirby, D., & DiClemente, R.J. (1994). School-Based Interventions to Prevent Unprotected Sex and HIV Among Adolescents. In R. J. DiClemente & J. Peterson (Eds.),*Preventing AIDS: Theories and Methods of Behavioral Interventions* (pp. 117-139). New York, NY: Plenum Publishing Corporation.

Klepp, K.I., Halper, A., & Perry, C.L. (1986). The Efficacy of PeerLeaders in Drug Abuse Prevention. *Journal of School Health, 56,* 407-411.

Leviton, L.C., Valdiserri, R.O., Lyter, D.W. Callahan C.M., Kingsley, L.A., Huggins, J. & Rinaldo C.R. (1990). Preventing HIV Infection in Gay and Bisexual Men: Experimental Evaluation of Attitude Change From Two Risk Reduction Interventions. *AIDS Education & Prevention, 1,* 96-107.

Mays, V.M., & Cochran, S.D. (1990). Methodological Issues in the Assessment and Prediction of AIDS Risk Related Sexual Behaviors Among Black Americans. In B. Voeller, J. Reinisch & M. Gottlieb (Eds.), *AIDS and Sex - An Integrated Biomedical and Behavioral Approach.* New York: Oxford University Press Inc.

Mays, V.M., & Cochran, S.D. (1988). Issues in the Perception of AIDS Risk and Risk Reduction Activities by African-American and Latino Women. *American Psychologist,43,* 949-957.

McNeil, J.G., Brundage, J.F., Gardner, L.I., Wann, Z.F., Renzullo, P.O., Redfield, R.R., Burke, D.S., & Miller, R.N. (1991). Trends of HIV Seroconversion Among Young Adults in the US Army, 85-89. *Journal of the American Medical Association, 265,* 1709-1714.

Melton, G.B. (1988). Adolescents and Prevention of AIDS. *Professional Psychology Research and Practice, 19,* 403-408.

Morales, E.S. (1987). AIDS and Ethnic Minority Research. *Multicultural Inquiry and Research on AIDS,* 1, 2.

Perry, C.L., & Grant, M. (1988). Comparing Peer-Led to Teacher-Led Youth Alcohol Education in Four Countries. *Alcohol Health Research World, 12,* 322-326.

Peterson, J., & DiClemente, R.J. (1994). Lessons Learned from Behavioral Interventions: Caveats, Gaps and Implications. In R.J. DiClemente & J. Peterson (Eds.), *Preventing AIDS: Theories and Methods of Behavioral Interventions* (pp.

319-322). New York, NY: Plenum Publishing Corporation.

Richman, R.L., Lodico, M., DiClemente, R.J., Morris, R., Baker, C., & Huscroft, S. (1994). Sexual Communication is Associated With Condom Use by Sexually Active Incarcerated Adolescents. *Journal of Adolescent Health, 15,* 383-388.

Robinson, T.N., Killen, J.D., Taylor, B., Telch, M.J., Bryson, S.W., Saylor, K.E., Maron, D.J., Maccoby, N., & Farquhar, J.W. (1987). Perspectives on Adolescent Substance Abuse. *Journal of the American Medical Association, 258,* 2072-2076.

Romer, D., Black, M., Ricardo, I., Feigelman, S., Kalijee, L., Galbraith, J., Nesbit, R., Hornik, R., & Stanton, B. (1994). Social Influences on the Sexual Behavior of Youth at Risk for HIV Exposure. *American Journal of Public Health,* 84, 977-985.

Schinke, S.P., Botvin, G.J., Orlandi, M.A., Schilling, R.F., & Gordon, A.N. (1990). African-American and Hispanic-American Adolescents, HIV Infection, and Preventive Intervention. *AIDS Education & Prevention, 2,* 305-312.

St. Lawrence, J.S., Brasfield, T.L., Jefferson, K.W., Alleyne, E., O'Bannon, III, R.E., & Shirley, A. (1995). Cognitive-Behavioral Intervention to Reduce African-American Adolescents' Risk for HIV Infection. *Journal of Consulting and Clinical Psychology, 63,* 221-237.

St. Lawrence, J.S. (1993). African-American Adolescents' Knowledge, Health-related Attitudes, Sexual Behavior, and Contraceptive Decisions: Implications for the Prevention of HIV Infection. *Journal of Consulting and Clinical Psychology, 61,* 104-112.

St. Louis, M.E., Conway, G.A., Hayman, C.R., Miller, C., Petersen, L.R., & Dondero, T.J.(1991). Human Immunodeficiency Virus Infection in Disadvantaged Adolescents. *Journal of the American Medical Association, 266,* 2387-2391.

Telch, M.J., Miller, L.M., Killen, J.D., Cooke, S., & Maccoby, N. (1990). Social Influences Approach to Smoking Prevention: The Effects of Videotape Delivery With and Without Same-age Peer Leader Participation. *Addictive Behavior, 15,* 21-28.

Thomas, S.B. & Quinn, S.C. (1991). The Tuskegee Syphilis Study, 1932 to 1972: Implications for HIV Education and AIDS Risk Education Programs in the Black Community.*American Journal of Public Health, 81,* 1498-1505.

Vermund, S.H., Hein, K., Gayle, H.D., Cary, J.M., Thomas, P.A., & Drucker, E. (1989). Acquired Immunodeficiency Syndrome Among Adolescents. *American Journal Diseases of Children, 143,* 1220-1225.

Vincent, M.L., Clearie, A.F. & Schluchter, M.D. (1987). Reducing Adolescent Pregnancy Through School and Community-based Education. *Journal of the American Medical Association,* 257, 3382-3386.

Walter, H.J., & Vaughan, R.D. (1993). AIDS Risk Reduction Among Multi-ethnic Urban High School Students. *Journal of the American Medical Association, 270,* 725-730.

Walter, H.J., Vaughan, R.D., Gladis, M.M., Ragin, D.F., Kasen, S., & Cohall, A.T. (1992). Factors Associated With AIDS Risk Behavior Among High School Students in an AIDS Epicenter. *American Journal of Public Health, 82,* 528-532.

Wight, D (1992). Impediments to Safer Heterosexual Sex: A Review of Research With Young People. *AIDS Care, 4,* 11-21.

Wingood, G.M., & DiClemente, R.J. (1992). Cultural, Gender and Psychosocial Influences on HIV-related Behavior of African-American Female Adolescents: Implications for the Development of Tailored Prevention Programs. *Ethnicity &*

Disease, 2, 381-388.

Wulfert, E., & Wan, C.K. (1993). Condom Use: A Self-efficacy Model. *Health Psychology, 12,* 346-353.

Wyatt, G.E., Strayer, R.G. & Lobitz, W.C. (1976). Issues in the Treatment of Sexual Dysfunctioning Couples of Afro-American Descent. *Psychotherapy, 13,* 44-50.

Yankauer, A. (1986). The Persistence of Public Health Problems: SF, STD and AIDS. *American Journal of Public Health, 76,* 494-495.

Part Two

Epidemiological Issues

INTRODUCTION

HIV/AIDS was first manifested in the USA among homosexual men and IV drug users. The epidemiological pattern of HIV has since changed. HIV/AIDS is now found within all strata of the human community. The spread of HIV now occurs more frequently through heterosexual contact. The infection has spread to women, children and adolescents. Prostitution, unsafe sexual behavior, poverty, IV drug use and infected blood are factors that influence the spread of HIV in different parts of the world.

In "Plan to Control AIDS: A Profile of India," Minakshi Tikoo discusses the epidemiological trend of HIV/AIDS in India. She emphasizes that the National AIDS Control Organization predicts that by the year 2000, five million people will be infected and that the number of AIDS cases will exceed one million in India. The number of AIDS cases has increased from 2.5 per 1,000 in 1986 to 11.2 per 1,000 in 1992. The spread of HIV in reality is still a concern for only a few people in India. According to Tikoo, the government has a lackadaisical attitude toward planning to educate the masses about AIDS and human sexuality.

Frank Machlica, in "HIV/AIDS Epidemiology Affecting Special Population Groups," reviews the current epidemiology of HIV/AIDS among specific groups in New York City which have a very large ethnically diverse population. The data illustrate the need for specific culturally and linguistically appropriate HIV-related mental hygiene services that could be adapted to traditional, non-traditional, and intrinsic mental health approaches being used by service providers.

Jerome Okafor, in "AIDS Campaign in Nigeria: The Efforts of the Federal Government," describes the spread of HIV infection in Nigeria. He further investigates the activities of the Nigerian government toward effective control of the spread of HIV/AIDS. He points to the problems that militate against effective execution of HIV/AIDS prevention programs in Nigeria.

Gina Wingood and Ralph DiClemente in "Prevention of Human Immunodeficiency Virus Among African-American Women..." identify AIDS as a public health problem for women, particularly African-American women. They emphasize that prevention programs for African-American women must address the realities of life for them in heterosexual relationships. Research indicates that powerlessness, abuse, lack of negotiation skills, traditional gender roles supporting women's passiveness, sex ratio imbalances, in addition to the constraints of being economically disenfranchised make practicing safer sex a difficult reality for many African-American women in heterosexual relationships. HIV prevention programs that apply Social Cognitive Theory and address gender specific risk factors, such as relational influences, power imbalances and stressors specific to women in their design and implementation are more efficacious at reducing women's risk to HIV than programs that fail to address these larger socio-cultural factors.

Plan to Control AIDS: A Profile of India

Minakshi Tikoo

The worldwide Acquired Immune Deficiency Syndrome (AIDS) epidemic and the resulting loss of lives makes it important for countries of the world to research human sexuality and to seek ways to prevent the spread of HIV. Ripples created by the threat of AIDS in industrialized countries are now being felt by the third world countries. The International Conference on Population Development 1994 in Cairo (ICPD 94, Newsletter) made population control an agenda item to address the rights of women to reproductive information, since women comprise the population in which the number of AIDS cases is growing exponentially. With the exception of Thailand most south-east Asian countries do not have governmental policies regarding the inclusion of a comprehensive sexuality education curriculum in schools. Many of these countries are planning and working on developing policies to help combat HIV/AIDS through education.

Since gaining independence in 1947, the Indian government has followed a series of five-year plans to map out the future growth and development of the country. Population control and family planning have been priority areas since the first five-year plan. The Indian population has increased from 342 million in 1947 to 900 million in 1993, and the government allocation (budget) increased from Rs 6.5 million in 1952 to Rs 10,104.1 million in 1992 (FPAI, 1992) (U.S. $1=Rs 31.00). The present period is covered by the eighth five year plan (1992—1997), which emphasizes the role of information, education, and communication (IEC) and the importance of women's status and education in family planning and population growth reduction.

The ratio of boys to girls is 1000:927. The number of girls per thousand boys continues to decline steadily. The rural population is 74% of the total population. The urban literacy rate was higher (73%) than the rural literacy rate (45%). Although, Kerala has achieved 100% literacy, most states have not, and child marriages, bride burning, dowry and malnutrition continue to be major problems in Madhya Pradesh, Rajasthan, Bihar, and Uttar Pradesh. It is important to understand the context in which India is trying to educate the youth about human sexuality and AIDS. Table 1 provides a brief demographic summary of India.

Table 1 Demographics of India

Population mid-1993 (million)	900
Income per head 1991 (US $)	330
Infant mortality rate (deaths per 1,000 live births)	91
Population growth (% per annum)	2.1%
Annual population increment (`000)	17,652
Agricultural population density per km	441
Adult literacy 1990 (%)	M-62 F-34
Total fertility rate (no. children per woman)	3.9
% birth to teenagers	9
Maternal mortality (deaths per 100,000 live births)	340
Crude birth rate (per 1,000)	31
Crude death rate (per 1,000)	10
Contraceptive prevalence rate (%couples)	49
Under-five mortality by sex 1991 (death per 1,000 live births)	M-123 F-125
Life expectancy (years)	M-58 F-59

As cited in International Planned Parenthood Federation, South Asia Strategic Plan 1994—2002.

History of AIDS in India

In India traditional family norms still hold, talk of sexuality is taboo and very few authentic, accurate sources of information regarding sexuality exist. India officially reports 310 cases of AIDS (NACO, 1993). The World Health Organization (WHO) predicts that by the year 2000, the Asian continent is going to lead the world in the number of AIDS cases. For India, the future looks bleak for its 900 million people, growing at the rate of 2.1% annually.

The first case of AIDS in India was reported in 1986. There are now 310 documented AIDS cases (NACO, 1993). Ninety percent of the cases reported were among those below the age of 50 and more than two-thirds of these persons were between 20 and 40 years of age. Heterosexual contact is mainly responsible for the spread of HIV in India except in the northeastern region, where intravenous drug use is the primary cause. (NACO, 1993). The reason for these unusually low numbers could be the lack of diagnostic capabilities in addition to lack of systematic record keeping.

Although AIDS is not among the ten leading causes of death in India (Census, 1991) if the disease keeps growing at the present rate, before long India will have a staggering number of cases reaching an unmanageable proportion in the population. Prevention is always better than cure and this is especially true for countries like India because of limited resources. In addition, the prevalent rate of the spread of HIV in a climate lacking comprehensive sexuality education and reliable sources of information makes AIDS an even deadlier disease.

The primary cause for the spread of HIV and other sexually transmitted infections is prostitution. Failure to practice contraception, though use is promoted, is a secondary cause. Most women do not have any choice in the matter. Whether they want safe sex is immaterial because men make most of the decisions. The philosophy of the government has been like a pendulum swinging from either complete lack of initiative or lukewarm efforts, to forcefully sterilizing people. To control the population the government is promoting the one- or two-children norms, population clocks[1], and using media to provide information, so that people have choices available to make responsible decisions regarding their sexuality.

India at present practices a social system of medicine, but the kind of resources needed to tackle the demands of HIV/AIDS are just not available. The sheer numbers which are being projected are mind-boggling and the expertise required to help in the care of HIV/AIDS patients would put a tremendous strain on the existing resources (health care plan), which the system would be unable to bear. AIDS continues to be an enigma in the medical community in India as many doctors fear AIDS themselves.

Plan to Combat AIDS

The Family Planning Association of India (FPAI) is a non-government organization (NGO) which formulates national plans for family planning and reproductive health. During the last 25 years the association has expanded the range of activities through programs of population education for the younger generation, both school and college students, out-of-school youth and young workers, in rural, semi-urban and urban areas. These programs also include family life and sexuality education. A more recent initiative has been the establishment of Sex Education, Counseling, Research, Training and Therapy

Centers (SECRT) to meet the contemporary need for specialized counseling in marital, sexual and other related issues including sexually transmitted infections (STI) and AIDS (FPAI, 1992).

The goal set for the year 2000 by the Family Planning Association of India is to reduce the population growth rate to 1.25% annually. The mission to control population may become a reality if AIDS and HIV transmission continue to spread at present rates. The number of AIDS cases being reported has increased from 2.5 per 1000 in 1986 to 11.2 per 1000 in 1992. If this rate of transmission continues, by the year 2000 about five million people would be infected and the number of AIDS cases would exceed one million (NACO, 1993).

The government of India through its Ministry of Health and Family Welfare in collaboration with WHO has established The National AIDS Control Organization (NACO) which has developed an action plan regarding how to deal with the burgeoning AIDS epidemic. NACO has been operational since 1987, but it is only since 1992 that much stricter comprehensive plans to combat AIDS have been developed.

The broad *objectives* of this program are: 1) Establishment of effective program management mechanisms at the National and State levels, and 2) Provision of technical, financial, and operational support to the staff and organizations implementing program activities. *Four* strategies have been developed to accomplish these objectives.

Strategy I

a) National AIDS Committee (NAC): This is a forum of ministry officials, non-governmental organizations (NGOs), and other private voluntary organizations with a view to coordinate program activities.

b) Multi-sectoral Committee: This committee has been set up under the chairmanship of the secretary of health to assist in the development of coordinated policies to prevent and control the spread of HIV/AIDS in the country.

Strategy II

I National Level

a) National AIDS Control Board: Approves policies and the programs of NACO.

b) NACO: A conglomeration of dedicated staff under the Ministry of Health and Family Welfare. This organization exercises all the financial and administrative powers vested in the Department of Health, Government of India.

II State Level:

a) Organizing state AIDS cells to strengthen the program management at the state level.

b) State AIDS cell.

Strategy-III

To strengthen the technical and research capabilities of the program at both the national and the state level.

Strategy IV

Monitoring, review, and evaluation of the programs. Monthly reports are sent to NACO where they are compiled to map the progress of the epidemic in India.

To implement all these plans and strategies effectively and to achieve the noble objectives of the organization, the first and foremost need is to compile baseline data against which progress and achievements can be measured. Currently there is a dearth of relevant studies researching behavior, knowledge, and attitudes of people regarding AIDS and human sexuality. To bridge this gap, NACO has funded 65 risk behavior studies, mainly through local initiatives, NGOs, and social institutions (personal communication, Dr. P. R. Dasgupta, August 26, 1994).

AIDS has a unique position in relation to any of the other diseases because of its fatal prognosis. HIV/AIDS education and prevention programs are being given top priority and have been incorporated in future planning for all nations, and especially the third world countries which have neither the resources nor the research climate to tackle an AIDS epidemic. The survival method for these countries is education.

Research Findings

Information regarding the adolescent age group is required as studies show a tremendous increase in the number of AIDS cases reported in the 21-44 year age group. Given the long incubation period (10 years) of the AIDS virus, it is possible that these young people testing Human Immunodeficiency Virus (HIV) positive were most likely infected in early adolescence. Adolescent sexuality can be defined as the adoption of certain beliefs and forms of behavior in response to their sexual desires (Sorenson, 1973). It is important to learn about adolescent sexuality because it influences all aspects of development. There is a need to understand the modus operandi of the adolescents before successful programs targeted at this population can be developed. Great inroads into gaining information about human sexuality in general and adolescent sexuality in particular have been made through research by Kinsey

(1948) in the 1940s-50s on male and female sexual behavior; followed by the first systematic study carried out by Robert C. Sorenson in 1970 that focused on adolescent sexuality and explored the relationship between sexual behavior and sexual values. More recently *The Janus Report* (1993) documented an increase in premarital and extramarital sex, and continued the interest in the area of sexuality. *Sex in America* (Michael, Gagnon, Laumann, & Kolata, 1994) has presented findings that are in contradiction with the earlier findings. They report "...(that) America may not be as sexy a place as it is often portrayed, most people are satisfied with the sexual lives they have chosen or that were imposed upon them" (p. 246).

Despite a number of studies being undertaken to understand adolescent behavior in America, a gap in knowledge about adolescent sexual behavior still remains. This is even more true for India where there are only a few documented studies, even though seminars debating the need for sex education have been ongoing since 1968.

In India, and most other countries in the world, the spread of HIV is in the heterosexual population, as opposed to the popular belief that AIDS is a homosexual disease in the United States. Other problems among teenagers are those of drug and alcohol abuse and pregnancy. In the United States, teenage pregnancy increases the chances for an individual not to finish high school, to have a low paying job, or to end up on welfare. India, in contrast has the problem of teenage pregnancies as a result of early marriages. Both countries share the problem, even though the origin of the problem is not the same.

Some of the questions that need answers in the context of planning for human sexuality and HIV/AIDS education are:

1. What is the present level of knowledge among adolescent boys and girls regarding human sexuality and AIDS in India?

2. What are the general attitudes of adolescent boys and girls regarding human sexuality in India?

3. What are the general behaviors of adolescent boys and girls regarding human sexuality and AIDS in India?

This information will benefit the people of India but will be of special use to educators, ministry officials, and policy planners looking for research evidence to support their plans for India's future. A survey (SCERT, 1988) of 3,850 unmarried young men and women (15-29 year old) revealed no significant differences in the attitudes of the young people regarding marriage and sex across regions. Liberal attitudes towards sexual behavior were found among urban youth and both young men and women were looking for equality in marriage. However, a need for knowledge about reproductive health and a need for more in-depth studies to explore the area of reproductive health were indicated.

The All India Institute of Medical Sciences (AIIMS) has been fairly instrumental in spearheading research and setting up a clearing house of information for AIDS and other STIs. So far only one documented study has been reported on knowledge, beliefs, and attitudes regarding AIDS, STIs, and human sexuality among senior secondary students (11th and 12th grade) in Delhi (Chowdhury & Gill, 1993). The results of the study indicated that students:

1) have high knowledge regarding AIDS;

2) have misconceptions regarding masturbation;

3) obtain knowledge about sex from books (53.8%), friends (47.3%), cinema (20.7%), or parents (8%);

4) friends (44%) and doctors (42%) were the preferred choices while parents (14%) and teachers (2%) were the least likely sources of information regarding sex.

The study recommended that schools should devise ways to open up more effective communication with students in relation to education on sex, AIDS, and STIs.

Preliminary findings of a study (Chowdhury & Gill, 1994) of 17-22 year old students from 13 colleges in Delhi indicated:

1) general level of knowledge about AIDS is high and was obtained from newspapers, magazines, television, and friends. Boys were more knowledgeable than girls;

2) sex workers and foreigners were thought to be the primary cause for the spread of AIDS;

3) sexual experience was reported by 16.8% of the students. Of these, 92% of the boys (n=195) and 78% of the girls (n=32) admitted heterosexual experience. Nineteen percent of the boys and 43.8% of the girls reported homosexual experience;

4) premarital sex with a person with whom they were in love was favored by 64% of the boys and 20.5% of the girls;

5) among the students, 9.3% of the boys and 3.7% of the girls knew of a person suffering from AIDS;

6) the protective value of a condom was known to a majority of the students;

7) among the students, 10.7% of the boys and 1.6% of the girls knew somebody in their class who injected drugs. These students also reported a higher amount of sexual activity (13.2%) in comparison to those who had not used drugs (2.3%).

AIIMS has another research study underway, exploring the behavior of urban slum populations (personal communication, Dr. Chowdhury, August 20, 1994). These studies will help to fill the existing gap in information, establish baseline data, strengthen and further improve the efforts of the NGO cells in education, delivery, and implementation of the prevention programs.
Tikoo (1995) reported that, overall, Indian adolescents had very limited knowledge regarding AIDS and human sexuality. The situation is grim given the evidence that students who use parents and teachers as sources of information about sexuality scored lower on scales measuring their knowledge about AIDS and Human Sexuality. This lends support to the fact that inaccurate information is being disseminated which, in itself, provides reason enough for implementing a well thought out sexuality education curriculum. Some of the other salient findings of the study were:

1) The mean score on the knowledge scale was 4.19 (maximum=15) and the AIDS scale was 3.08 (maximum=7). No one scored full points on the knowledge scale. However, on the AIDS scale 33 people scored full points. The boys scored somewhat higher than the girls.

2) Adolescents who reported getting along with their parents scored higher on these scales.

3) Adolescent expression of sexuality as defined by their attitude toward premarital sex tended more towards neutral (neither agree nor disagree). A large number of both boys and girls agreed with the statement that sex is okay only if you are married which is in keeping with the traditional values of India.

4) There was a lack of sexual activity and experimentation. Most boys and girls reported not being attracted to others, using drugs or alcohol, or having sexual intercourse.

5) Helpful sources of information in the descending order by preference were: books/magazines/newspapers, teacher, mother, friends/classmates, father and siblings, and movies/videos/television.

6) If given a choice girls would prefer to get information from doctor or friends followed closely by parents. Boys chose a doctor

over friends and the parents were very low in priority.

7) Most people rated their own knowledge of human sexuality as average or good and recommend a mean age of 15.55 years to begin sexuality education. Both boys and girls supported sex education in schools.

The results of the existing few studies suggest the need for a comprehensive sexuality education program. Ironically, in India, the teachers are the biggest hindrance to the delivery of the program. "Teachers feel that discussion of human sexuality vis-à-vis AIDS will harm their self-esteem among students," said Mahesh Mahalingam, national consultant of NACO (Times of India, 1993). This fact was also supported by the AIIMS study. One of the long-term goals of NACO is to establish inter-sectoral collaboration (public and private), so as to hasten the process of policy formulation.

Conclusion and Discussion

It becomes important in light of the increase in the number of AIDS cases, adolescent pregnancies and sexually transmitted infections, that India should educate her adolescents regarding safer sex practices to enable them to make responsible decisions based on accurate information. With no vaccine available for preventing HIV infection, special attention needs to be aimed at behavior modification. Change in the normative sexual behavior patterns of the adolescents may be the only safe and successful route to saving nations from losing their youth and having imbalanced populations (missing generations) with far-reaching consequences. To prevent such a scenario there is a need for researching the adolescent population to understand their views regarding human sexuality and AIDS before any programs can be formulated.

So far in India there is no directive nor policy that makes sexuality education mandatory in schools. Efforts are ongoing to formulate a sexuality curriculum which would be named the "adolescent curriculum," so as to be culturally acceptable. The National Council of Education for Research and Training (NCERT) is working with NACO to develop the adolescent curriculum, which would make AIDS awareness an integral part of the curriculum. NACO is hopeful of getting the curriculum pilot-tested and revised by January 1995, so that it could be implemented at the beginning of the next academic school year in July 1995 (personal discussion with Dr. P.R. Dasgupta, 1994).

Though implementing sexuality education is one small part of the larger picture, it is a crucial and essential part. Once the children and the youth of the country are educated, India would have prepared the coming generations to take care of themselves and their country. By delivering comprehensive sexuality education, India will reap the harvest of youth who not only will be able to make the right decisions for themselves, but also will be equipped with the correct information and decision-making skills that are an asset in any situation. The delivery of a sexuality education program makes sure that those youth not in schools are also able to educate themselves by organizing activities through the Nehru Yuva Kendras (community youth clubs) which are part of each district. Plans are also underway to tap youth organizations such as the Bharat scouts and guides, National Cadet Corps (NCC), Youth Hostel Association of India, YMCA and YWCA to help with the delivery of education and prevention programs.

In the past, India or any country in the world did not have to fight against an unknown enemy on limited time. Strategic planning is the only way out in this otherwise no win situation. Mr. Dasgupta (1994) aptly summed up India's efforts for health, "... (we) have lacked holistic planning because we think in terms of disease and not health." It is true that AIDS is forcing us to think in terms of disease again, but the NACO plan goes a long way toward improving the general health of an average Indian by providing education.

Notes

1. These are electronic clocks which give the current population of India, accounting for the number of children born every minute and are displayed at major intersections where people can see them while waiting for the lights to change.

References

Cairo Conference Maps Out Path to a Better Reality. (ICPD, September, 1994). 19, 1-6.

Chowdhury, S., & Gill, F. P. T. (1993). *A Study of Knowledge, Beliefs, and Attitudes Regarding AIDS, STDs and Human Sexuality Among Senior Secondary Students in Delhi*. Unpublished manuscript.

Chowdhury, S., & Gill, F. T. P. (1994). *Knowledge of College Students Regarding AIDS*. Unpublished manuscript.

Family Planning Association of India (FPAI). Challenges Strategic Plan 1992-2000, 3.

International Planned Parenthood Federation (IPPF), South Asia, Strategic Plan 1994-2002 (U.K., 1993), 4.

Janus, S. S., & Janus, C. L. (1993). *The Janus Report on Sexual Behavior*, (pp.40-43). New York: John Wiley & Sons Inc.

Michael, R. T., Gagnon, J. H., Laumann, E. O., & Kolata, G. (1994). *Sex in America*. New York: Little, Brown and Company.

Ministry Of Home Affairs, Survey of Cause of Death (rural), Annual Report 1990. Series 3, No. 3, Office of the Registrar General, India, (New Delhi).

National AIDS Control Program India, Country Scenario an update, April, 1993.

National AIDS Control Organization, Ministry of Health and Family Welfare, Government of India, 1.

Sex Education Counselling Research Training and Therapy Department of FPAI.

(1988). *Attitudes and Perceptions of Educated, Urban Youth to Marriage and Sex.*

Sorenson, R. C. (1973). *Adolescent Sexuality in Contemporary America.* New York: World Publishing.

Tikoo, M. (1995). *Survey of Adolescent Knowledge, Attitudes, and Behaviors Regarding Human Sexuality and AIDS in India.* Unpublished doctoral dissertation, Kansas State University, Kansas.

Taboos Hinder AIDS Education. (Dec. 4, 1994). *Times of India*, p. 8.

HIV/AIDS Epidemiology Affecting Special Population Groups

Frank Machlica

As the Human Immunodeficiency Virus (HIV) and Acquired Immune Deficiency Syndrome (AIDS) pandemic continues to accelerate worldwide, New York City still has the largest number of AIDS cases (70,880) nationwide (New York City Department of Health [NYC DOH], October, 1994b; Centers for Disease Control and Prevention [CDC], 1994). In addition, HIV/AIDS has affected special population groups in New York City more than the general population. This article addresses the need for culturally competent mental hygiene services for the large ethnically and culturally diverse mosaic that exists in New York City. As the special population groups affected by HIV/AIDS have shifted, mental hygiene services have not adequately addressed the needs of uninsured and under-insured HIV-infected individuals, communities of color, women, children, adolescents and young adults, the homeless, mentally ill chemical abusers, detainees and recently released inmates, recent immigrants and undocumented residents, and those with the dual infection of TB/HIV, in addition to men who have sex with men and alcohol and other drug users. It is important for mental hygiene services to respond to these emerging affected populations while continuing to expand and provide care to the existing affected populations.

Men, Gay Men, Gay Men of Color and Men of Color

According to the NYC DOH (October, 1994b), men comprise 79% (55,942) of the 70,880 AIDS cases in New York City. Of these cases, 39% are black, 30% are white, 30% are Hispanic and less than 1% are Asian and Pacific Islanders, Native American, or Alaskan. Men of color are disproportionately affected by AIDS. Regarding transmission categories among males, 46% have or have had sex with other men, 43% are injecting drug users, and 4 percent are injecting drug users who have or have had sex with other men. In looking at transmission categories by race, 74% of white men, 32% of Hispanic men and 31% of black men have or had sex with other men. However, because of societal and cultural taboos against homosexuality, these numbers may not be very accurate due to under-reporting.

Thus, the stigmatization of men who have sex with men, coupled with the above epidemiological data illustrate the need for more HIV/AIDS mental hygiene services for men, gay men, gay men of color and men of color in New York City.

Women, Gay Women, Gay Women of Color and Women of Color

Women constitute the fastest growing number of people with AIDS nationwide (Osborn, 1990; Lerner, 1994). In New York City, AIDS is the primary cause of death for women between the ages of 25 to 34 (Perez, 1990). According to the NYC DOH (October, 1994b), women comprise 19% (13,519) of the 70,880 AIDS cases in the city. Of these cases, 53% are black, 33% are Hispanic, 13% are white and less than 1% are Asian and Pacific Islanders, Native American, or Alaskan. Regarding transmission categories, 61% of the women were infected through IV drug use, and 28% through heterosexual activity.

Women with AIDS who are lesbian are not specifically identified in any Federal, State or city surveillance data exposure categories. Only four references on female-to-female transmission have been reported in mainstream medical journals (Cole, et al., 1990). Many lesbians with AIDS have identified themselves as being in "known risk" categories. There is no surveillance data related to women-to-women transmission. In New York City, 11 percent of all women with AIDS are in the "Other/no-known risk" category. Furthermore, the percentage of "no-known risk" for women (11%) is almost double that of men (six percent) indicating less is known about HIV risk regarding women (NYC DOH, October, 1994b). There exist tremendous gaps in knowledge related to women and lesbians with AIDS, yet women account for the highest growth rate of any group.

Children and Adolescents

It should be noted that, given the expanded CDC definition of AIDS and recent epidemiological trends, the increased level of cases reported in women and children is expected to continue and will result in greater need for mental health services on all levels. HIV/AIDS is a leading cause of death among young women in New York City. Adolescents, who are prone to acting out and impulsivity, may be left to care for younger siblings or end up homeless when a parent dies. Many children are orphaned by HIV/AIDS or may have siblings and family members who are HIV-infected. They may end up in an already overburdened foster care system. Children can react to the loss of a parent, relative or friend through depression, anger, fighting in school, and difficulty in peer relationships.

While only 3% of the nation's adolescents live in New York City, as of June, 1994, there are 161 cumulative reported adolescent AIDS cases in New York City, representing 1/3 of the adolescent AIDS cases nationwide (NYC DOH, October, 1994a). Furthermore, due to the incubation period of HIV infection, most of the cases in the 20-29 age range, representing 19% of all AIDS cases, were infected during adolescence (Health Systems Agency of New York City, Inc. [HSA], 1993). Young people are at risk for HIV infection due to their risk-taking behaviors. Youth who drink and/or use drugs are less likely to engage in safer sex activities. Many adolescents contract sexually transmitted diseases and/or become pregnant. In addition, the deficiency of mental health and health support services for young people has resulted in youth lacking motivation, information and resources to prevent them from contracting HIV and taking care of themselves if infected.

The HIV-related needs of adolescents in New York City have increased significantly, particularly among gay and lesbian youth, "street kids," young women, youth who have been sexually abused, youth who have been involved in the criminal justice system, and adolescents in HIV-affected families. HIV-related mental health issues such as prevention, treatment, alcohol and other drug treatment, bereavement and suicide prevention become greater needs as the rate of infection rises in this population throughout the city.

The Severely and Persistently Mentally Ill (SPMI)

Clients who are Severely and Persistently Mentally Ill (SPMI) are at a higher risk for HIV infection than the general population. Seroprevalence studies of chronic psychiatric patients in New York City have indicated that the rates of HIV infection range from 4.0% to 19.4% (Cournos, June, 1993; HSA, September, 9 1994). In the mentally ill population, it has been reported that women were as likely as men to be infected and African-Americans had higher rates of infection than non-African-Americans (Cournos, et al., 1991). Several authors have indicated that about 50% of the chronic psychiatric patients studied reported engaging in high risk behaviors (injection drug use, unsafe sex) during the past one to five years (Kelly, et al., 1992; Sacks, et al., 1990).

Mentally Ill Chemical Abusers (MICAs).

HIV disease is also affecting mentally ill chemical abusers (MICAs) and the homeless mentally ill who represent a significant percentage of the severely and persistently mentally ill (HSA, September, 1994). Over 50% of all psychiatric inpatient admissions in New York City are for MICA clients; and "hospitals in selected low income communities report that MICAs represent 75-80% of all admissions" (Landsberg, 1994, pg.3). Cournos, et al. (1991) studied 200 state psychiatric hospital patients (with schizophrenia and other psychotic disorders) many of whom had multiple prior admissions. Two thirds (2/3) of these patients had a lifetime DSM-IIIR diagnosis of either alcohol or drug abuse or dependence. Twenty percent (20%) had injected drugs at least once since 1978. Therefore, a majority of chronic psychiatric patients have primary substance abuse problems. Since a significant number of HIV-positive SPMIs reported drug injection, Cournos (June, 1993) suggests "this risk factor is significantly related to the impressive rate of HIV infection among the severely mentally ill" (pg.4).

Immigrants

Since the beginning of the pandemic, people of color have been affected by HIV/AIDS. In 1982, a little under 50% of the males, over 75% of the females and about 66% of the children diagnosed with AIDS in the U.S. were African Americans and Latinos. During the 1980s, New York City's five largest immigrant source countries were the Dominican Republic, Jamaica, China, Guyana, and Haiti. Of all recent immigrants to the United States, about 61% of Dominicans, 45% of Jamaicans, 20% of Chinese, 70% of Guyanese and 37% of Haitians settled in New York City. Additionally, the neighborhoods with the highest concentrations of immigrants are Elmhurst, Queens, Central Brooklyn, and Washington Heights (New York City Department of City Planning [NYC DCP], 1992). Due to the fastest rate of increase of AIDS among Asians and Pacific Islanders (A&PIs), and the large influx of Caribbean immigrants to New York City in the 1980s, there is a need for more specialized services for these populations (Chin, et al., 1994; Rey, 1993).

Asian and Pacific Islanders (A&PIs).

The HIV/AIDS pandemic has been spreading rapidly in Malaysia and Singapore where prostitutes are 15 to 60 years old, come from poverty, and have difficulty negotiating condom use. In Thailand, where HIV has reached epidemic proportions among prostitutes, up to 20% of military recruits are HIV-positive. In addition, Thai prostitutes have been leaving their homeland in droves because the sex tourism industry has declined due to foreigners' fear of HIV/AIDS. In the Philippines, as a result of U.S. Military base closures, prostitutes lowered their fees and HIV is spreading rapidly among the working class (Garrett, 1994). Therefore, as South and Southeast Asia become epicenters of HIV/AIDS, and as the heterosexual rate of transmission increases, it is essential to target prevention efforts to immigrant women (Mangaliman, 1994).

Although Asian and Pacific Islanders (A&PIs) account for about 7% of the total population of New York City, they account for less than 1% of all AIDS cases in the city. However, in the 1980s, Asian born immigrants represented 25% of all immigrants to New York City and about 46% of Asians nationwide. Relative to the 1970s, Asian immigration to the United States during the 1980s increased by about 70 percent (NYC DCP, 1992).

Thus, the rapid spread of AIDS in Asia, and the increase in Asian immigration to the U.S. (including sex workers) may explain why the incidence of AIDS is increasing the fastest among A&PIs than among any other racial group in the city. To date, there have been 414 A&PIs diagnosed with AIDS (NYC DOH, October, 1994b); recent estimates suggest that there are 129 A&PIs living with AIDS in New York City and that 1,082 additional A&PIs are HIV+ (Chin, et al., 1994; HSA, September, 1994). Currently, among A&PIs, 30-39 year olds have accounted for approximately 30% of all AIDS diagnoses while persons aged 40-49 years old have accounted for about 40% of all diagnoses. With an incubation period of approximately 10 years between infection and onset of symptoms, 70% of all AIDS diagnoses among A&PIs in New York City may be the result of exposure occurring between the ages of 20 to 30. While the proportion of HIV transmission among A&PI men who have sex with men (currently 71%) has been decreasing steadily, there has been a continuous increase in the proportion of diagnoses attributed to transmission through IV drug use (Chin, et al., 1994; NYC DOH, October, 1994b).

Caribbean Populations.

"Some Caribbean countries... have some of the highest per capita rates of reported AIDS cases in the world. This, perhaps, together with the high rate of occurrence in Haiti, has led to the description of the Caribbean as an area of 'high risk' in some of the earlier reports" (Livingston, 1992, pg.5). Given its proximity to, trade relationships with, and travel (vacationing and migrant work) to and from North America, these are important reasons contributing to the increase in HIV/AIDS in the Caribbean.

The Caribbean Epidemiology Center (CAREC) has reported that outside of North America, the Caribbean has produced over 10% of the AIDS cases in the Americas (Livingston, 1992). Haiti has reported the largest number of cases in the Caribbean region (Rey, 1993). Regarding the distribution of cumulative adult AIDS cases in the Caribbean by transmission category: 53% was by heterosexual contact, 38% by homosexual and bisexual contact, seven percent by intravenous drug use, and one percent by blood transfusions (Livingston, 1992).

In New York City, as of July, 1994, people born in the U.S. and its possessions account for 46,197 (or 70%) of the 65,703 reported AIDS cases. Haitian-born individuals account for 1,205 AIDS cases, which represents 1.84% of *all* reported AIDS cases in New York City, and 12% of all of the reported AIDS cases *among immigrants* in New York City. Haiti accounts for the highest number of AIDS cases in New York City among people who were not born in the U.S. or whose country of origin is unknown (NYC DOH, August, 1994). Other than the aforementioned data, there has been little to no epidemiological research in the United States of Haitian-Americans due to language and cultural barriers. Most epidemiological research and statistical reports merge Haitians with other black Americans (Rey, 1993).

Given the large number of Caribbean immigrants in New York City, these populations require culturally-specific programs addressing the full range of HIV-related mental health problems. Planning and development of these programs must take place in close partnership with these communities that include undocumented as well as documented immigrants and refugees. Access and service utilization patterns of newly established programs as well as of existing traditional service networks must be assessed and strengthened through the funding of community-based organizations (CBOs) and the provision of technical assistance.

Latino Populations.

According to the CDC (1994), there were 68,903 Latinos with AIDS in the United States as of June, 1994, representing 17% of the 401,749 total U.S. AIDS cases. Of the 68,903 Latinos with AIDS, 49,300 (or 72%) of the men, and 8,865 (or 13%) of the women were between the ages of 25 and 49 years.

In looking at cases in New York City, Latinos account for 20,827, or 30% of the 69,461 total documented adult AIDS cases. This makes Latinos the group with the second highest incidence of AIDS, after the 27,362 Blacks representing 39 percent. Regarding transmission categories, in New York City, 12,088 (58%) of Latino men and women obtained AIDS through intravenous drug use, 5,266 (32%) of Latino men were infected through sex with a male partner, and 1,492 (33%) of the 4,501 Latina women with AIDS were infected through heterosexual transmission (DOH, October, 1994b).

Given the high incidence of AIDS among the Latino communities in New York City, culturally and linguistically relevant HIV/AIDS mental hygiene programs are essential. Workers must learn to acknowledge and address the conservative and religious Latino family structure that is hesitant to discuss sexuality, homosexuality, and drug use and abuse issues. The machismo aspect of the Latino culture which discourages condom use must also be recognized in the treatment of this population.

In summary, traditional mental health modalities implemented for persons living with AIDS (PLWAs) do not always address the needs of immigrants, particularly with respect to language and culture. Many HIV infected immigrants and their families are isolated, even within their own communities. The majority of these individuals do not speak English as a primary language, if at all. Mental health services must be available in languages representing the various immigrant/refugee communities.

Middle-Aged and Older People

Individuals who are age 60 and older are the fastest growing group of the U.S. population. One in nine Americans is over 60 years old. By the year 2000, the median age of America's total population will increase to 37 years, and by year 2020 to 42 years. As a result, by the year 2030, one in four persons, or 25% of our population will be over age 60 (Rey,1994).

Nationwide, over 10% of the AIDS cases are reported in people age 50 and older, and were primarily transmitted through unprotected sex (both homosexual and heterosexual) or blood transfusion (Scharnhorst, 1992). In New York City, over 11% of the cumulative AIDS cases are among those aged 50 and above. Regarding transmission categories among men and women age 50 and older in New York City, 49% were HIV infected due to unprotected (homosexual and heterosexual) sex, 34% due to intravenous drug use, and 1.4% from blood transfusions (DOH, October, 1994b). These numbers do not include the many people over age 50 who are HIV positive, or have AIDS but are undiagnosed or misdiagnosed with other illnesses. There are many illnesses affecting the aging population with symptoms similar to HIV/AIDS including opportunistic infections, neoplasms, lymphomas, and AIDS dementia (Grossman, 1994).

HIV disease has affected middle-aged and older individuals in multiple ways. After being diagnosed with HIV/AIDS, as well as other serious or life-threatening illnesses, the elderly must face "Living with AIDS" when little is known about the parameters of HIV/AIDS for the elderly, especially women. Many older gay men and lesbians, like the immigrant population, have experienced social stigmatization and are very fearful of others finding out about their sexual orientation and HIV status. Many are reluctant to obtain mental hygiene treatment because of their experience with "anti-gay, reversal treatments" when they were younger. Because of HIV infection, the gay and lesbian elderly must face the loss of gay-families, whole social groups, and the decimation of a developing gay culture that has been a sole source of support amid the discrimination. In addition, older people must deal with grieving the loss of adult children to HIV/AIDS and/or substance abuse. Moreover, their children, grandchildren and extended family members may require them to be supportive even as they deal with their own untimely losses.

People with Disabilities

Greater awareness of the special mental health needs of disabled individuals and those who are HIV positive is required not only on the part of the public and social institutions, but also on the part of provider agencies. Additionally, agencies that serve the developmentally and physically disabled, and the visually and auditorially impaired require technical assistance to deal with the multiple problems associated with HIV infection among these populations.

Risks and concerns raised about HIV/AIDS in the general population are magnified for the mentally retarded and developmentally disabled populations. People with mental retardation and developmental disabilities may have cognitive limitations or poor impulse control which may impede their decision-making in potential HIV risk situations such as unsafe sex with prostitutes, or housemates, roommates or friends in communal living situations. This population is also vulnerable to being persuaded or manipulated into engaging in high risk behaviors because they are accustomed to having others (such as parents or agency staff) make decisions for them. In addition, the developmentally disabled are at risk of becoming intravenous drug users and thus would be at risk of contracting AIDS through needle sharing (Jacobs, et al., 1991). With the increasing integration of persons with developmental disabilities into the mainstream of community life, it is imperative that both the program staff and those responsible for caring for the developmentally disabled client be given concrete, specific instruction in HIV/AIDS risk reduction behavior. Equally as important is the reinforcement of risk reduction techniques in the home or residence of the developmentally disabled person, making the training of the caretaker/caregiver essential. There is an absence of HIV/AIDS mental hygiene services for people with disabilities, especially for the auditorially impaired and deaf.

Criminal Justice Population

The forensic population has a broad range of HIV-related mental health and health needs. Adults with serious mental illness are becoming increasingly involved with the criminal justice system. In New York City, 25% of newly admitted inmates require some level of mental health services. About 75% of the mentally-ill incarcerated in local jails are MICA clients (HSA, September, 1994). Many inmates are diagnosed or undiagnosed with HIV and/or AIDS dementia. Prevention and treatment is essential in a population with a 90% rate of alcohol and other drug abuse (S. Lamon, personal communication, March 21, 1995). In addition, tuberculosis and tuberculosis in combination with HIV disease, disproportionately affect this population.

A plan is needed specifically to examine, assess and determine this population's eligibility for alternatives to incarceration related to these mental health and health problems. Linkages between CBOs and the mental health system for these individuals must become a systematic component of forensic services. Similarly CBOs, mental health and health providers need to be sensitized to the needs of the forensic population. Training of jail and prison staff, guards, doctors, parole officers and others around HIV related issues is essential. In general, increased mental health service to this population is imperative. HIV/AIDS prevention and education could easily be implemented in the New York City Correctional System which has a captive population of 120,000 people a year. The majority of whom, men and women, are alcohol and other drug users.

HIV and Tuberculosis Infected Individuals

In New York City, TB infections have reached almost epidemic proportions. Blacks and Hispanics in the 20-50 year age range have the fastest growing incidence of tuberculosis. A higher incidence of HIV-related TB has been found in inner-city areas. Co-infection of HIV and TB seems to be related to high HIV risk behaviors and poor socioeconomic conditions (Sutton, et al., 1993). Populations at risk for tuberculosis include persons at risk for HIV, foreign-born individuals from countries where TB is common, medically underserved low income populations, alcohol and other drug users, and residents of correctional and psychiatric institutions, shelters for the homeless, and nursing homes (NYC DOH, November, 1992).

The HIV-infected population and people living with AIDS are 500 times more likely than the general population to develop tuberculosis (Birenbaum, 1994). According to the NYC DOH (October, 1994b), about 5,577 (8%) of the 70,880 cumulative AIDS cases in New York City have some form of tuberculosis. HIV/AIDS pre- and post-test counseling should include information about tuberculosis and its link to HIV infection. HIV positive individuals should be screened for TB every 6 months if they live in areas endemic for tuberculosis (World Health Organization, January, 1994). Among both the hard-to-reach and underserved populations with TB, mental health services and support (especially in hospital and prison settings) are necessary to maintain long-term self administration of TB treatment and to stem the tide of this disease.

Conclusion

In the continuum of care to HIV-affected individuals, there has often been a deficiency in HIV/AIDS mental health services. Limited funds and problems in program design have restricted the availability of needed services for persons suffering from the neuropsychiatric consequences of HIV infection such as depression and adjustment disorders. Another obstacle has been the language and cultural barriers to care. In order to increase access for the aforementioned HIV-affected special population groups in New York City to existing mental hygiene services, several steps must be taken. First, in-house, cultural competency trainings of mental hygiene providers should be developed for both the established and new immigrant populations in the city. Second, traditional, non-traditional and indigenous provider networks utilized by these communities to provide supportive services must be included in the planning and establishment of service delivery. Additional issues to be addressed include: HIV/AIDS denial, stigmatization, somatization of mental health symptoms, and resistance to traditional mental health services. It is essential for mental hygiene workers serving HIV-affected populations to continue to evaluate existing service mechanisms and develop and implement new strategies for the future.

References

Birenbaum, E. (1994, October). *Tuberculosis and HIV: Dual Epidemics*. Presentation at The Lower Manhattan AIDS Task Force General Membership Meeting, New York, New York.

Centers for Disease Control and Prevention. (1994). *HIV/AIDS Surveillance Report*, 6(1), 5-13.

Chin, J., Eckholdt, H., & Lee, Y. (1994). *HIV/AIDS and the Needs of Asians and Pacific Islanders in New York City: Re-centering Families in Caregiving*. Paper presented at the annual conference of the Association of Asian American Studies, Ann Arbor, MI.

Cole, R., & Cooper, S. (December, 1990). Lesbian Exclusion From HIV/AIDS Education: Ten Years of Low-risk Identity and High-risk Behavior. *SIECUS* Report, 19(2), 40-45.

Cournos, F., Empfield, M., Horwath, E., McKinnon, K., Meyer, I., Schrage, H., Currie, C., & Agosin, B. (1991). HIV Seroprevalence Among Patients Admitted to Two Psychiatric Hospitals. *American Journal of Psychiatry*, 148(9), 1225-1230.

Cournos, F. (June 25, 1993). *HIV Seroprevalence and Sexual Risk Behavior*. Paper presented at the HIV/AIDS and the Mentally Ill Conference (pp. 1-6). Columbia University College of Physicians & Surgeons, New York, NY.

Garrett, L. (August 16, 1994). Covert Sex Practices Put Asians at Risk. *Newsday*, p. B31.

Grossman, A. (Ed.) (1994). *Reaching Out to Middle Age and Older People: The Challenge of HIV/AIDS*. New York: New York University, AIDS/SIDA Mental Hygiene Project, pp. 9-22.

Health Systems Agency of New York City, Inc. (October 8, 1993). *HIV/AIDS Needs Assessment* (Draft).

Health Systems Agency of New York City, Inc.(September, 1994). *Preliminary HIV/AIDS Strategic Plan for the City of New York (Volume II)*, pp. 157-175.

Jacobs, R., Samowitz, P., Levy, J.M., & Levy, P.H. (1989, August). Developing an AIDS Prevention Education Program for Persons with Developmental Disabilities. *Mental Retardation*, 27(4), 233-237.

Jacobs, R., Samowitz, P., Levy, J.M., Levy, P.H., & Cabrera, G. (1991). Young Adult

Institute's Comprehensive AIDS Staff Training Program. In A. C. Crocker, H. J. Cohen, & T.A. Kastner (Eds.), *HIV Infection and Developmental Disabilities* (pp.161-169). Baltimore, MD: Paul H. Brooks Publishing Company.

Kelly, J.A., Murphy, D.A., & Bahr, G.R. (1992). AIDS/HIV Risk Behavior Among the Chronically Mentally Ill. *American Journal of Psychiatry*, 149, 886-889.

Landsberg, G. (January, 1994). *Planning for Mental Health Services for HIV Impacted Populations*. A Work Paper Prepared for the New York City Health Systems Agency, pp. 3-4.

Lerner, S. (June/July, 1994) Microbicides: A Woman-controlled HIV Prevention Method in the Making. *SIECUS Report*, 10-13.

Livingston, I.L. (1992). AIDS/HIV Crisis in Developing Countries: The Need for Greater Understanding and Innovative Health Promotion Approaches. *AIDS Reference Guide*. Washington, D.C: Atlantic Information Services Inc., 218, 1-16.

Mangaliman, J. (August 22, 1994). Nailing AIDS: Disease Battlefront Enters Multicultural Beauty World. *Newsday*, p. A-12.

New York City Department of City Planning. (June, 1992). *The Newest New Yorkers: An Analysis of Immigration into New York City During the 1980s*, pp. 23-31.

New York City Department of Health. (November, 1992). *City Health Information* (CHI), 2(5), 1-4.

New York City Department of Health, Bureau of HIV Program Services-HIV Prevention Planning Group. (August 22, 1994). *Recommendations of the Immigrant Work Group*, Appendix 5.

New York City Department of Health, Bureau of HIV Program Services. (October, 1994a). *HIV Prevention Plan*, p. A- 21.

New York City Department of Health, Office of AIDS Surveillance. (October, 1994b). *AIDS Surveillance Update.*

Osborn, J. (December, 1990). Women and HIV/AIDS: The Silent Epidemic. *SIECUS Report*, 19, 23-26.

Perez, E. (December, 1990). Why Women Wait to be Tested for HIV Infection. *SIECUS Report*, 19, 28-29.

Rey, K. (May 7, 1993). *Cultural Beliefs Affecting AIDS Education in the Haitian Community*. Paper presented at an Inter-Agency Meeting regarding the Guantanamo Bay refugees, New York City Department of Mental Health, Mental Retardation & Alcoholism Services, New York, NY.

Sacks, M.H., Perry, S., & Graver, R. (1990). Self Reported HIV-related Risk Behaviors in Acute Psychiatric Inpatients: A Pilot Study. *Hospital and Community Psychiatry*, 41, 1253-1255.

Scharnhorst, S. (August, 1992). AIDS Dementia Complex in the Elderly. *Nurse Practitioner*, 17(8), 37-43.

Sutton, G., Adler, L., Allen, B., Anastos, K., Fletcher, C., Reichman, L., Remien, R., & Zorrilla, C. (July, 1993). HIV and Tuberculosis in the Correctional System. *AIDS Reference Guide*. Washington, D.C.: Atlantic Information Services, Inc., 1715, 1-16.

World Health Organization (WHO) Tuberculosis Programme. (January, 1994). Tuberculosis Preventive Therapy in HIV-infected Individuals. *AIDS Reference Guide*. Washington, D.C.: Atlantic Information Services Inc., 206, 1-4.

AIDS Campaign In Nigeria: The Efforts of the Federal Government

Jerome O. Okafor

Introduction

Acquired Immune Deficiency Syndrome (AIDS) is one health problem that has created a tremendous amount of concern the world over, including Nigeria. Ever since its discovery in Nigeria in 1986, numerous reports have been written about HIV/AIDS. The prevention of the disease is recognized to require a multi-sectorial approach. The Federal Government, in recognition of this fact, has taken a number of steps to control the spread of HIV. These steps include the involvement of non-governmental and private organizations in the process of HIV/AIDS education and prevention programs.

In this paper therefore, efforts were made to describe the activities of the Federal Government of Nigeria toward effective AIDS campaign programs in the country. Finally, problems militating against the effective execution of HIV/AIDS programs in Nigeria are also listed.

Acquired Immune Deficiency Syndrome, known as AIDS, is one disease whose origin, control and total implication are yet to be fully understood but, like many mysterious diseases, it has brought misery to its victims, communities and nations. The Nigerian government was reluctant to admit the presence of HIV/AIDS. Even more reluctant were the preparations to get

Nigerians ready to avoid the onslaught of the worldwide plague that has enmeshed itself in the bloodstream of millions of people worldwide. Evidence available shows that by 1987, the disease had already killed over 42,000 people in different parts of the world (Orere, 1987).

Nigerians were informed in 1985 that HIV/AIDS had killed some people. However, in 1986, the Federal Government regarded the threat of HIV/AIDS as unworthy of any serious attention. After a number of health professionals claimed in 1985 that they had diagnosed symptoms similar to AIDS disease, the World Health Organization (WHO) set up a committee to investigate Nigeria for HIV-infected cases. Dr. Christopher Williams of the University College Hospital (UCH), Ibadan, was the chairman of the WHO research committee. UCH was to provide the committee assistance, but funds for the jobs came from the WHO. The research report of the committee and those of other private individuals showed that some of the patients tested presented some symptoms of AIDS. These reports in 1986 prompted some media publications on HIV/AIDS in Nigeria.

The Federal Health Authorities consistently denied the claims that HIV/AIDS was affecting people in Nigeria. Several times, the then health minister, Professor Olikoye Ransome-Kuti told the public that he would not be distracted from his goal to provide a sound Primary Health Care (PHC) System for Nigeria. He thought that the reports about HIV/AIDS were false. He did not understand how he could give more attention to a disease that did not exist than preventable diseases that kill or maim hundreds of thousands of Nigerian children daily.

That was the minister's position on June 25, 1986, before he set up a 19 member Expert Advisory Committee on AIDS in Nigeria. In those early days of the Expert Committee, blood samples screened in the few hospitals (usually university teaching hospitals) that had reagents were sent to West Germany, later Kenya, for confirmatory tests of sero positive cases. About 59 days after the inauguration of the Expert Committee, it released its first report that no AIDS case nor the presence of the virus had been found in the country. Nevertheless, the committee advised Nigerians to restrict their sexual activities to only known partners while the search for the presence of the elusive virus continued.

In March, 1987, Professor Ransome-Kuti, the health minister, announced positive proof that there were Nigerians who suffered from AIDS (Olojede, Ezekiel, Lufadeju and Aguiyi-Ironsi, 1987). Ever since then, many reports have been released about AIDS in Nigeria, such as: 83,000 Nigerians may die of AIDS by the year 1995 and an additional 69,000 cases of AIDS would occur in the country between 1990 and 1995 (Health minister, 1991); AIDS kills 32 in Nigeria (Ulasieme, 1991). Also, the Global Program on AIDS (GPA), an international body in Geneva, Switzerland set up to liaise with governments and other bodies to control the AIDS disease, said that Nigeria was not serious in the fight to contain the spread of the dreaded disease

(Oladepo, 1991). GPA, after giving a gloomy report about the AIDS problems in Nigeria, further said that HIV was spreading very fast in Nigeria because the Federal and State Governments lacked the political will to take positive steps.

The GPA officials finally warned that it was up to Nigeria to decide whether the spread would be allowed to continue or whether they, through an intensified and effective campaign, would be able to stop the spread, and create awareness among the people on how to change their behavior toward being infected. These and many other startling revelations about the AIDS situation in Nigeria made the Federal Government start the AIDS Campaign Program (ACP) in the country. There was a Short Term Plan (STP) which was succeeded by a Medium Term Plan (MTP) in 1990. All these strategies were put together by the Federal Ministry of Health, WHO/GPA and all the states of the federation including Abuja. In preparation for the Medium Term Plan, national and state's AIDS Program Secretariats were established in the Health Ministries and these were made responsible for AIDS control at the Federal and State levels, while the committees would remain advisory. Local governments were also advised to establish AIDS Units. This Medium Term Plan has four main components, namely:

1. Program Management;
2. Information, Education and Communication (IEC);
3. Blood and Blood Products; and
4. Epidemiology, Clinical Management, and Counseling.

It is therefore the aim of this paper to review the efforts of the Federal Government of Nigeria to control the spread of HIV infection in line with its ACP objectives as discussed below.

Initial Efforts of the Government

AIDS is one health problem that has defied all medical solutions at present. Because of this, the government started expanding efforts aimed at reducing the spread of the disease immediately after its presence was announced in 1986 (Okoro, 1987). Thereafter, the Federal Ministry of Health, through investigations, revealed that about 90 people were affected by HIV. This sudden revelation prompted the Federal Ministry of Health to establish a National Expert Advisory Committee on AIDS (NAECA) in 1987. The committee was succeeded in January, 1989 by the National AIDS Committee chaired by the then health minister (Eloike, 1992). They established HIV testing centers nationwide, set up a national expert committee on sexually transmitted diseases (STDS) and a national policy on blood transfusions (Okoro, 1987). By 1987, the Federal Government had set up nine centers which would test for AIDS at a government-subsidized rate of N5 per blood sample. These centers are:

1. University of Maiduguri Teaching Hospital (UMTH)
2. The Federal Ministry of Health's Vaccine Manufacturing Laboratory,

Yaba, Lagos;

3.Obafemi Awolowo University Teaching Hospital Complex (OAUTHC) Ile-Ife;

4.Lagos University Teaching Hospital (LUTH);

5.University of Calabar Teaching Hospital (UCTH);

6.University of Nigeria Teaching Hospital (UNTH) Enugu;

7.University of Jos Teaching Hospital (JUTH);

8.Ahmadu Bello University Teaching Hospital (ABUTH) Zaria; and

9.Uthman Dan Fodio University Teaching Hospital (UDFUTH) Sokoto.

The arrangement then was such that both UCH and UMTH were to serve as referral laboratories for all AIDS cases.

As a result of this initial step by the government, by 1991, many government HIV testing centers and facilities offering safe blood for transfusion were established (Table 1). By November 1991, these HIV testing centers sent returns of the following data to the Federal Ministry of Health: the different groups of people screened for AIDS, the number screened, the number positive and the prevalence rate in percentages (Table 2). Data was also provided on HIV prevalence in the country showing among other things, the number of blood samples screened, the number of positive on ELISA WB or Dual ELISA/one ELISA, prevalence in percentages; and the number of AIDS cases for each state of the federation (Table 3). The returns also included a projection of HIV sero-prevalence and progression in Nigeria from 1986 to 1995. The projection was based on the survey conducted with prostitutes and Sexually Transmitted Disease (STD) patients and pregnant women in some cities (African Science Monitor, 1992).

TABLE 1
Number of Health Facilities that Have HIV Screening Facilities in the States and Number of Those Providing Safe Blood are thus:

S/NO.	STATE	NO. OF HIV SCREENING FACILITIES PER STATE	FACILITIES OFFERING SAFE BLOOD
1.	ABUJA	1	1
2.	PLATEAU	5	5
3.	RIVERS	4	3
4.	SOKOTO	2	1
5.	KADUNA	3	2
6.	BAUCHI	2	2
7.	TARABA	1	1
8.	ADAMAWA	1	1
9.	KANO	5	5
10.	DELTA	1 BUT NOT YET INSTALLED	-
11.	LAGOS	9	9
12.	ANAMBRA	8	2
13.	EDO	5	5
14.	AKWA IBOM	3	2
15.	IMO	4	3
16.	CROSS RIVER	1	1
17.	ONDO	3	1
18.	OSUN	2	1
19.	OYO	4	4
20.	ENUGU	4	4
21.	KWARA	2	1
22.	KOGI	NONE	NIL
23.	KATSINA	4	2
24.	JIGAWA	1 BUT NOT YET INSTALLED	NIL
25.	BENUE	2	1
26.	ABIA	3	2
27.	OGUN	4	2

SOURCE: STATISTICS DIVISION OF FEDERAL MINISTRY OF HEALTH, LAGOS, 1992

TABLE 2
HIV SCREENING RETURNS (UP TO NOVEMBER 18, 1991)

GROUPS	NO. SCREENED	NO. POSITIVE	PREVALENCE (%)
BLOOD DONORS: (80.08%)	66,139	569	0.86
ANTE NATAL CLINIC MOTHERS: (4.52%)	3,731	18	0.33
SEXUALLY TRANSMITTED DISEASES PATIENTS: (3.50%)	2,894	44	1.58
FEMALE COMMERCIAL SEX WORKERS: (3.23%)	2,671	225	8.42
PATIENTS: (5.33%)	4,406	88	1.99
OTHERS: (3.33%)	2,750	31	1.13
TOTAL:	82,591	975	118

SOURCE: STATISTICS DIVISION OF FEDERAL MINISTRY OF HEALTH - LAGOS, 1992.

HIV/AIDS EDUCATION IN NIGERIA

Given its characteristics, HIV is transmissible only under specified conditions. Therefore, its control and management become feasible if necessary adjustments in people's lifestyles can be achieved. At this point, the Federal Government recognized that health education constituted a credible vehicle for combating the spread of HIV/AIDS. The recognition was based on the assumption that, with adequate enlightenment of the society, appropriate attitudes and practice of healthful living could be cultivated and maintained. Anderson and May (1995) emphasized that "targeting education and condom distribution at high risk groups will always be beneficial in the early stages of the epidemic, when infection in the general population is limited. Such a policy would clearly be beneficial in countries, such as Nigeria, where the levels of HIV infection in high risk groups such as prostitutes and their male clients are low to moderate and the levels are very low in pregnant women."

Beyond the litany of public health education, according to the editor of the Sunday Champion (1992), the government had installed a primary health care scheme, which was to sensitize the public towards healthy living. It is in this light that the Federal Minister of Health and Human Services designed the HIV/AIDS campaign for the community level, through the facilities of the Primary Health Care (PHC) scheme. Essentially, this initiative has the advantage of integrating the AIDS Campaign with the public health care program. This approach will reduce the cost of informing the public about HIV/AIDS.

TABLE 3
HIV PREVALENCE IN NIGERIA: NOVEMBER, 1991

	STATE (OLD STRUCTURE)	NO. OF BLOOD SAMPLES SCREENED	NO. POSITIVES ON ELISA WB OR ELISA/ONE ELISA	PREVALENCE (%)	NUMBER OF AIDS CASES
1.	AKWA-IBOM	2,407	4	0.17	1
2.	ANAMBRA	27,434	648	2.36	3
3.	BAUCHI	1,715	5	0.29	-
4.	BENDEL	5,121	32	0.62	-
5.	BENUE	5,587	34	0.95	-
6.	BORNO	13,098	83	0.88	7
7.	CROSS RIVER	11,750	103	0.63	20
8.	GONGOLA	2,524	31	3.41	3
9.	IMO	2,312	79	3.41	4
10.	KADUNA	10,138	72	0.71	7
11.	KANO	15,134	195	1.29	-
12.	KATSINA	-	-	-	-
13.	KWARA	2,292	6	0.26	-
14.	LAGOS	20,525	107	0.52	31
15.	NIGER	2,673	21	0.79	-
16.	OGUN	18,315	154	0.84	-
17.	ONDO	3,000	2	0.07	-
18.	OYO	34,609	186	0.54	13+9
19.	PLATEAU	10,071	35	0.35	5
20.	RIVERS	2,977	14	0.47	-
21.	SOKOTO	6,336	78	1.23	-
22.	FCT ABUJA	106	3	2.83	-
23.	FOBTAC	1,645	4	0.24	-
	TOTAL:	199,663	1,896	0.97	91

SOURCE: FEDERAL MINISTRY OF HEALTH - LAGOS, 1992

On Friday, August 23, 1991, the then President of Nigeria, General Ibrahim Babangida, launched the War Against AIDS (WAA) in Nigeria. During the launching, Babangida (1992) made it clear that the Federal Government alone would not be expected to tackle all health problems, even with the best inten-

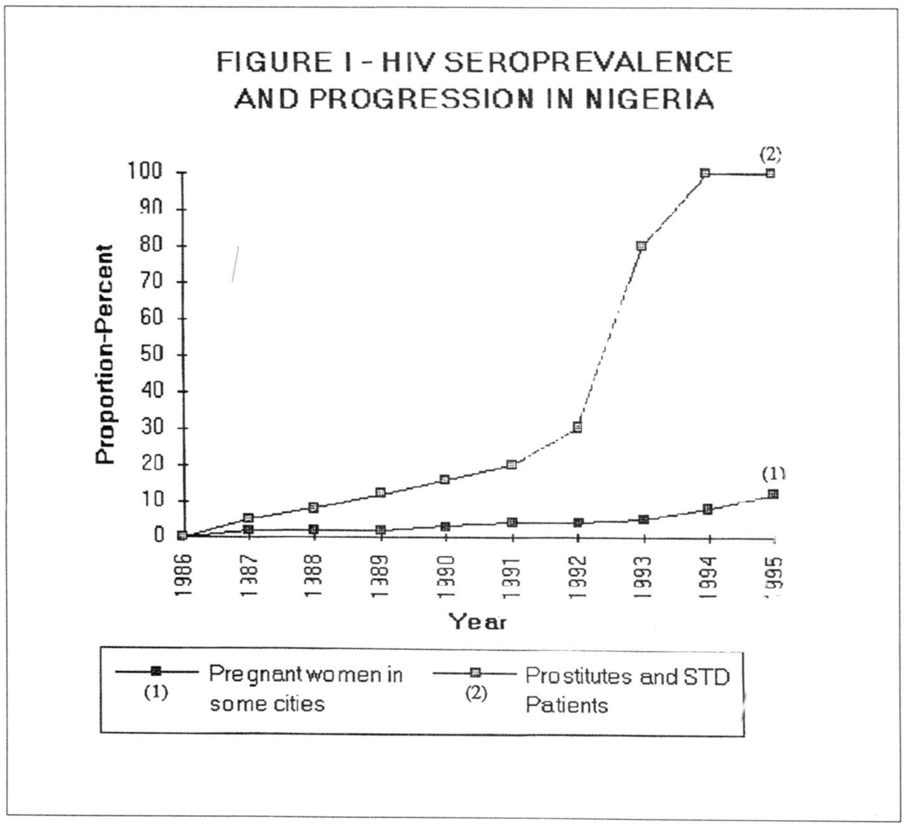

tions. Therefore, he urged the state and local governments; and the Federal Capital Territory to recognize AIDS as their problem, and initiate their own chapters of WAA by December 1, 1991. Non-governmental organizations and the private sector were also requested by the President to be more involved in educating people about AIDS, as well as the care of persons infected with Human Immunodeficiency Virus (HIV).

President Ibrahim Babangida also directed each state and local government to provide a yearly budgetary provision of not less than N1 million and N500,000 respectively toward their AIDS Control Programs. The Federal Government on its part, demonstrated its commitment to the prevention of HIV/AIDS by providing N20 million in the 1992 fiscal year towards the National AIDS Control Program (NACP). Table 4 shows:

a.States that have provided annual statutory allocation for AIDS control activities;

b.States without annual statutory allocation for AIDS control activities;

c.States that have established financial mechanisms toward AIDS control; and

d.States without financial mechanisms as of December, 1993.

TABLE 4

S/ NO	STATES THAT HAVE PROVIDED ANNUAL STATUTORY ALLOCATION FOR AIDS CONTROL ACTIVITIES		STATES WITHOUT ANNUAL STATUTORY ALLOCATION FOR AIDS CONTROL ACTIVITIES	STATES THAT HAVE EST. FINANCIAL MECHANISMS	STATES WITHOUT FINANCIAL MECHANISMS
	STATES	AMOUNT			
1.	BENUE	N1,000,000	KANO	DELTA	BENUE
2.	DELTA	1,000,000	RIVER	KWARA	EDO
3.	EDO	1,000,000	BAUCHI	OGUN	PLATEAU
4.	PLATEAU	130,000	ABIA	LAGOS	SOKOTO
5.	SOKOTO	1,000,000	ANAMBRA	ONDO	KOGI
6.	KOGI	200,000	ABUJA	ENUGU	OYO
7.	OGUN	20,000	KADUNA	KANO	OSUN
8.	LAGOS	1,000,000	KATSINA	RIVER	JIGAWA
9.	ONDO	1,000,000	CROSS RIVER	ABUJA	ADAMAWA
10.	OYO	250,000	-	-	BAUCHI
11.	OSUN	1,000,000	-	-	ABIA
12.	KWARA	-	-	-	ANAMBRA
13.	ENUGU	1,000,000	-	-	AKWA IBOM
14.	JIGAWA	500,000	-	-	KADUNA
15.	ADAMAWA	1,800,000	-	-	TARABA
16.	AKWA IBOM	1,000,000	-	-	IMO
17.	TARABA	1,000,000	-	-	KATSINA
18.	IMO	1,000,000	-	-	-

SOURCE: STATISTICS DIVISION OF FEDERAL MINISTRY OF HEALTH - LAGOS, 1993

For the program to succeed, the Federal Government recognized that there must be inter-sectoral and inter-ministerial collaboration. It therefore directed the Ministry of Education to ensure that HIV/AIDS education was incorporated in all schools curricula. Similarly, the Ministry of Information was directed to waive all air-time charges for HIV/AIDS education messages. Also, the private sector and other non-governmental organizations were requested to make substantial contributions towards federal, state and local government AIDS Control Programs. These measures were taken because the incidence of the disease was regarded as a national emergency where the lives of all members of the society was at stake.

Problems of AIDS Control in Nigeria

The problems of HIV infection control in Nigeria span from the inception to date in all ramifications. The problems encountered in the political, economical, educational, religious and industrial systems have affected the success of the AIDS Control Program (ACP). These problems include:

1.No acceptable local language or terminology for AIDS.

2.Increased prostitution among Nigerian women in Nigeria and when they travel abroad. Various sources (Mukasa, 1992; Ransome-kute, 1992; Aghanya, 1992 and Yusuf, 1991) indicated that Nigerian girls travel to New York, France, and Saudi Arabia to prostitute for foreign currencies.

3.Nigerian men, due to cultural beliefs, refuse to use condoms. This behavior creates an impediment to HIV/AIDS education in Nigeria.

4.The poor economy of Nigeria, together with malnutrition, famine, and the presence of many epidemic diseases, have forced Nigeria to give inadequate attention to spending on HIV/AIDS programs. As a result of the poor economy, there is a low standard of blood screening for transfusion.

5.The Nigerian culture of privacy and non-discussion of STDs including AIDS has also slowed down the rapid spread of information on HIV/AIDS.

6.The poor health care facilities in Nigeria have also caused Nigerians to ignore the present impact of AIDS. Nigeria is not presently involved in HIV/AIDS research. She lacks the equipment and adequate laboratories to engage in sophisticated HIV/AIDS research. Most laboratory work on HIV/AIDS in Nigeria is at the level of screening and diagnosis.

7.Problems of personal dedication or lack of resolve to serve humanity. It is not an envious task to work on the HIV/AIDS control program. Many people in the program have some selfish interests, including the desire to take vantage positions.

8.HIV/AIDS education is not yet well-integrated in the school curriculum at all levels. Hence, people, especially adolescents, have not understood adequately the causes, modes of transmission, prevention, signs and symptoms of the disease and its effects on the individual, nation and society in general.

Summary

The Acquired Immune Deficiency Syndrome (AIDS) is giving the Nigerian government great concern. As a result, the government is expanding efforts aimed at reducing the spread of HIV/AIDS. However, the sole effort of the Federal Government will not be enough to effectively eradicate the widespreading nature of HIV infection. The government requires the concerted efforts of everyone to control HIV/AIDS.

The Nigerian Government has recognized that AIDS is not only a health problem; but has ramifications that affect other sectors of the society. Hence, the National AIDS Program is guided by a high level multi-sectorial committee with representation from many sectors of the government ministries of planning, social welfare, information, education, youth and industry, as well as representatives from the private sector and non-governmental organizations. All of these sectors have been mobilized in the preventive efforts against HIV/AIDS.

References

Aghanya, C. (August, 1992). Fight Against AIDS: Anambra State Government to Release 1 Million Naira, *Daily Star*, p.2.

Anderson, R. M. and May, R. M. (1995). Understanding the AIDS Pandemic. In E. R. Bethel (Ed.), *AIDS: Readings on a Global Crisis* (pp. 320-324). Boston: Allyn and Bacon.

Babangida, I. (1992). AIDS Patients Need Care and Love. *The Road Journal*, 2(4). p.10

Editor. (1992). HIV/AIDS Prevalence in Nigeria. *African Science Monitor*, 2(5), pp 14-15.

Editor. (August, 1992). AIDS Campaign. *Sunday Champion*, p.12.

Eloike, T. (1992). *AIDS Control in Nigeria: Problems and Prospects*. Paper presented at National Conference on AIDS in Nigeria, Enugu.

Health Minister. (1991). 83,000 Nigerians May Die of AIDS. *The Stateman*, 7(99), p. 8.

Mukasa, P. (Feb. 7,1992). Using Education to Fight AIDS Among Youth. *Daily Star*, p. 12.

Okoro, S. (Dec. 10, 1987). AIDS: A Multi-sectorial Disease. *Daily Star*, p.12

Oladepo, W. (March, 1991). AIDS Body Indicts Nigeria. *Newswatch*, p.25.

Olojede, D., Ezekial, M. E., Lufadeju, S. & Aguiyi-Ironsi, L. (March, 1987). Battle the AIDS Scourge. *Newswatch*, pp. 26-27.

Orere, O. (March/April, 1981). Nigeria Finally Accepts the Challenge of AIDS. *Home Doctor*, pp. 14-15.

Ransome-Kute, O. (August 4, 1992). AIDS Campaign to Reach Community Levels. *Daily Champion*, p. 9.

Ulasieme, O. (December 10, 1991). AIDS Kills 32 in Nigeria. *Daily Star*, p. 8.

Prevention of Human Immunodeficiency Virus Infection among African-American Women: Sex, Gender and Power and Women's Risk for HIV

Gina M. Wingood and Ralph J. DiClemente

Introduction

In 1981, when AIDS first appeared in the United States, it was considered a disease of homosexual men. However, as a result of the changing demographics of the disease, AIDS has emerged as a serious public health problem for women. In 1992, the World Health Organization (WHO) reported that worldwide, women are infected about as often as men, and it is predicted that, by the year 2000, most new infections would be among women (Altman, 1992). In the United States, the fastest growing sector of people with AIDS are women between the ages of 18 and 44 (Centers for Disease Control and Prevention, 1990). As of February 1995, the Centers for Disease Control and Prevention reported that 58,448 women had AIDS, accounting for 13% of all AIDS cases nationally (Centers for Disease Control and Prevention, 1994a).

Efforts to tailor prevention programs towards women, particularly African-American women, have emphasized designing ethnic and gender sensitive HIV risk-reduction messages. However, tailoring HIV prevention efforts to African-American women must go beyond these fundamental steps and address the sociocultural and power imbalances that define the realities of life for African-American women in heterosexual relationships. In this chapter we will first review the epidemiology of HIV/AIDS among African-American women, discuss behavioral factors that increase African-American women's risk for HIV, explore the sociocultural, gender and relational factors that are often ignored in prevention interventions tailored for this population, discuss models that may facilitate the design of more appropriate gender-sensitive interventions, and review HIV sexual risk-reduction interventions conducted among predominantly African-American women.

Epidemiology of AIDS in Women

AIDS is the fourth leading cause of death among women aged 25-44 years in the United States (Centers for Disease Control and Prevention, 1994b). In 1994, of the 79,674 persons older than 13 years of age reported with AIDS, 18% were women, nearly threefold greater than the proportion (7%) reported in 1985. Most women with AIDS are young. The median age of women living with AIDS is 35 and women between the ages of 15-44 accounted for 84% of all cases (Centers for Disease Control and Prevention, 1994a).

African-American women are disproportionately represented among AIDS cases as of 1996. The majority, sixty percent of AIDS cases were reported among African-American women. In contrast, white and Latina women account for only 22% and 20%, respectively, of all AIDS cases among women in the United States. Furthermore, during this same time period, AIDS rates for African-American women were 16 times higher than those for white women. Though infected women have been identified in all 50 states, they are more likely to live in the northeast, the District of Columbia, or Puerto Rico. However, between 1988 and 1991, the most rapid increase in AIDS cases among heterosexually infected persons occurred among persons from the south (Chu & Wortley, 1995).

The proportion of AIDS cases reported in women that are attributed to injection drug use and heterosexual contact are almost comparable, 41% and 38%, respectively. Only two percent of women were infected from contaminated blood or blood products; and 19% had no specific HIV risk exposure category reported. However, women with AIDS who initially reported no risk, were later re-classified, the majority, 66%, were re-classified as having heterosexual contact with a high risk partner and 27% were re-classified as having a history of injection drug use (Centers for Disease Control and Prevention, 1992a). Among women who reported acquiring HIV from heterosexual contact, the majority 53%, reported sexual intercourse with a partner who had documented HIV infection or AIDS but whose risk was unspecified while 38% reported having a male partner who was an injection drug user.

Epidemiology of HIV Among Women

Seroprevalence data on HIV infection predict increasing numbers of women with AIDS in the coming years. Using findings from the HIV Survey in Childbearing Women, from 1989 through 1993, the prevalence of HIV infection among childbearing women remained relatively stable at 1.7 per 1000 women (Gwinn et al., 1991). However, seroprevalence rates vary by region, in the northwest, prevalence rates decreased from 4.1 to 3.4 per 1000; in the south prevalence rates increased from 1.6 in 1989 to 2.0 in 1991 and remained stable through 1993 (Centers for Disease Control and Prevention, 1993).

Serosurveys in 54 drug treatment centers in 28 cities also confirm the strong association between HIV infection and injection drug use among women (Chu & Wortley, 1995). Seroprevalence rates among women in drug treatment programs ranged from 0% to 44.6%, with a median of 3.7% (Allen et al., 1990). Serosurveys of 107 STD clinics in 44 cities report substantially lower median seroprevalence rates for women not reporting intravenous drug use (0.7%). Among applicants for military service between 1985 and 1989, seroprevalence rates among 17- and 18-year-old women exceeded those among male applicants of the same age (Burke et al., 1990). This study reported that HIV seroprevalence has decreased among 17- to 19-year-old male military applicants, though less so among African Americans. However, the seroprevalence rates increased over time among African-American female applicants of the same age.

The number, as well as the proportion of women infected through heterosexual transmission, regardless of the partner's risk, is expected to continue to rise. Key epidemiologic factors in this continuing heterosexual transmission to women are the greater effectiveness of HIV transmission from men to women than from women to men (European Study Group on Heterosexual Transmission of HIV, 1992; Padian et al.,1991) and the greater probability for women to encounter an HIV-infected partner than for men (Chu & Wortley, 1995). Other data indicative of the heterosexual spread of AIDS, are the increasing rates of gonorrhea and syphilis, particularly among African-Americans in U.S. cities (Aral & Holmes, 1991). As STDs facilitate the transmission of HIV, the higher incidence of STDs among African-Americans may contribute to the higher incidence of AIDS in this ethnic population (Rolfs & Nakashima, 1990; Holmberg et al., 1989). Additionally, the National Survey of Family Growth has shown that women are becoming sexually active at younger ages (Anderson & Dahlberg, 1992). Younger age at sexual intercourse is associated with a greater number of sexual partners and increased risk for STDs, including HIV (Centers for Disease Control and Prevention, 1990). These findings corroborate other national surveys explaining the significant increase in AIDS cases among women infected as adolescents. HIV will continue to escalate among women, until they adopt safer sex practices (Catania et al., 1992).

Prevalence of Consistent Condom Use Among African-American Women

A primary HIV prevention strategy for sexually active persons is to use condoms on every episode of sexual intercourse. Studies of sexually active persons demonstrate that condoms, when used correctly and consistently, effectively prohibit the transmission of viral pathogens, including HIV (Roper, Peterson & Curran, 1993). In particular, evidence from prospective epidemiologic studies of HIV-discordant couples indicate that consistent condom use is a highly effective prevention strategy (Cates & Stone, 1992; Saracco et al., 1993; Laurian, Peynet, Verrout, 1989). Recent findings from the European Study Group on Heterosexual Transmission of HIV identified a markedly higher seroconversion rate among the seronegative partner of HIV-discordant couples who used condoms inconsistently relative to couples who used condoms consistently. Among couples who reported inconsistent condom use, a seroconversion rate of 4.8 per 100 person years was observed (De Vincenzi, 1994).

While the use of latex condoms can substantially reduce the risk of sexually transmitted infections including HIV, many sexually active African-American women do not use condoms consistently. Furthermore, many women never use condoms when engaging in sexual intercourse. Several studies have examined the prevalence of consistent condom use and non-condom use among African-American women. While epidemiologic data suggests that condoms can be an effective HIV preventive strategy, the prevalence of consistent condom use is relatively low, ranging from 8% to 35% of the studies reviewed. A high degree of individual compliance is necessary for condoms to be used consistently during sexual intercourse. For economically disadvantaged African-American women, numerous behavioral, social, cultural and gender-related factors may reduce their compliance with consistent condom use, explain their non-use of condoms and, thus, elevate their risk of HIV exposure (Wingood & DiClemente, 1992).

Social, Cultural and Gender-Related Factors That Increase African-American Women's Risk for HIV

HIV prevention research has excelled in identifying behaviors associated with risky sexual practices and transmission of HIV. However, behavioral variables often fail to provide insight into the influence of the pervasive cultural, economic, gender-specific, and relational factors that mediate risky sexual and drug-related behaviors. When conducting research with African-American women, it is important to understand their risk and HIV risk-reduction efforts in a gender-specific manner. Clearly, understanding the social influences that shape sexual relationships for African-American women is critical to the development and implementation of tailored and more efficacious programs designed to reinforce the adoption and maintenance of HIV preventive behaviors among African-American women (Wingood & DiClemente, 1992).

These studies are presented in Table 1 below.

Table 1.
PREVALENCE OF CONDOM USE AMONG AFRICAN-AMERICAN WOMEN

	TRIAL SAMPLE	NEVER USE	CONSISTENT USE
DICLEMENTE & WINGOOD (1995)	128 WOMEN RECRUITED FROM A COMMUNITY BASED SAMPLE IN SAN FRAN., CA	45.0	28.1
PETERSON ET AL.(1992)	230 WOMEN RECRUITED FROM A COMMUNITY BASED HOUSE HOLD PROBABILITY SAMPLE IN SAN FRAN., CA	73.0	8.0
JOHNSON ET AL. (1992)	165 FEMALE COLLEGE STUDENTS	—	28.0
MAYS & COCHRAN (1988)	98 FEMALE COLLEGE STUDENTS	17.0	35.0

African-American Women's Socioeconomic Vulnerability

Socioeconomic status (SES) is an important correlate of behavior that affects health, access to health services, the risk of disease, the risk of an adverse outcome once disease occurs, and mortality (Antonovsky, 1967; Adler et al., 1993; Pappas et al., 1993; Rice et al., 1991; Jacobsen & Thelle, 1988; Gittelsohn, Halpern & Sanchez, 1991). When HIV and AIDS rates have been adjusted by SES, both HIV prevalence and AIDS incidence rates have been found higher in areas where populations have lower SES (Morse et al., 1991; Fife & Mode, 1992). A recent study characterized the SES profiles of individuals living with AIDS (Diaz et al., 1994). Significant differences in educational attainment were noted between African-American and white women with AIDS regardless of their risk exposure. Notable income differences were also reported between races. African-American injection drug using women were more likely to have household incomes less than $10,000 (91%) compared to white women (76%). Additionally, among women who acquired HIV heterosexually, 81% of African-American women reported having an income of less than $10,000 compared to 49% of white women. African-American women's SES constraints may exacerbate their risk of infection and impede access to optimal and quality care. African-American women's vulnerability for HIV is further elevated due to their lack of confidence and power to implement and sustain HIV risk reduction practices.

Power Inequities in African-American Heterosexual Relationships

Power is a fundamental element of all human relationships, particularly intimate heterosexual relationships (Gillespie, 1971). Numerous studies indicate that women are psychologically, economically and socially the more dependent partners in heterosexual dyads (Kelley & Thibaut, 1978). Often the male partner brings more assets (i.e. money, status, security) to the relationship and the female partner becomes dependent on these resources. The dynamics in these relationships evolve into an imbalance of power whereby the male wields the power and the female lacks the power. Women in these power imbalanced relationships are defenseless against males' use and abuse of power. The consequence of women's powerlessness in relationships is their inability to negotiate condom use to protect themselves from the acquisition of sexually transmitted infections, including HIV.

Inability to Negotiate Condom Use

Sexual negotiation is the process of bargaining for safer sex in light of the social cost of such negotiations (Worth, 1990; Wingood, Hunter & DiClemente, 1993). Therefore, the decision to negotiate condom use is based on the women's perceptions of the costs of and benefits to a particular relationship and the relationship's role in the woman's economic, social, physical survival and goals. Women's inability to negotiate condom use is one of the strongest correlates of never having used a condom (Peterson et al., 1992). In one study, African-American women who failed to assertively demand that their partner use a condom, were 6.2 times more likely to report having a sexual partner who never used a condom compared with women who were assertive with their demands to use a condom (95% CI = 2.1 - 16.2) (Wingood & DiClemente, in press). Power inequalities in relationships strongly influences women's confidence to negotiate safer sex by depriving them of opportunities that would enable them to feel efficacious. Asserting her needs for safer sex undermines the trust in relationships (Wingood, Hunter & DiClemente, 1993) and challenges traditional male power roles such as having authority over the relationship and exerting control over using condoms. The resulting conversation escalates into an argument and ends with both partners feeling anxious and threatened. Negotiating safer sex is even more difficult for women in abusive relationships.

Violence against Women Increases their Risk for HIV

Power inequalities in heterosexual relationships are evident in the prevalence, severity and continuity of physical, sexual and emotional abuse against women. HIV risk-taking behaviors have been associated with women who are victims of rape (Irwin et al., 1995), and with women who are in physically abusive relationships (Wingood & DiClemente, in press). Recent findings from a study conducted among African-American women indicated that 17.6% of women were in physically abusive relationships (Wingood & DiClemente, in press). Women with physically abusive partners were less likely to use condoms (P.04), seven times more likely to experience verbal abuse when they asked their partner to use condoms, nine times more likely to have a partner who threatened to physically abuse them when he was asked to use a condom, and four times more likely to believe that their physical partner might verbally abuse them when he was asked to use condoms, compared to women not in an abusive relationship.

Qualitative research exploring social influences on African-American women's attempts to negotiate safer sex with their partners also reports findings of women enduring threats of abuse while trying to negotiate condom use (Wingood, Hunter & DiClemente, 1993). In one study a woman's partner responded in the following manner when she tried to negotiate condom use.

> B——, I'll beat you a—! Don't do me like that [don't ask me to wear a condom].

> Another woman expressed fear about negotiating safer sex. She stated: I never have [asked my partner to use a condom]. I'm scared to tell him to use one, he ain't been using no condom..., you don't know my man, honey.

Sex-Ratio Imbalances May Affect African-American Women's Sexual Risk Taking

Power inequities within heterosexual relationships are complicated by the perceived and actual limited availability of African-American men. For African-American women who are considering marriage there are fewer marriageable men, that is, males who are heterosexual, employed and not incarcerated, than there are marriageable females. In a recent study, conducted among economically disenfranchised African-American women, 80% of women believed that there was a limited number of eligible African-American men (Wingood & DiClemente, in press). This sex-ratio imbalance, or difference between the genders in number of eligible partners with whom to establish a relationship, can have adverse psychological and behavioral consequences that may elevate African-American women's risk for HIV (Mays & Cochran, 1990). African-American women may be more likely to tolerate objectionable behavior and be less likely to demand that condoms be used during sex. Furthermore, African-American men may exhibit greater power within relationships, feel less pressure to develop commitments and engage in higher rates of sexual activity outside of the relationship, increasing their own and their female partners' exposure to HIV.

These findings suggest that powerlessness, abuse, a lack of negotiation skills and traditional gender roles supporting women's passiveness, in addition to the constraints of being economically disenfranchised make practicing safer sex a difficult reality for many African-American women in heterosexual relationships. Furthermore, these social and gender-related constraints are rarely addressed in social psychological theories that guide the design and delivery of many HIV risk reduction interventions for African-American women.

Limitations of Social Psychological Theories for HIV Prevention among African-American Women

In the field of social psychology, several attitude-behavior models have been useful in predicting health-related behavior changes. Some of these models including the Health Belief Model (Rosenstock, Strecher & Becker, 1994), the Theory of Reasoned Action (Fishbein, Middlestadt & Hitchcock, 1994), and the Social Cognitive Theory (Bandura, 1994) have been used specifically in the area of HIV prevention for African-American women. However, these models fail to consider the social contextual issues of gender, class, and ethnicity that may exert considerable influence on key theoretical constructs (Cochran & Mays, 1993). Several limitations exist when applying these aforementioned models to predict HIV risk-reduction practices among African-American women.

First is the reliance on models whose assumptions are based on individualistic, rational choices determining behavior. African-American women place less value on an individualistic focus and place more emphasis on familial responsibilities and community norms (Gasch, Poulson, Fullilove & Fullilove, 1991). For many African-American women, safer sex practices are complicated by the more proximate influence of securing safety and food for themselves and their children. In the African-American community, perceptions of behavior as indicating a sense of belonging to the community may function to endorse different patterns of behavior (Mays & Comas-Diaz, 1988). Certain behaviors that are associated with African-American woman are important to the individual's survival and emotional wellbeing and if not engaged in may leave the individual without a solid sense of belonging to or identification with particular parts of the African-American community.

Second, these models fail to acknowledge socioeconomic factors as influencing safer sex practices, particularly for African-American women. Earlier, we discussed that among women with AIDS, African-American women are less likely to complete the twelfth grade and more likely to have household incomes less than $10,000 compared to white women (Diaz et al., 1994). The influence of economic factors must be given greater consideration when designing interventions to reduce the risk of HIV among African-American women.

Third, these models fail to incorporate ethnicity in a meaningful and useful manner. Historically, the African-American culture has been portrayed as deviant or pathological (Clark, 1947). However, recent research on African-Americans has challenged this cultural bias (McKenry, 1989). A recent trend in the literature has been the attempt to move beyond the pathology model to an exploration of the sources and mechanisms underlying "positive" African-American's social and psychological functioning. Currently, much of this research is focusing on acknowledging and understanding positive racial identity, adaptive coping styles, healthy role modeling and high self esteem. This "emerging" model views the positive and adaptive features of African-Americans as products of an interaction between their culture and their environment (Fine, Schwevbel & James-Myers, 1987).

The fourth limitation of these models is the failure to acknowledge gender as an independent variable influencing safer sex practices. Gender-blind models implicitly assume static "sex roles" and often obscures potentially modifiable social processes that influence women's risk of HIV infection (Wingood & DiClemente, 1994). This approach to risk reduction fails to recognize the importance of social sexual relationships between women and men and how these relationships may adversely affect women's abilities to adopt and maintain HIV-preventive behaviors. Relational factors, such as having a physically abusive partner, having poor sexual communication skills, and having a long-term relationship, have been repeatedly cited as major determinants of women's high-risk sexual behavior (Wingood & DiClemente, in press; Plichta et al., 1992; Peterson et al., 1992). Effective HIV prevention efforts will need to change gender-based relational norms to support women's role in practicing safer sex.

Without incorporating these gender, cultural, and psychosocial influences, attempts at program development, by necessity, will lack the cultural and contextual cohesiveness which often determines whether or not programs are accepted, adopted and effective as the threat that HIV poses for women is considerable and growing (Wingood & DiClemente, 1992; Airhihenbuwa et al.,1992). Only an orchestrated and integrated social sexual research agenda can hope to identify and understand the cultural, gender and psychosocial influences within the African-American community. Recent research on HIV risk-reduction interventions conducted with African-American women are incorporating these contextual factors.

Gender Specific Theories

The convention in epidemiological studies is to ascribe "gender" on the basis of biological sex and to use the term "sex differences" rather than "gender differences" (Gold, 1984). However, differences between women and men are not essentially biological or behavioral but are the result of prevailing socially defined societal norms that dictate appropriate sexual conduct for women (Bem, 1993). Precisely because AIDS is a condition that links sex, gender, and disease, a social structural framework such as the Theory of Gender and Power that addresses norms governing social sexual relations may serve as a useful heuristic for designing HIV interventions for women (Connell, 1987). The Theory of Gender and Power incorporates three overlapping, but distinct structures that serve to explain and constrain the culturally-bound roles between men and women. As women's vulnerability to HIV infection is closely intertwined with her gender roles, understanding theories that examine gender relations is crucial in order to understand women's risk and risk-reduction practices in a gender-related manner. According to the Theory of Gender and Power, the division of labor, the structure of power and the structure of cathexis are the major tenets that characterize relationships between men and women.

The sexual division of labor is an allocation of particular types of work to certain categories of people. The social context is attributed to the allocation which becomes a constraint on human behavior. The sexual division of labor is manifested in the segregation of unpaid work namely housework and childcare to women, and inequalities in wages and educational attainment between the sexes. The sexual division of labor explains African-American women's socioeconomic vulnerability to HIV. African-American women living with AIDS are less likely than white women to complete their high school education and more likely to earn less than $10,000 per year compared to white women (Diaz et al., 1994). Additionally, African-American women are less likely to access and use STD services, and have markedly higher STD rates than white women (Aral & Holmes, 1991).

The association of power with the demarcation between men and women's work also serves to constrain gender relations. Inequalities in power between the sexes forms the basis for the sexual division of power. This structure deals with issues such as control, authority and coercion within heterosexual relationships. The structure of power explains why African-American women who have physically and sexually abusive partners are at increased risk for sexually acquired HIV. The constraints of power are evident in the difficulty women have in negotiating safer sex. The permanence of this structure helps us to understand why women with a history of child sexual abuse are more likely to engage in high risk sexual practices. This structure is illustrated in the sexual politics of the inaccessibility of condoms in schools, the inordinate time to develop a female-controlled device that protects women from HIV, and norms supporting male control over condom use.

The structure of cathexis localizes the social norms that govern appropriate sexual behavior for women, and characterizes the erotic and affective influences in sexual relationships. The structure of cathexis, explains why relationships between men and women are often called social sexual relationships. This structure rationalizes that women fail to negotiate safer sex because it undermines the trust and intimacy in relationships. This structure explains why the sex-ratio imbalance in the African-American community makes it difficult for African-American women to exert control over her partner by asking him to use a condom. The structure of cathexis illustrates why women's concern for securing food, shelter and money for her children take priority over practicing safer sex. Furthermore, this structure creates the norms for women's passivity in sexual relationships, normalizes men having multiple sexual partners and disapproves of women engaging in the same practices. This structure is also evident by women's attraction to older men, even if these relationships are characterized by power imbalances.

The Theory of Gender and Power provides an understanding of why economically disadvantaged women are at increased risk for HIV infection, by identifying gender-specific risks. However, this theory is less informative at providing methods that promote and maintain behavior. The Social Cognitive Theory addresses both the psychosocial dynamics underlying health behavior and the mechanisms for modifying behavior.

A Review of Theory-Based HIV Sexual Risk-Reduction Interventions Involving Predominantly African-American Women

As the heterosexual spread of HIV continues to rise in women, the design, implementation and evaluation of HIV sexual risk-reduction interventions will be a necessity. Presently, four theoretically-based HIV sexual risk-reduction interventions have been conducted that assess changes in HIV risk-taking. Each of these interventions utilized Social Cognitive Theory (SCT) to guide program design and implementation. Furthermore, each of these interventions have taken into account the broader contextual issues that influence HIV risk-taking among African-American women. While only one intervention actually applies a gender-specific theory (Wingood & DiClemente, 1995), these interventions address assertiveness skills, negotiation skills, power imbalances and stressors specific to women.

El-Bassell and his colleagues conducted an HIV-prevention intervention for females 21 to 42 years of age, the majority of whom where either African-American or Hispanic recruited from a methadone maintenance program in Bronx, New York (El-Bassell & Schilling, 1992). Women were randomly assigned to either a skills-based intervention condition (n=48) or an information only control condition (n=43). Participants randomized to the peer-led skills based intervention condition received training in AIDS education, proper condom use, assertiveness and communication skills as well as identifying personal barriers to implementing safer sex practices. The theoretical framework guiding the intervention was Social Cognitive Theory. The study reported a significant increase in the mean frequency of condom use 15 months post-intervention (P.01).

While this study has numerous strengths, including random assignment to treatment conditions and the use of a social psychological model which has proven useful in guiding the development of HIV prevention programs with other risk populations, it has several methodological limitations. This investigation did not blind interviewers to subjects' group assignment, increasing the potential for interviewer bias at follow-up assessment. The investigation also failed to provide data assessing pretest equivalence between treatment groups on sociodemographic, behavioral and psychological variables and lacked a measure of variability for the designated effect size.

Hobfoll and his colleagues conducted an HIV sexual risk reduction intervention for single pregnant women 16 to 29 years of age, the majority of whom where either African-American or Caucasian, recruited from three inner city obstetric clinics in Akron, Ohio (Hobfoll et al., 1994). Women were randomly assigned to one of three conditions: a four-session AIDS prevention condition (n=68), a health promotion comparison condition (n=77) or a control condition (n=61). Participants randomized to the four-session peer-led AIDS prevention condition received AIDS education, assertiveness skills, negotiation skills, planning skills, skills in cleaning drug works and relapse prevention. Peer leaders utilized role playing to refine participants' sense of mastery, positive expectations of success, problem solving skills and sense of vulnerability. The theoretical models underlying the intervention were the Social Cognitive Theory and Conservation of Resources Theory (COR). The COR theory posits that an intervention must increase both a woman's personal and social resources in order to combat her increased threat of AIDS. The COR theory further suggests that target groups must see the intervention as both adding new resources and building on their current strengths. Participants randomized to the intervention demonstrated favorable changes in mean scores on a composite measure of spermicide and condom use over a six-month time period compared to the no-intervention control conditions (X2 = 2.44, P .05). While this investigation has numerous strengths, including random assignment to treatment conditions and the use of social psychological models, it has several methodological limitations. Perhaps the major limitation is non-use of an intention-to-treat protocol in conducting data analyses. Specifically, while women were assigned to the four-session intervention, the investigators only included women who completed three or more of the treatment sessions in the analysis. Thus, women who completed only two or fewer treatment sessions were excluded for the data analysis. Excluding participants from the experimental intervention on the basis of the number or proportion of treatment sessions attended clearly violates the intent-to-treat principle. The intention-to-treat analytical approach is the only one that preserves the full value of randomization, providing a more valid assessment of treatment efficacy. Thus, while the findings from this study might appear promising, the failure to conduct intention-to-treat analyses may result in spurious conclusions regarding treatment effects. Further, the investigation did not use interviewer blinding procedures, failed to provide retention rates by study condition, failed to provide pretest equivalence data on sociodemographic behavioral and psychological variables and did not provide a measure of variability for the designated effect size.

Kelly and his colleagues conducted an HIV sexual risk-reduction intervention among women 18 to 40 years of age recruited from a primary health care clinic in Milwaukee, Wisconsin (Kelly et al., 1994). The majority of women were African-American with multiple male sexual partners who had diagnose of sexually transmitted infections or had sex with high risk male partners. Participants were randomized to either a five-session peer-led HIV/AIDS intervention condition (n=100) or a comparison condition (n=87). Women randomized to the intervention condition received five-sessions which emphasized AIDS education, attitudinal and social factors affecting safer sex, proper condom use skills, identifying personal triggers, such as involvement in coercive or power imbalanced sexual relationships, peer support elements (i.e. endorsing the norm that men can be denied sex unless condoms are used). As in the other theoretically-based interventions, Social Cognitive Theory was used to guide intervention development. Women randomized to the intervention condition demonstrated increased frequency of condom use; from 26% at baseline to 56% of all intercourse occasions in the three-months post-intervention assessment (p .001). The comparison group showed little change in condom use at follow-up assessment.

While the study has a number of design and methodological strengths, it also has several methodological limitations which may affect internal validity. The investigation did not provide any data on the study participation rate, failed to use procedures to blind interviewers to subjects' group assignment and did not use the standard intention-to-treat protocol. Moreover, there was no assessment of pretest equivalence between treatment groups on sociodemographic, behavioral and psychological variables. And, finally, a measure of variability for the designated effect size was not calculated.

DiClemente and Wingood (DiClemente & Wingood, 1995) conducted an HIV sexual risk-reduction intervention among African-American women 18-29 years of age recruited from the Bayview Hunter's Point neighborhood in San Francisco, California. Participants were randomized to either a five-session peer-led HIV/AIDS intervention condition (n=53), an HIV education only condition (n=35) or a delayed HIV education control condition (n=40). Women randomized to the five-session peer led HIV/AIDS intervention received five sessions which emphasized ethnic and gender pride, HIV risk-reduction information, sexual self-control, sexual assertiveness and communication skills, proper condom use skills, and developing relationship norms supportive of consistent condom use. The theoretical frameworks guiding intervention development were the Social Cognitive Theory and Theory of Gender and Power. The Theory of Gender and Power posits that difficulties arise in following safer sex practices because self-protection often is swayed by feelings of intimacy, abusive partners, economic factors, and norms supporting women's passive behavior within sexual relationships. The Theory of Gender and Power addresses the influence of these larger social structures that can compromise the sexual health of women. Women randomized to the intervention condition, compared to the delayed HIV education control condition, demonstrated increased consistent condom use (adjusted odds ratio = 2.1, 95% CI 1.03-4.15; p=.04). No statistically significant differences in condom use were observed between the HIV education-only condition relative to the delayed HIV education control condition.

In general, behavioral interventions that are theory-driven utilized a randomized controlled design, used peers to implement the intervention, addressed gender relations and used multiple sessions are effective at promoting the adoption of condom use during sexual intercourse. Further studies are needed to corroborate and extend the findings reported here using rigorous methodological research designs, appropriate data analytic techniques and longer follow-up intervals to evaluate programmatic efficacy; in particular, the stability of program effects over time.

Conclusion

This chapter has highlighted the epidemiology of AIDS in African-American women, the behavioral and social forces that increase the risk of HIV infection for African-American women and existing HIV-prevention interventions that demonstrate changes in women's high-risk sexual behavior. A continuing challenge is to understand the implications of previous research for the development of more tailored gender-relevant behavioral interventions. For instance, while Social Cognitive Theory has provided a promising theoretical framework for developing skills training interventions which have proven to be effective in enhancing women's condom use, this model does not entirely address the role of contextual and sociocultural variables such as gender, class and ethnicity and their influence on sexual behavior. These social structures shape the reality of risk for HIV infection and potential for adopting HIV-preventive strategies by African-American women.

Gender roles, cultural values and partner attitudes, for example, are highly influential in affecting the behavior of African-American women and the nature of their heterosexual relationships in which sexual activity occurs (Gasch et al., 1991). Understanding the interpersonal and sexual dynamics within African-American heterosexual relationships and how these dynamics influence behavior remains an understudied area that offers potential insights into how to design more targeted interventions. Thus, there is a need to apply gender-specific theories and construct HIV prevention strategies that address the structure of gender relations (Wingood & DiClemente, 1995).

Controlling the HIV epidemic among African-American women requires designing interventions that address the larger social contextual issues that characterize the daily hardships and gender-specific risks of African-American women. Only by addressing the larger structural issues will African-American women's vulnerability to HIV diminish. The urgency of the HIV epidemic demands that the development and evaluation of HIV-prevention interventions tailored towards women remain a public health priority.

References

Adler, N.E., Boyce, T., Chesney, M.A., Folkman, S. & Syme, L. (1993). Socioeconomic Inequalities in Health, No Easy Solution. *Journal of the American Medical Association*, 269, 3140-3145.

Airhihenbuwa, C.O., DiClemente, R.J., Wingood, G.M. & Lowe, A. (1992). HIV/AIDS Education and Prevention Among African-Americans: A focus on Culture. *Journal of AIDS Education and Prevention*, 4, 251-260.

Allen, D.M., Onorato, I.M., Sweeney, P.A. et al. (1990). *Seroprevalence of HIV Infection in Intravenous Drug Users (IVDUs) in the United States*. Abstract presented at the Sixth International Conference on AIDS, San Francisco.

Altman, L.K. (1992). Women Worldwide Nearing Higher Rate for AIDS Than Men. *The New York Times*, July 21, C1, C3.

Anderson, J.E. & Dahlberg, L.L. (1992). High-risk Sexual Behavior in the General Population: Results From a National Survey, 1988-1990. *Sexually Transmitted Diseases*,19, 320-325.

Antonovsky, A. (1967). Social Class, Life Expectancy and Overall Mortality. *Milbank Memorial Fund Quarterly*, 45, 31-73.

Aral, S.O. & Holmes, K.K. (1991). Sexually Transmitted Diseases in the AIDS Era. *Scientific America*, 264, 62-69.

Bandura, A. (1994). Social Cognitive Theory and Exercise of Control Over HIV Infection. In R. J. DiClemente & J. L. Peterson (Eds.), *Preventing AIDS: Theories and Methods of Behavioral Interventions* (pp. 25-54). New York, NY: Plenum Press.

Bem, S.L. (1993). *The Lenses of Gender: Transforming the Debate on Sexual Inequality*. New Haven, Conn: Yale University Press.

Burke, D.S., Brundage, J.F., Goldenbaum, M., Gardner, L.I., Peterson, M., Visintine, R., Redfield, R.R., & the Walter Reed Retrovirus Research Group. (1990). Human Immunodeficiency Virus Infections in Teenagers: Seroprevalence Among Applicants for US Military Service. *Journal of the American Medical Association,* 263, 2074-2077.

Catania, J.A., Coates, T.J., Kegeles, S., et al. (1992). Condom Use in Multi-ethnic Neighborhoods of San Francisco: The Population-based AMEN (AIDS in Multi-ethnic Neighborhoods) Study. *American Journal of Public Health*, 82, 284-287.

Cates, W. & Stone, K.M . (1992). Family Planning, Sexually Transmitted Diseases and Contraceptive Choice: A Literature Update - part I. *Family Planning Perspectives,* 24, 75-84.

Centers for Disease Control and Prevention. (1994). *Annual Summary of Births, Marriages, Divorces, and Deaths: United States, 1993*. Hyattsville, Maryland: US Department of Health and Human Services, Public Health Service, CDC, 18-20.

Centers for Disease Control and Prevention. (1994). Mid-year edition. *HIV/AIDS Surveillance Report*, 6, 5-10.

Centers for Disease Control and Prevention. (1992). 1993 Revised Classification System for HIV Infection and Expanded Surveillance Case Definition for AIDS Among Adolescents and Adults. *Morbidity & Mortality Weekly Report*, 41, (no. RR-17).

Centers for Disease Control and Prevention. (1992). Selected Behaviors that Increase Risk Among High School Students-United States, 1990. *Morbidity & Mortality Weekly Report*, 41, 236-240.

Centers for Disease Control. (1991). Premarital Sexual Experience Among Adolescent Women-United States, 1970-1988. *Morbidity & Mortality Weekly Report*, 39, 929-931.

Centers for Disease Control and Prevention. (1990). AIDS in Women-United States. *Mortality & Morbidity Weekly Report*, 39, 845-846.

Chu, S.Y. & Wortley, P.M. (1995). Epidemiology of HIV/AIDS in Women. In H. Minkoff, J.A. DeHovitz, A. Duerr (Eds.), *HIV Infection in Women*. New York, New York: Raven Press.

Clark, K.B. & Clark, M.K. (1947). Racial Identification and Preference in Negro Children. In T. Newcomb & E. Hartley (Eds.), *Readings in Social Psychology*, (pp. 602-611). New York, NY: Henry Holt.

Cochran, S.D. & Mays, V.M. (1993). Applying Social Psychological Models to Predicting HIV-related Sexual Risk Behaviors Among African-Americans. *Journal of Black Psychology*, 19, 142-154.

Connell, R.W. (1987). *Gender and Power*. Stanford, Calif: Stanford University Press.

De Vincenzi, I. (1994). A Longitudinal Study of Human Immunodeficiency Virus Transmission by Heterosexual Partners. *New England Journal of Medicine*, 331, 341-346.

Diaz, T., Chu, S.Y., Buehler, J.W. et al., (1994). Sociodemographic Differences Among People With AIDS: Results From a Multistate Surveillance Project. *American*

Journal of Preventive Medicine, 10, 217-222.

DiClemente, R.J. & Wingood, G.M. (1995). A Randomized Controlled Trial of a Community-based HIV Sexual Risk Reduction Intervention for Young Adult African-American Females. *Journal of the American Medical Association*, in press.

El-Bassel, N., & Schilling, R.F. (1992). 15-Month Follow-up of Women Methadone Patients Taught Skills to Reduce Heterosexual HIV Transmission. *Public Health Reports*, 107, 500-504.

Fife, D. & Mode, C. (1992). AIDS Incidence and Income. *Journal of Acquired Immune Deficiency Syndrome*, 5, 1105-1110.

Fine, M., Schwevbel, A.I., & James-Myers, L. (1987). Family Stability in Black Families: Values Underlying Three Different Perspectives. *Journal of Comparative Family Studies*, 13, 1-23.

Fishbein, M., Middlestadt, S.E. & Hitchcock, P.J. (1994). Using Information to Change Sexually Transmitted Disease-related Behaviors: An Analysis Based on the Theory of Reasoned Action. In R. J. DiClemente & J. L. Peterson (Eds.), *Preventing AIDS: Theories and Methods of Behavioral Interventions (61-77).* New York, NY: Plenum Press.

Gasch, H., Poulson, D.M., Fullilove, R.E., & Fullilove, M.T. (1991). Shaping AIDS Education and Prevention Programs for African-Americans Amidst Community Decline. *Journal of Negro Education*, 60(1), 85-96.

Gillespie, D. (1971). Who Has the Power? The Marital Struggle. *Journal of Marriage and the Family*, 33, 445-458.

Gittelsohn, A.M., Halpern, J. & Sanchez, R.L. (1991). Income, Race, and Surgery in Maryland. *American Journal of Public Health*, 81, 1435-1441.

Gold, E. (1984). *Changing Risk of Disease in Women: An Epidemiological Approach.* Lexington, Mass: Colbamore-Press.

Gwinn, M., Pappaioanou, M., George, J.R. et al. (1991). Prevalence of HIV Infection in Childbearing Women in the United States. *Journal of the American Medical Association*, 265, 1704-8.

Hobfoll, S.E., Jackson, A.P., Lavin, J., Britton, P.J. & Shepherd, J.B. (1994). Reducing Inner-city Women's AIDS Risk Activities: A Study of Single, Pregnant Women. *Health Psychology*, 13, 3979-403.

Holmberg, S.C., Horsburgh, C.R., Ward, J.W. & Jaffe, H.W. (1989). Biologic Factors in the Sexual Transmission of Human Immunodeficiency Virus. *Journal of Infectious Diseases*, 160, 116-125.

Irwin, K.L., Edlin, B.R., Wong, L. et al. (1995). Urban Rape Survivors: Characteristics and Prevalence of Human Immunodeficiency Virus and Other Sexually Transmitted Infections. Multicenter Crack Cocaine and HIV Infection Study Team. *Obstetrics & Gynecology,* 85, 330-336.

Jacobsen, B.K. & Thelle, D.S. (1988). Risk Factors for Coronary Heart Disease and Level of Education. The Tromso Heart Study. *American Journal of Epidemiology*, 127, 923-932.

Johnson, E.H., Gant, L., Hinkle, Y.A., Gilbert, D., Willis, C., & Hoopwood, T. (1992). Do African-American Men and Women Differ in Their Knowledge, About AIDS Attitudes About Condoms and Sexual Behavior. *Journal of the National Medical Association*, 84, 49-64.

Kelley, H.H., & Thibaut, J.W. (1978). *Interpersonal Relations: A Theory of Interdependence*. New York, NY: John Wiley & Sons.

Kelly, J.A., Murphy, D.A., Washington, C.D., Wilson, T.S., Koob, J.J., Davis, D.R., Ledezma, G. & Davantes, B. (1994). The Effects of HIV/AIDS Intervention Groups for High-risk Women in Urban Clinics. *American Journal of Public Health*, 84, 1918-1922.

Laurian, Y., Peynet, J., Verroust, F., (1989). HIV Infection in Sexual Partners of HIV Seropositive Patients with Hemophilia. *New England Journal of Medicine*, 320, 183.

Mays, V.M. (1989). AIDS Prevention in Black Populations: Methods of a Safer Kind. In V.M. Mays, G.W. Albee & S.F. Schneider (Eds.), *Primary Prevention of AIDS* (pp. 264-279). Newbury Park, CA: SAGE Publications.

Mays, V.M., & Comas-Diaz, L. (1988). Feminist Therapy with Ethnic Minority Populations: A Closer Look at Blacks and Hispanics. In M.A. Douglas & L. Walker (Eds.), *Feminist Psychotherapies: Integration of Therapeutic and Feminist Systems* (pp. 228-251). Norwood, NJ: Ablex.

Mays V.M. & Cochran S.D. (1990). Methodological Issues in the Assessment and Prediction of AIDS Risk-related Sexual Behaviors Among Black Americans. In B. Voeller, J.M. Reinish, M. Gottlieb (Eds.), *AIDS and Sex: An Integrated Biomedical and Biobehavioral Approach* (pp. 97-120). New York, New York: Oxford University Press.

McKenry, P.C., Everett, J.E., Ramseur, H.P. & Carter, C.J. (1989). Research on Black Adolescents: A Legacy of Cultural Bias. *Journal of Adolescent Research*, 4(2), 254-264.

Morse, D.L., Lessner, L., Medvesky, M.G., Glebatis, D.M. & Novick, L.F. (1991). Geographic Distribution of Newborn HIV Seroprevalence in Relation to Four Sociodemographic Variables. *American Journal of Public Health*, 81, 25-29.

Padian, N.S., Shiboski, S.C. & Jewell, N.P. (1991). Female-to-Male Transmission of Human Immunodeficiency Virus. *Journal of the American Medical Association*, 266, 1664-1667.

Pappas, G., Queen, S., Hadden, W., Fisher, G. (1993). The Increasing Disparity in Mortality Rates Between Socioeconomic Groups in the United States, 1960 and 1986. *New England Journal of Medicine*, 329, 103-109.

Peterson, J.L., Grinstead, O.A., Golden, E, et al., (1992). Correlates of HIV Risk Behaviors in Black and White San Francisco Heterosexuals: The Population-based AIDS in Multiethnic Neighborhoods (AMEN) study. *Ethnicity & Disease*, 2, 361-370.

Plichta, S.B., Weisman, C.S., Nathanson, C.A., Ensminger, M.E., & Robinson, C.J. (1992). Partner-specific Condom Use Among Adolescent Women Clients of a Family Planning Clinic. *Journal of Adolescent Health*, 13, 506-511.

Rice, R.J., Roberts, P.L., Handsfield, H.H., Holmes, K.K. (1991). Sociodemographic Distribution of Gonorrhea Incidence: Implications for Prevention and Behavioral Research. *American Journal of Public Health*, 81, 1252-1258.

Rolfs, R.T. & Nakashima, A.K. (1990). Epidemiology of Primary and Secondary Syphilis in the United States, 1981 Through 1989. *Journal of the American Medical Association*, 264, 1432-1437.

Roper, W.L., Peterson, H.B. & Curran, J.W. (1993). Commentary: Condoms and HIV/STD Prevention—Clarifying the Message. *American Journal of Public Health*, 83, 501-503.

Rosenstock, I.M., Strecher, V.J. & Becker, M.H. (1994). The Health Belief Model and HIV Risk Behavior Change. In R. J. DiClemente & J. L.Peterson (Eds.), *Preventing AIDS: Theories and Methods of Behavioral Interventions* (pp. 5-22).

New York, NY: Plenum Press.

Saracco, A., Musicco, M., Nicolosi, A., et al. (1993). Man-to-Woman Sexual Transmission of HIV: Longitudinal Study of 343 Steady Partners of Infected Men. *Journal of Acquired Immune Deficiency Syndromes*, 6, 497- 502.

Wingood, G.M. & DiClemente, R.J. Consequences of Having a Physically Abusive Partner on Condom Use and Sexual Negotiation of Young Adult African-American Women. *American Journal of Public Health;* (in press).

Wingood, G.M. & DiClemente, R.J. Correlates of Non-condom Use Among Young Adult African-American Women. *American Journal of Community Psychology*; (in press).

Wingood, G.M. & DiClemente, R.J. (1995). HIV Sexual Risk Reduction Interventions for Women: A Review. *American Journal of Preventive Medicine.*

Wingood G.M., DiClemente R.J. (1995). Understanding the Role of Gender Relations in HIV Prevention Research. *American Journal of Public Health.* 85(4), 592.

Wingood, G.M. & DiClemente, R.J. (1992). Cultural, Gender and Psychosocial Influences on HIV-related Behavior of African-American Female Adolescents: Implications for the Development of Tailored Prevention Programs. *Ethnicity & Disease*, 2, 381-388.

Wingood G.M. Hunter D. & DiClemente R.J. (1993). A Pilot Study of Sexual Communication and Negotiation Among Young African-American Women: Implications for HIV prevention. *Journal of Black Psychology*, 19, 190- 203.

Worth, D. (1990). Sexual Decision Making and AIDS: Why Condom Promotion Among Vulnerable Women is Likely to Fail. *Studies in Family Planning*, 20, 297-307.

Zierler, S., Feingold, L., Laufer, D., Velentgas, P., Kantrowitz-Gordon, I. & Mayer, K. (1991). Adult Survivors of Childhood Sexual Abuse and Subsequent Risk of HIV Infection. *American Journal of Public Health*, 81, 572-575.

Part Three

Ethical Issues

Introduction

HIV/AIDS has raised a lot of ethical issues. There has been considerable discussion on issues of confidentiality and informed consent, individual and collective rights, the mother's right and the rights of her unborn child, mandatory testing for HIV, and policies to protect the rights of people who are either HIV positive and/or have full blown AIDS. These vexing questions on HIV/AIDS have continued to generate varied opinions from politicians, researchers, students and AIDS activists. An increased understanding of HIV/AIDS will limit the varied ethical arguments that engulf the real issues militating against effective prevention of HIV/AIDS in the society.

In "AIDS and Sports Participation: Knowledge and Opinions of Male and Female Athletes," Davidson C. Umeh examines students' views on sports participation. He administered a questionnaire to 134 student athletes in a four year college. The results show that although athletes know the basic methods of HIV transmission, some misconceptions still exist. There were no gender differences in knowledge; however, female athletes were more tolerant of participation of HIV-positive athletes in sports competition than male athletes. More tolerant attitudes were positively associated with knowledge of HIV/AIDS. There were no differences in knowledge and attitudes between athletes in contact and non-contact sports.

In "AIDS: A Community Answers the Call," Marietta Federici-LaFargue discusses the efforts of a community to give people with AIDS support and assistance necessary to overcome the predicament of their illness. Her discussion explores the activities that can be organized to help AIDS patients live and die with dignity. The article emphasizes that there is still life after HIV infection or AIDS disease. An understanding of the virus/disease can help alleviate the fears that prevent people from providing support for individuals who are living with AIDS.

Tim Rodgers in "A Case Study of a Long Term Survivor of HIV Infection," chronicles the discovery of his infection and the emotional roller coaster he experienced as he came to grips with his social environment, interaction with rural health workers and the realization of his impending death. He attributes much of his good health to excellent social support, commitment to completion of his graduate studies and a personal adoption of practice of a healthy lifestyle.

McDaniel, et. al., in "Delivering Culturally Sensitive AIDS Education in Rural Communities," provide an overview of challenges and strategies useful to AIDS education in rural communities. The authors draw attention to the need to extend AIDS education into rural areas of the United States which have previously not experienced the full impact of the AIDS pandemic.

In "Protocol 076: A New Look at Women and Children with AIDS," Nora K. Bell examines some of the ethical and political considerations inherent in evaluating proposals for mandatory testing of all pregnant women as against policies that recommend voluntary testing.

Lynn Morrison and Sepali Guruge, in "We Are a Part of All That We Have Met: Women and AIDS," focus on the historical antecedents that put women at risk for HIV today. They examine the roots of sexually transmitted diseases and how women have been portrayed as the "vectors" of diseases in the past and compare this to the role of women in the HIV/AIDS epidemic. Morrison and Guruje include graphic images from earlier decades to illustrate the similarities of recurrent themes which stereotype women.

AIDS and Sports Participation: Knowledge and Opinions of Male and Female College Athletes

Davidson C. Umeh

The increase in the number of HIV-positive and AIDS cases has created concern for sports organizations and athletes. This concern was manifested when Ervin "Magic" Johnson of the Los Angeles Lakers basketball team announced that he was HIV-positive. According to Hamel (1992), since Magic Johnson's retirement, athletes as well as sports organizations are taking more interest in HIV and AIDS. Many athletes seek answers from physicians about the risk of HIV transmission through athletic competition and the rights of HIV-positive players. Magic Johnson's announcement raised many questions concerning HIV infection and sports participation: Should athletes who are HIV-positive be allowed to continue playing? Should there be mandatory HIV testing for athletes? Should an athlete be informed about the HIV status of other athletes? Are other athletes comfortable playing with athletes who are HIV-positive? These questions demand urgent answers as the number of athletes who are HIV-positive increases. Greg Louganis, Olympic medalist, announced that he had AIDS. "His admission ignited a debate about whether athletes should be tested for HIV and whether he should have admitted he was HIV-positive at the 1988 Summer Olympics, where he hit his head on the diving board and got a scalp wound that required stitches" (Longman, 1995).

Perhaps the most controversial question relating to HIV/AIDS and sports participation is whether to allow athletes who are HIV-positive to continue to engage in contact sports. Some experts believe that participation in sports presents a very low risk in the transmission of HIV although there are proponents for the development of precautionary policies. According to one editorial, (AIDS in sports, 1993) contact sports are relatively safe in terms of HIV transmission; however, it is still important to adopt precautionary measures.

Krucoff (1992) stated that numerous sports and health organizations have developed guidelines on AIDS and athletics since experts' predictions indicate that more athletes may become HIV-positive in coming years due to sexual promiscuity and intravenous drug use. Some athletes believe that individuals who are HIV positive should be prevented from participating in contact sports. The Associated Press (1992) reported the Australian Olympic Federation had planned to boycott sports competition against the United States basketball team if Magic Johnson was allowed to participate. As a result, mandatory testing of athletes for HIV has been advocated by some individuals as a measure to prevent the spread of HIV during sports participation. Springer (1991) stated that Jim Wahler of the Phoenix Cardinals believes HIV testing in football is necessary for the safety of players and due to evidence of bloodshed in the sport.

A different point of view is shared by others. For example, Donald Fehr, executive director of the Major League Baseball Players Association believes that mandatory HIV testing is an infringement on the players' privacy (Springer,1991). Fehr contended that compulsory HIV testing of professional athletes may lead to demand by employers for other forms of testing. According to the American Academy of Pediatrics (1991), infected athletes should not be involuntarily excluded from sports. Routine testing is not justified and physicians should respect the infected athlete's right to confidentiality.

Will athletes accept the concept of voluntary testing? If yes, this awareness raises new issues. If an athlete tests positive for HIV, should he or she inform other teammates? For the athlete, there are obvious conflicts having to do with rights and responsibilities. Ethically, it is only fair for a player who is HIV-positive to inform members of the team. A knowledge of one another's HIV status may help teammates to adopt correct preventive measures on the playing field. On the other hand, the divulging of one's HIV status is an infringement on individual privacy. It may also result in discriminatory behavior from coaches and other players.

The National Collegiate Athletic Association and other professional organizations established guidelines in an effort to prevent the spread of HIV in sports arenas. Game officials are required to stop play when an athlete is bleeding to enable the athlete to leave for treatment of a bleeding wound. HIV/AIDS education programs for athletes have been established by some colleges and professional sporting organizations. Despite efforts by sporting organizations to prevent the spread of HIV during sports participation, athletes still express concern about contracting HIV in the sports arena. Krucoff (1992) stated that despite increased education and awareness that the virus is transmitted in body fluids primarily through sexual intercourse and the sharing of dirty needles, some athletes are still concerned about playing against people who are HIV-positive.

While there is obvious controversy about the many aspects of HIV/AIDS and its relationship to participation in sports, there can be no controversy that AIDS is a relevant concern for college athletes, particularly in urban inner city schools with high minority student populations. James Allan, Director of the National AIDS Program at the Public Service, reports that compared to the total population, the newly infected are likely to be people of color and residents of inner cities (Eckholm, 1991). Curran et al. (1988) stated that one-fifth of all reported cases of AIDS occur in individuals 20-29 years of age. Given the long incubation period of the illness (seven to 10 years), it may be logical to assume that many were infected during the college age years.

There is also other evidence to suggest that college aged individuals may be at particular risk for contracting HIV. During the college years, there is a high degree of alcohol and drug use and sexual experimentation. Because college aged individuals are generally in prime health and rarely, if ever, encounter a peer visibly stricken with AIDS, they are likely to view themselves as invincible and not at risk.

One might even argue that the college athlete may be at increased risk of infection. There is the obvious potential of blood exchange through physical injury during competition, particularly in contact sports. Also, athletes often boast of their popularity and the ease with which sexual encounters are likely to occur. They describe parties where peer pressure for alcohol and drug use present themselves with regularity.

As a coach of a varsity team at an urban university, this researcher has become increasingly concerned about players' health and safety. It has also been my experience that athletes harbor fears and anxieties about HIV infection in sports competition. How well informed about HIV/AIDS are our college athletes? What are their concerns and opinions about participating in contact sports given the potential of HIV transmission?

This study will explore the following questions:

1.What is the knowledge level of athletes about HIV/AIDS?

2.How do athletes feel about the inclusion of HIV-positive athletes in competition?

3.Is there any significant difference in knowledge about HIV/AIDS and attitudes toward HIV-positive athletes in sports participation between male and female athletes?

4.Is there any significant difference in knowledge about HIV/AIDS and attitudes toward HIV-positive athletes in sports participation between athletes in contact and non-contact sports?

5.What is the relationship between knowledge about HIV/AIDS and attitudes toward AIDS in sports participation?

Methods

Sample

The questionnaire was administered to 87 male and 47 female athletes in a four year college in a Northeastern city. The participants were selected based on membership in the intercollegiate teams of the college.

Instrumentation

The study used a 28 item questionnaire constructed by the researcher that included some original questions and some questions used in similar surveys. Twenty-two items covered a wide range of knowledge about HIV/AIDS. Six items covered the athletes opinion about HIV/AIDS and sports.

The knowledge items were listed as statements, such as, "AIDS virus may be contracted through giving a blood donation," to which the respondents were to indicate whether they agreed, disagreed, or were not sure. All "Not sure" responses were coded as incorrect. Agreement to the above statement was scored as incorrect, while disagreement was scored as correct. Correct responses were summed over the 22 items. The knowledge items were tested for internal consistency reliability, achieving a Spearman-Brown split half coefficient of .69, and a coefficient alpha of .74. A copy of the knowledge items are in Appendix A.

The attitude survey contained six items related to HIV/AIDS and contagion through sports activities. A typical item was , "I would be afraid to compete in contact sports with athletes who are HIV positive." Each item was anchored to a five-point Likert-type response mode using the following categories: Strongly agree, agree, not sure, disagree, and strongly disagree. High scores on the scale indicated greater permissiveness. Therefore, in the example above, strongly disagree was scored 5 and strongly agree was scored 1. The theoretical range of scores was from 6 to 30. The Attitude toward HIV/AIDS in Sports Scale (AHASS) was tested for internal consistency reliability using Cronbach's coefficient alpha, which was .81. A copy of the attitude items is in Appendix B.

Data Collection

The questionnaire was administered to the athletes either before practice or during the team's meeting period. The coach of each sport was informed about the study and they granted permission for the questionnaire to be administered to the athletes. The researcher informed the students of the purpose of the study, advised them of their rights to confidentiality and refusal, and passed out the survey instruments. A total of 134 completed surveys were returned that were adequately completed for data analysis.

Table 1 AIDS Knowledge and Attitude towards AIDS in Sports Participation by Sex

Group	n	M	SD	$t_{[132]}$
	Knowledge			
Males	87	16.40	3.71	-0.54
Females	47	16.74	3.14	
TOTAL	134	16.52	3.51	
	Attitude			
Males	87	16.48	5.28	2.60*
Females	47	18.93	5.06	
TOTAL	134	17.34	5.32	

*p.01

Results

The first research question relates to the level of knowledge of athletes about HIV/AIDS. The mean score on the 22-item scale was 16.52, indicating that the average student was incorrect on five or six items. The average score was about 75%. More than half wrongly thought that HIV could be contracted through the giving of blood or that blood transfusions were unsafe because of HIV contamination, and half wrongly thought that HIV could be transmitted through mosquito bites. Other items that had more than 25% incorrect responses were: Acquired Immune Deficiency Syndrome (AIDS) is caused by human immunodeficiency virus, homosexuals are responsible for spreading HIV and AIDS, HIV is transmitted through the saliva of a person who is HIV positive, a person can get AIDS from someone who is HIV positive through their perspiration, and HIV can be transmitted by kissing someone who has AIDS. Each of these responses is an error in which a supposed method of transmission is false, indicating that fear may be motivating respondents to err on the side of caution. Two items that had less than 10% incorrect responses were: Unprotected sex with several people makes a person susceptible to contracting HIV, and Sharing of intravenous needles and syringes is a risky behavior because of HIV, indicating that the vast majority knew the two most common methods of transmission.

The second research question concerned the attitudes of the respondents toward participation by HIV-positive athletes in sports. The data on the AHASS indicate that the mean item score was 2.89 on a scale from one to five, that, in general, the athletes studied were highly ambivalent about playing with HIV-positive athletes. Most athletes indicated that they were hesitant to allow HIV-positive athletes to play or were fearful of infection. For example, 30.6% of the respondents either agreed or strongly agreed that an athlete who is HIV positive should be barred from participation in contact sports like basketball, wrestling, football, or soccer, and an additional 25.4% were not sure. Similarly, 38.1% of the respondents agreed or strongly agreed that they would be afraid to compete in contact sports with athletes who are HIV positive, and an additional 24.6% were not sure.

Research question 3 asked if there were any gender differences in knowledge about HIV/AIDS or attitudes toward HIV infection and sports participation. There were no significant differences between male and female athletes on knowledge of HIV/AIDS. However, on the attitude survey (AHASS), the data indicated that female athletes were more permissive in their attitudes toward playing with HIV-positive athletes than were male athletes (t[132] = 2.60, p .01).

The fourth research question concerned whether differences in knowledge or attitudes existed between athletes in contact sports and non-contact sports. Persons involved in soccer and basketball were considered participants in contact sports, while respondents who did not participate in those two sports, but who played baseball, softball, volleyball, tennis, or ran cross-country were considered participants in non-contact sports.

Table 2 presents the results of the comparisons of the two groups. There were no significant differences between athletes who participated in contact sports and non-contact sports on knowledge or attitudes.

Research question 5 speculated on the relationship between knowledge about HIV/AIDS and attitudes toward AIDS in sports participation. A Pearson correlation was computed between knowledge scores and attitude scores. The result was r = .27, p .01, indicating that higher knowledge scores were associated with more tolerant views of sports participation by HIV-positive individuals.

Table 2
AIDS Knowledge and Attitude towards AIDS in Sports Participation by Participation in Contact Sports

(N =134)

Contact Sports Participation	n	M	SD	$t_{[57]}$
	Knowledge			
Yes	69	16.07	3.95	1.54
No	65	17.00	2.93	
	Attitude			
Yes	69	17.46	5.53	0.25
No	65	17.23	5.14	

Discussion

The results indicate that the athletes in this study know the two major ways in which HIV is transmitted. However, there is a general trend that suggests that the athletes in this study think that HIV is transmitted in more ways than it actually is. On the one hand, the fear of transmission through mosquito bites, kissing, blood donations, or saliva may indicate a high level of caution. However, these pieces of misinformation along with the belief that homosexuals are responsible for spreading HIV, suggest that a substantial number of the athletes surveyed may base their attitudes toward HIV/AIDS on misinformation and hysteria. Surprisingly, half of the athletes sampled thought that there was a cure available.

Although a substantial minority of between 20-30% of the athletes thought AIDS to be a "gay" disease and blamed homosexuals for its spread, these results indicate a decline in numbers since Goodwin and Roscoe (1988) reported that college students viewed AIDS as a gay disease and blamed homosexuals for its spread.

Although the findings suggest that athletes have a significant level of knowledge about AIDS, there was evidence that the athletes sampled were not accurately informed about all aspects of HIV/AIDS. For example, a substantial number of athletes reported that HIV could be contracted through blood donation. One might speculate that athletes' responses were influenced by their perceptions of the blood donation process which utilizes syringes and needles. Also, the athletes indicated that blood transfusion is unsafe because of the risk of contracting HIV. Clearly, athletes must be helped to understand the blood screening regulations that were put into effect in 1985 which have helped to eliminate HIV infected blood from the pool for transfusion (Hochhauser & Rothenberger, 1992).

The athletes polled in this study were hesitant to allow HIV-positive persons to participate in sports, or indicated that they were afraid of their participation. Some of this hesitancy may be based upon misinformation such as fears that saliva or perspiration can transmit the HIV.

The more permissive views of women athletes about sports participation by HIV-positive athletes suggests that women athletes may be less likely to discriminate against HIV-positive athletes. Whether the more permissive attitudes of female athletes is due to a lower level of homophobia, their experience of being discriminated against as females, or some other factor is beyond the scope of this study, but should perhaps be an object of study by future researchers.

Although it would be expected that participants in contact sports might be more restrictive in their views of playing with HIV-positive athletes, there were no differences between them and non-contact sport athletes. Contact sports athletes would have greater possibilities of direct contact with the blood of other athletes, yet their views were no more restrictive than non-contact athletes. These data suggest that attitudes toward HIV-positive athletes may be based on something other than fear of contact and possible infection, perhaps on more generalized attitudes toward HIV-positive individuals. The findings on the positive relationship between knowledge scores and more tolerant attitudes toward HIV-positive athletes' participation in sports suggests that part of the fear of participation by HIV-positive athletes is based on ignorance and misinformation.

Given these findings, it is recommended that colleges and universities begin to formulate or review their policies regarding HIV/AIDS as it is applied to sports participation. HIV/AIDS programs geared to the athletes on campus must move beyond providing only basic information about the disease and its transmission. Programs must be designed to focus on the obvious fears and anxieties that the athlete harbors with respect to risk of infection. Well-designed HIV/AIDS education programs for athletes must allow them the opportunity to identify and express their concerns about sports participation. The counseling staff within each institution should be called upon to facilitate programs that encourage open dialogue regarding this sensitive and complex issue, with its primary goal to reduce fears and anxieties. Emphasis should be placed on instructing athletes about the known methods of HIV transmission and the methods of protection from infection. It is important that student athletes be disabused of mistaken notions about how HIV is transmitted, since they may lead to counter-factual concepts of methods and carriers of HIV. It is also important for educators to point out that becoming infected with HIV is extremely unlikely in sports competition. The potential risk for transmitting blood-borne pathogens during sporting activity is extremely low (Mast, Goodman, Bond, Favero & Drotman, 1995). HIV-positive athletes became infected because of unprotected sexual intercourse or the sharing of drug paraphernalia, not through intercollegiate competition. Finally, it is recommended that athletes be encouraged to become actively involved in formulating college policies on this issue, since they are the individuals subjected to the potential risk.

This study has revealed a number of questions that need to be considered by subsequent researchers. First, why do female athletes seem to have more tolerant attitudes toward HIV-positive athletes than do men? Second, what is the basis for restrictive attitudes toward HIV-positive athletes? What is the relationship between homophobia and restrictive attitudes toward HIV-positive athletes in sports competition? Since this researcher is suggesting increased and coordinated efforts by colleges and universities to educate athletes about HIV/AIDS, it is important that such programs be evaluated in terms of changes in knowledge and attitudes resulting from such instruction.

References

"AIDS in Sports." (1993). *The Physical Education Journal of Sports Medicine*, 2(2), 7.

American Academy of Pediatric Committee on Sports Fitness.(1991). Human Immunodeficiency Virus [Acquired Immunodeficiency Syndrome(AIDS) Virus] In the Athletic Setting. *Pediatrics*, 88(3), 640-641.

Associated Press. (1992, January 23). Australians Consider Boycott if Magic Plays. *Los Angeles Times*, p. C1.

Curran, J., Jaffe, H., Hardy, A. M., Morgan, W. M., Selik, R. M. & Dondero, T. (1988). Epidemiology of HIV Infection and AIDS in the United States. *Science*, 239, 610-616.

Eckholm, E. (1991, November 17). More than Inspiration Is Needed To Fight AIDS. *New York Times*, p. E1.

Goodwin, M. P., & Roscoe, B. (1988). AIDS: Students' Knowledge and Attitude at a Midwestern University. *American Journal of College Health*, 36, 214-222.

Hamel, R. (1992). Assessing the Risk Among Athletes. *The Physician and Sports Medicine*, 20(2), 139-146.

Hochhauser, M. & Rothenberger, J. H. (1992). *AIDS Education*, Dubuque, IA: Wm. C. Brown Publisher.

Krucoff, C. (1992). AIDS Time Out: Assessing the Risk of HIV Transmission in Sports. *Washington Post*, p. 20.

Longman, J. (1995, February 26). Debate About HIV Tests Sparked by Diver with AIDS. *New York Times*, p. E2.

Mast, E. E., Goodmwn, R. A., Bond, W. W., Favero, M. S. & Drotman, P. (Feb. 15, 1995). Transmission of Blood-borne Pathogens During Sports: Risk and Prevention. *Annals of Internal Medicine*, 122(4), pp. 283-285.

National Collegiate Athletic Association Committee on Competitive Safeguards and Medical Aspects of Sports. (1992). *AIDS and Intercollegiate Athletics: NCAA*

Sportsmedicine Handbook, Overland Park, KS. NCAA.
Springer, S. (1991, November 9) Testing Not Mandatory in Pros. and NCAA. *New York Times*, p. C7.

Appendix A

Knowledge Items

1. Acquired Immune Deficiency Syndrome (AIDS) is caused by human immunodeficiency virus. (T)
2. AIDS virus may be contracted through giving a blood donation. (F)
3. Homosexuals are responsible for spreading HIV and AIDS. (F)
4. Unprotected sex with several people makes a person susceptible to contracting HIV. (T)
5. Proper use of condom can serve as a preventive measure against HIV infection. (T)
6. AIDS is manifested by the inability of the body to fight off diseases. (T)
7. HIV is transmitted through the saliva of a person who is HIV positive. (F)
8. Sharing of intravenous needles and syringes is a risky behavior because of AIDS. (T)
9. HIV can be contracted through anal sex. (T)
10. A person can get AIDS from someone who is HIV positive through their perspiration. (F)
11. A cure has been found for AIDS. (F)
12. HIV can be transmitted through mosquito bites. (F)
13. HIV can be transmitted by kissing someone who has AIDS. (F)
14. A person can get AIDS by sharing a towel or cup with someone who has AIDS. (F)
15. A pregnant woman can transmit HIV to her baby. (T)
16. AIDS is a disease for gay people. (F)
17. People who are HIV positive cannot transmit the virus until they have AIDS. (F)
18. HIV is transmitted through vaginal sexual intercourse. (T)
19. Receiving a blood transfusion is unsafe because of the risk of contracting HIV. (F)
20. People who are HIV positive die from other diseases rather than from AIDS. (T)
21. AIDS can be prevented by douching with bleach immediately after vaginal sexual intercourse. (F)
22. AIDS can be prevented by urinating immediately after sexual intercourse. (F)

Appendix B

Attitude Items

1. HIV can be spread through contact in sports like basketball, wrestling, football or soccer.
2. There should be mandatory HIV testing for all athletes in contact sports like bas-

ketball, wrestling, soccer or football.

3. An athlete who is HIV positive should be barred from participation in contact sports like basketball, wrestling, football or soccer.
4. I would be afraid to compete in contact sports with athletes who are HIV positive.
5. It would not bother me to compete in contact sports against an athlete who is HIV positive.
6. It is ethical to inform other athletes of any athlete who is HIV positive.

AIDS — A Community Answers the Call

Marietta Federici-LaFargue

In September of 1983 my phone rang and the security guard at the entrance desk announced, "Uncle Lionel is here and wants to come up." "Send him up," I told him. He replied; "Are you sure?" "Of course," I said, "send him up!"

"Uncle Lionel" had been a part of our extended family since my husband and I first met in 1970, a rotund, boisterous, black, activist and writer who was gay. He was a very central figure in his East Village community and in our lives. I called him "sister-in-law."

On this particular evening, when I opened the door I saw before me a filthy, gaunt, frightened man, who was under-dressed and holding a cucumber in one hand and a quart of milk in the other. He rushed into my apartment as if it were an oasis in the middle of a desert.

I was stunned to see him in this condition and stood gaping until I gathered my wits about me. He was making small talk to comfort himself and me. I could see that he was very sick. I sent my children to neighbors to play and called my husband at work. Then I made him strip off his clothes, helped him into a hot bath, put his clothes in the washer and prepared a meal for him. He hadn't eaten in days. He was so weak I had to physically carry him out of the bath tub. Wrapped in blankets, comfortable on the sofa, he ate the meal as if it were the last one he would ever eat. It probably was close to the last.

One month later, tied to a city hospital bed, he died of complications from AIDS. We had no idea what was happening, what AIDS was, or what to do. Lionel had no living relatives; we were his only family. We just didn't have the information or facilities to take care of him at home, and we were scared. At his memorial service I made a vow never to allow any friend or relative to die in this manner.

In April of 1984 I had the opportunity to test my vow. "Uncle Kenny," another long-time extended family friend, called in the middle of the night gasping for breath. He lived several floors down from us so I rushed down to see what was wrong. He was running a high temperature and seemed agitated because he couldn't get a deep breath. Since we both meditated and I was teaching Yoga breathing at the time, I sat with him and guided him through a relaxation which calmed him and helped slow down his breathing. I took him to the emergency room of a local hospital. His doctor met us there. When I asked about his condition the doctor looked at me cautiously, then said Ken was in grave condition. Since Kenny was a gay man I asked if it was AIDS. The doctor said, "I can't tell you that." When I told him that I was a family member he said yes, but that I couldn't tell anyone that he had told me.

For the next three weeks another friend and I took turns sitting with him in Intensive Care as he struggled against Pneumocystis Carini Pneumonia, PCP. When he was out of danger and taken to a regular room we continued our vigil to be sure Kenny received proper treatment. Meals were left outside the door; hospital workers refused to come into the room for routine care. We provided the care he needed until he could be released. No one in the hospital ever interfered with our ministrations.

At the same time our drama was unfolding, several other members of our community were experiencing similar situations with their friends and neighbors. We needed help so we turned to the management of our building.

In 1977 Manhattan Plaza, two high-rise buildings on West 43rd street, opened to house 3,500 people. Seventy percent of this population were in the performing arts. The others came from the surrounding area and some were "fair market" tenants. The idea behind the buildings was that performing arts people in New York City brought large income into the city, via the Broadway stage, television and films. However, since their work was so tenuous their living situations were usually substandard. The two high-rise buildings had been built to entice people to move into the Hell's Kitchen/Clinton neighborhood, an area of high crime, drugs and prostitution. The Jacob Javits Center was due to open and the thinking was that monied people would move in and that gentrification would then ensue. It didn't happen quite in that way. Several years went by and the buildings remained empty. HUD stepped in with the urging of many New York politicians and offered a federal subsidy. It was a miracle for those of us struggling to stay in the arts and raise a family.

The management of our building enabled us to start family cooperatives, babysitting exchanges, health food coops, and even a pre-nursery school for young artists. This same management came through for us with offers of money and food when we appealed to them for help with the AIDS crisis.

In 1985 The Manhattan Plaza AIDS Project (MPAP) began. We were neighbors helping neighbors. At first we delivered meals, cleaned apartments, took people to the doctor/hospital, and sometimes just sat holding a frightened, sick or dying neighbor with AIDS. We advocated for persons with AIDS (PWA) in hospitals, called families and helped them understand what was happening to their relatives. We planned memorial services, scattered the ashes of the dead in their favorite places and wept at the loss of so many of our talented, beloved friends.

Since 1985 we have lost over 250 members of our community to AIDS; young men, older men, women, fathers and mothers. In 1990 Manhattan Plaza had the highest per capita death rate from AIDS in the country. What started as five volunteers has become a staff of over 60. We have ongoing education for our volunteers as well as information regarding new therapies and services provided for PWAs. Management also offered training to the maintenance staff to help them understand HIV/AIDS. Before the training these people were frightened to enter the apartments of PWAs. Since then two of the men offered their services to PWAs free of charge.

We learn about client advocacy and strategies to use in negotiating with health care systems. We have community forums; one included teenagers and their parents, as well as members of the surrounding community. We sponsor a booth at the Ninth Avenue Food Festival to distribute AIDS information and condoms. We have several of our own fund-raising events which raise thousands of dollars for MPAP each year. The surrounding community reached out and offered to help our clients with fifteen restaurants offering lunch and dinner daily to an average of seven PWA's a week, about 98 meals a week.

Manhattan Plaza Management has provided the complex with The Manhattan Plaza AIDS Project office and with a paid staff. There are weekly support meetings, both for PWAs and volunteers, as well as for family members. Part of our ongoing training comes at these meetings, including discussions of the following topics: Nutrition and HIV, Allowing Ourselves to Grieve, Practical Care Issues, HIV-Related Dementia, Writing Wills, Health Care Proxy and Power of Attorney and HIV Medical and Research Update. There is also a weekly meditation group for all, individual counseling, probono services from lawyers, nutritionists, CPAs and massage therapists. The Manhattan Plaza Health Club also provides reduced-rate memberships for PWAs.

In December of 1991 the AIDS project also started providing services to clients from Miracle House, located in a nearby apartment building. A large two-bedroom apartment is provided at an affordable rate to house out-of-town family members who are in New York visiting relatives with HIV/AIDS. Several apartments in Manhattan Plaza are available for homeless members of the performing arts community with AIDS, with the financial support of the Actor's Fund. These apartments are furnished by the project.

In order to be a volunteer with the MPAP you must undergo a short training session and strictly follow the confidentiality laws. There is no age limit for a volunteer; some of our members are in their eighties. A volunteer has a choice of tasks. The main idea is for volunteers to feel comfortable and empowered. Volunteers work in the project office, deliver meals, run errands, work on fund-raising events, and some do "one-on-one" care-partnering. This last commitment is not to be taken lightly, as it is a lifeline to the PWA. These volunteers are available to the PWA 24 hours a day and usually become like members of the family. Generally two or three volunteers will share this commitment as it can be very stressful.

I have been a care partner to five PWAs with the help of my daughter, who has been a volunteer with me since she was eight years old. Her presence, in all cases, has helped calm and bring joy to our friends with AIDS. We have hosted pot-luck suppers in our home and worked on fund-raising projects together.

Recently, at one of our fund-raising events, a group of volunteers sewed small celebrity quilts which were signed by members of the casts of several Broadway shows. The quilts were then sold in a lottery. Several thousand dollars were raised from this effort.

The Manhattan Plaza AIDS Project has been studied by several groups wishing to use it as a prototype for other communities. It is important to help PWAs stay at home and receive more personal care, with less financial burden. However, the project is difficult to duplicate since there are few communities bonded together through the common thread of the performing arts. Of the 3,500 members of the Manhattan Plaza community, 70% are in the performing arts. Members of the theatrical community have a history of supportive service to one another.

In 1993 I was invited to attend the World AIDS conference in Amsterdam after I submitted a paper written about our project. What I discovered when I attended the various workshops and seminars was that The Manhattan Plaza AIDS Project was the only community-based organization of its kind in the world. There were other groups with similar offerings but none had the ability to reach so many so effectively. The combination of management, volunteers and support of neighborhood services makes this project unique. For example, in May, our volunteers totalled 1150 hours of service (900 client hours and 250 program hours); in June, the total was 975 (875 client hours and 100 program hours). In December our volunteers set up booths in the lobbies of both buildings to recruit new volunteers. The staff then interviewed applicants and selected volunteers who then participated in a weekend training in February.

The primary objective of the Manhattan Plaza AIDS Project is to:

1. Help PWAs stay at home and remain integrated in community life.

2. Provide housing for performing artists who have become homeless due to AIDS.

3. Enhance the quality of life for PWAs and their families, prevent isolation and abandonment due to illness.

4. Ensure, through a case management system, that PWAs receive all

available support, benefits, entitlements and services from government and other programs.

5. Mobilize community human resources, including staff and resident volunteers, to assist and support PWAs and their families and meet other AIDS-related community needs.

6. Coordinate volunteer activities, including training and support programs and matching volunteer resources, with identified needs.

7. Increase community understanding of AIDS and AIDS prevention measures.

All MPAP programs and activities are provided free of charge and are open to those who are HIV+ as well as people diagnosed with AIDS in this performing arts community.

The current caseload is 65 clients, which is a 32% increase in cases over last year at the same time. There were 1,503 individual counseling sessions conducted during the period January 1, 1993—September 30, 1993. 75 support group sessions for people living with HIV disease were held, led by trained and certified therapists.

From January through September of 1993, volunteers provided over 12,000 hours of service to the clients and the organization. 74 support group sessions were conducted for family and friends.

References:

All information in this report is from personal experience and from the reports provided by James Kelley, Project Director, Manhattan Plaza AIDS Project.

A Case Study of a Long Term Survivor of HIV Infection in a Rural Community

Tim Rodgers

I am writing this paper from my hospital bed in Barnes Hospital in St. Louis (and later on from my home) during the summer of 1994. I am suffering the first major medical problem since I was diagnosed with HIV several years ago. At the time of this hospitalization I was a full-time doctoral student in health education at Southern Illinois University at Carbondale. In mid-July I was planning to complete my comprehensive examinations, whereupon I could start working on my dissertation.

In order for me to continue receiving my grants I must be enrolled for a minimum of six hours. I was planning on taking the last two courses of my program during the summer, but my illness prevented me from doing so. Fortunately, with the assistance of my doctoral advisor and his chair, I was able to register for three dissertation hours and a three credit independent study. My advisor has asked that I write about my experience as a long-term survivor of Acquired Immunodeficiency Syndrome (AIDS) and what recommendations I could provide to health care providers on how to deal with a person with AIDS (PWA). It is hoped that this paper will provide some assistance to those individuals who have not had the opportunity to work with an HIV infected individual.

Discovering I was Infected with HIV

Although I am unable to identify when I became infected with the Human Immunodeficiency Virus, I first discovered that I was infected in February 1991. I hesitated to become tested, perhaps due to the fact that most of the people who I knew with AIDS avoided being tested fearing impending doom. Although I had very strong suspicions that I was infected, I also rationalized on why I shouldn't disrupt my life and emotional well-being with this knowledge. In addition, as an active member of a small rural university community, I was not ready to face the opinions of others regarding my condition. I also had little idea how best to manage my need for confidentiality.

Most people that I have known who were infected with HIV discovered their status as the result of an opportunistic infection, such as Pneumocystis Carinii Pneumonia or Kaposi sarcoma. My initial health problem consisted of a two month long bout with bronchitis. The length of this illness suggested to me and my physician that, being in a high risk group (a gay male) I should be tested to allow proper treatment and prolong life if the test came back positive (Fee and Fox, 1992; Root-Bernstein, 1993).

The strongest association with the discovery of my infection was the expectation of an early death from AIDS. At first I felt hopeless, and then as I read more I became determined to fight this disease to my maximal strength. I began taking a prophylactic treatment to avoid Pneumocystis Carinii Pneumonia infection. Pneumocystis Carinii Pneumonia has been the major cause of death for most PWAs that I have known. Proper treatment has been highly successful in preventing the infection and has led to the most dramatic lengthening of life among PWAs. Respiratory infections contribute to half of all deaths (Hochhauser and Rothenberger, 1992).

A second intervention was proposed using 600 mg doses of AZT taken on a daily basis in order to increase my T-Cell count. According to my physician, those individuals with higher levels of CD4 T-cells were less likely to suffer opportunistic infections. AZT and other antivirals were designed to be a possible "cure" for AIDS. However, because of the high rate of mutation of HIV, a resistant strain soon continues to grow without reacting to the antiviral qualities of the new drugs. The new antivirals also have a variety of unpleasant side effects. Although there is little evidence that there are long term benefits from using these antivirals, many medical practitioners tend to have some faith in them anyway.

One of the most important aspects of my daily regimen is the implementation of the "Wellness" concept where attention is given to preventive health practices, such as no smoking or drinking alcohol, leading a low stress lifestyle, and eating a nutritious diet. My training as a health educator has been of tremendous help to me from that standpoint. I believe that these practices may be a critical difference between myself and other PWAs who die soon after a complete decline in CD4 T-cells. In addition, I found the use of the antioxidants, specifically Beta Carotene, Vitamin E, Vitamin B Complex, and occasional use of minerals such as iron, Selenium, and Zinc to be beneficial.

Above all, the most important issue to me is being able to maintain much control over my own needs. My recent hospitalization has confirmed this belief. Hospitals do nothing to make a person feel responsible for his/her health. This sense of having control has, in my opinion, provided me with good morale as I deal with this infection. Effective control has allowed me to remain relatively active, despite my declining CD4 T-cell count. Research has shown that good morale (more than just medical intervention) is known to be a major factor in maintaining good health (Eberst, 1984; Hochhauser and Rothenberger, 1992).

Despite my diligent efforts to follow good health practices and the advice of my physicians, the number of CD4 T-cells were finally reduced to zero in the summer of 1993. It is apparent that my good health practices allowed me to avoid being overwhelmed by any particular illness. However, it did not force the virus into abatement.

An important benchmark in the decline of these CD4 cells has been the inability to exercise properly. Even before my T-cell count declined to zero, the opportunity for fungal infections of the skin increased. Swimming in chlorinated water when my T-cells ranged between 35 to 50 (per liter of blood) would aggravate and open the skin to more serious yeast-like infections. Nevertheless, I still maintained a vigorous schedule of walking and light weight lifting two or three times a day.

At the same time as this depletion of CD4 T-cells, I started having severe bouts of fatigue. Weight loss (and probably muscle loss) took place. During the summer and fall months of 1993, I spent long periods in bed due to fatigue. It became a major force of will to fight against the virus. My two main physicians would tell me that this was a common — if not universal — development for people with advanced AIDS. They were not aware of ways to control the fatigue and they weren't willing to help me find ways to remedy it. In their experience this was merely part of the "last" stages of development in an advanced AIDS condition.

The fatigue persisted into 1994, with me literally begging my local physicians to consult colleagues and AIDS experts about what might be known about the fatigue syndrome. There might be therapies which could be tried without endangering my life. It appeared to me that the physicians were unwilling to explore this matter with colleagues — despite being aware that there are AIDS experts in places as close as Barnes Hospital in St. Louis, Missouri and AIDS hospitals in Chicago, Illinois.

My failure to motivate the physicians to pursue consultation and possible therapy became a major barrier to finding relief. The physicians' frame of reference strongly suggested that fatigue, weight and muscle loss were unavoidable or were not worth further consideration. Their reaction was that I would probably soon be dead and that I should accept the decline and prepare for the end.

Episodes of fatigue varied in an unpredictable way. Apples seemed to provide some energy. By the end of the spring semester of 1994 I had heard that an injection of testosterone might help. My doctors had never tried this before but agreed to give me a 400 mg dose on May 1, 1994. This probably gave me the energy to complete the last paper of the semester. It also enabled me to develop the energy for a vacation to New Orleans.

By the beginning of June 1994, an opportunity arrived which allowed me to greatly improve my housing situation. With friends from my support group I was able to move almost all of my property to a new apartment. Yet the energy it took to move may have contributed to the onset of HIV cardiomyopathy. HIV cardiomyopathy is a deterioration of the heart caused by the killing of heart cells by HIV. A week after the move I began experiencing tightness in the chest, shortness of breath, and a need for oxygen. One of the physicians X-rayed my heart and discovered it had enlarged over the past few months from 16 cm to 19 cm. Ultrasound investigation revealed there was a build up of fluid around the heart which might need to be drained. It was decided to transport me by helicopter to Barnes Hospital (St. Louis) to have a cardiologist and an infectious disease specialist diagnose and treat the condition. This was my first admission to a hospital for an HIV related condition—nearly a year after my CD4 cell count was at zero.

Advice to Health Care Professionals

Health care professionals may have opportunities to allow earlier interventions with PWAs and people at-risk for AIDS. Clients are likely to be uncomfortable discussing homosexual behaviors or IV drug abuse. The health care professionals can play a significant role in the HIV/AIDS prevention by encouraging individuals at risk to feel comfortable about discussing the disease. The involvement of clients in exploring at-risk issues can enhance their ability to manage the illness, prolong life and make a commitment to change risky behavior.

Clients should be educated to understand that having AIDS is not a death sentence. Physicians and health care professionals should view clients who test positive as *living* with AIDS rather than *dying* with AIDS. More and more evidence suggests AIDS should be viewed as a chronic condition where clients often have an opportunity to live an additional ten or fifteen years from the time of diagnosis (Root-Bernstein, 1993).

Knowledge and attitudes among health care professionals can make an important contribution in prolonging life and productivity years for PWAs (Chubon, 1988). Physicians and other health professionals may be overwhelmed, not only by lifestyle concerns, but by a vast array of possible opportunistic infections. The reality is more likely to be manageable within the bounds of accepted protocols and procedures for the most likely causes of infection before a person has "advanced" AIDS (defined here as a zero CD4 count). Attention to prophylactic treatments have been highly successful in allowing clients to avoid many of the most prevalent opportunistic infections. While media attention seems riveted on the failure to find a one shot "cure" for AIDS, incremental attempts to stop opportunistic infections have added years to people's life expectancy. This will no doubt affect people with advanced AIDS now as well as in the years ahead.

Health care professionals may often feel that clients who are homosexuals or drug addicts are wrong and immoral. Nevertheless, as professionals, health care providers are morally and ethically obligated to provide satisfactory services to their clients, without allowing their personal biases to affect their work. Treating homosexuals or IV drug users does not mean promoting or accepting their lifestyles, but it does mean attending to the health care needs of one's community.

Finally, health care professionals cannot ignore the importance of allowing PWAs to maintain as much control and dignity as possible. Many times I found that I was better informed of new advances and concepts related to AIDS than my primary care physicians. Being open to ideas will not diminish the respect one feels for a physician, instead it may enhance it. It is also important that health care workers have an AIDS expert as a contact person to ensure that the most up-to-date care can be given to a person with AIDS.

My Morale

According to my physicians I had beat most of the statistics on survival and could be regarded as a long-term survivor. Long-term survivors tend to be assertive in their lives and have good support groups and good morale. PWAs who are long-term survivors have no clear overall path to pursue in treatment opportunities—except on a personal level. On the personal level, a strong sense of independence and desire to live appear to be important in keeping a person's morale.

The person with AIDS experiences an immediate crisis over what makes life meaningful or meaningless. Why bother? Why even think of living (Beck, Carlton, and Allen. 1993)? Thoughts of my untimely death (with perhaps no way to predict when this might occur) were the most recurring worry that I had. Eventually, I have simply grown tired from thinking about it.

I am also constantly concerned about the reactions of others who find out about my illness. Most of these people have this pervasive concern about early death — largely due to the initial images of the epidemic when those living with AIDS were likely to die in less than six months after diagnosis. Unfortunately, many health care professionals and laymen feel the same way and expect an AIDS patient to just prepare for an early death.

Often the more typical reaction after surviving several months is coming to terms with the new condition, an adaptation to bring a new and more important understanding to the meaning of life. One tends to analyze and review many things about one's life. Often, beliefs such as sacrificing now for the future, or continuing to work on a job that is not liked, or of staying in unsatisfying relationships are challenged. The person with AIDS begins to think deeply about what might bring meaning to her or his life.

I very much felt this way. I've been lucky in that my life has really only changed dramatically since the summer of 1993 when the problems of fatigue and weight and muscle loss began affecting my abilities to maintain a normal lifestyle. I am happy with many of the long-term goals I am working towards in education. Being a scholar in an environment that a university provided has been enriching. This environment is definitely to my advantage since it helped me to maintain my life style. I am able to think of my academic career as a new concern to live for; I attempt to apply a scientific viewpoint to my situation. I use the scientific literature to investigate treatment options, understand the disease, and to find ways to prolong my life. A lot of this has been made possible because of the flexibility and support of important people in my academic pursuits and my support group of friends and family.

It is usually very important to the person with AIDS that they be allowed to manage the information about the disease in a way that is within their comfort level and disclosing information at their own pace. Early in my knowledge of my infection there was a withdrawal from participation in activities of the gay community and on the nearby college campus. There was a deep expectation that most members of these communities would not be supportive and only see my seropositive status as something to gossip about. I felt it necessary to withdraw inside an "AIDS closet" within the larger closet that many gay people use to survive in rural areas. The gay community has been panicked by the AIDS epidemic. In addition, there is a fear in the gay male "community" that the people around them might have the disease. Consequently, there is wild speculation and digging for information about members of this community. In many ways participation in the community is more trouble than it is worth. For me, there was constant fear of exposure to the public of my status of living with AIDS.

Issues of confidentiality are often extremely important to PWAs and I was no exception. There has been a deep feeling inside me that if information about my condition became public knowledge, problems of misunderstanding, fears of the general public, and other stigmatizing factors would overwhelm my life. I've seen firsthand how public exposure has led to one losing employment and housing, as well as "friends" who did not know previously of this person's "gay" lifestyle. Although there are laws that deal with the breaching of confidentiality and/or discriminating against PWAs, it nonetheless takes an enormous amount of energy to deal with such violations. Besides, the "damage" would already have taken place — monetary compensation means little at this time in life.

Related to issues of confidentiality is how the person with AIDS perceived his/her identity. This, to me, was one of the most important issues that

I had had to battle with. People identify themselves with their career, their family, and belief systems. I felt that as the disease progressed — particularly after the loss of all CD4 T-cells — my identity was increasingly overwhelmed by an "AIDS identity." I needed to discuss my health problems with more health care professionals. I also felt a need to be increasingly open about my condition with friends and family. Being associated with health education and public health individuals who are aware of the symptoms of AIDS, the weight loss I had been experiencing was a sure signal to them that something was wrong. It became distressingly apparent to me that many people around me would strongly suspect the truth about my condition and be curious about it. Though I felt secure in my support group and not stigmatized, there was the fear that thoughts of AIDS would absorb my attention and take over my identity. I wanted to be more than a person with AIDS. I fought to maintain other identities and considered these aspects of my life important in maintaining a healthy view of life and in avoiding being burnt out on the AIDS issues.

Issues of Support

There are a number of levels of personal or emotional support for myself. Many people cannot offer much more than words of sympathy. They probably have had limited, if any, contact with AIDS infected persons. As these people have spent more time with me, they have developed a greater understanding of my needs, my limitations, the ways I fight the disease through medication, exercise and state of mind.

Through trial and error, I have managed to build a support group that visits me on a daily basis (though not all at once). With a support group of approximately ten people I am able to avoid burning out any particular person with excessive demands. I recognize that supporters need to be able to carry on their own lives.

An informal support network is probably the most important element in maintaining morale. Also important is a formalized support network organized to provide educational opportunities and access to the larger AIDS community. In addition to educational opportunities, a formal support group for persons with AIDS has provided access to case managers who have knowledge about governmental bureaucracies such as state Public Aid, Medicaid, the State Department of Rehabilitation Services, and the Ryan White Act Consortium. This multitude of organizations can provide access to many of the financial resources necessary to pay for services, medication, and other benefits that a person needs to remain independent.

An important aspect of maintaining good health is monitoring clients' morale. In addition to building a meaningful life, it is imperative that the client build a good support network of friends and family. While health care professionals may not be qualified or have the time to pay attention to these matters in any detail, it is important that clients be informed of resources available in their community or nearby communities. In addition to friends and family, joining an AIDS support network can be helpful and beneficial. Health care providers should be willing to consult other professionals with knowledge of AIDS and PWAs (Beck, Carlton, and Allen, 1993). In addition to regular consultation much is available in the scientific literature and through on-line computer services.

Summary

I acknowledge that I am not the typical person with AIDS. I have had the ability to understand and act on my own needs. Most PWAs are likely to be less well-educated, and likely to have debilitating addictions such as smoking, drinking, or IV drug addiction — all of which contribute to a loss in ability to cope with the changing needs caused by AIDS. Most people are likely to die much sooner in the progression of the disease.

So far, I have defied the odds and have become a long-term survivor. I have maintained a high morale, good health, a good sense of identity, and confidence which engendered my chances of maintaining a happy, independent life. More research into how long-term survivors maintain themselves is needed to contribute to the fight against AIDS. The potential for examination of long-term survival strategies may hold more benefit than pursuing the much more expensive research on antiviral and other drugs purporting to be curative.

[After recovering from his bout of HIV cardiomyopathy in early summer, Mr. Rodgers completed and passed his comprehensive examinations in July, 1994 with exceptionally high marks. In August Tim celebrated with family and friends the passing of those comprehensive exams. During September Tim worked closely with his advisor in preparing to defend his dissertation prospectus. In late September Tim suffered his first bout of Pneumocystis Carinii Pneumonia. In mid-October, 1994 Tim died. For reprints of this article, please contact Tim's doctoral advisor—Dr. Mark J. Kittleson, Health Education Programs, Mailstop 4632, Southern Illinois University, Carbondale, IL 62901-4632]

References

Beck, R., Carlton, T., Allen H.(1993). Understanding and Counseling Special Populations with HIV Seropositive Disease. *America Rehabilitation*, 19(3), 20.

Chubon, R.A. (1988). Psychosocial Impact of Terminal Chronic Illness. *Journal of Applied Rehabilitation Counseling*, L19L:(3), 9-11.

Eberst, R.M. Defining health: A Multidimensional Model. *Journal of School Health*, 54 (3), 99-104.

Fee, E. and Fox, D.M. (Eds.) (1992). *AIDS: The Making of a Chronic Disease.* Berkeley: University of California Press.

Havranek, J.E. (1991). The Social and Individual Costs of Negative Attitudes Toward Persons with Physical Disabilities. *Journal of Applied Rehabilitation Counseling*, 22(1), 15.

Hochhauser, M. and Rothenberger, J. (1992). *AIDS Education*. Dubuque, IA: William C. Brown, Inc.

Root-Bernstein, R. (1993). *ReThinking AIDS: The Tragic Cost of Premature Consensus*. Toronto: The Free Press.

Delivering Culturally Sensitive AIDS Education in Rural Communities

J. Stephen McDaniel, Deborah J. Isenberg,
Debra G. Morris and Robin Y. Swift

With over 440,000 AIDS cases reported in the United States through 1994, what has become painfully clear in the AIDS pandemic is that the spread of HIV infection has not slowed (CDC, 1994). In fact, the pandemic now shows further expansion into populations which previously experienced low seroprevalence rates. Notably, those infected with HIV are increasingly heterosexual, men and women who are drug addicted, African American and Hispanic, poor, rural, or the offspring or sexual partners of members of these groups (Bell, 1991). In the south, a disproportionate number of African Americans, especially African American women and children, are among those currently HIV-infected (Ellerbrock et al, 1991). In exploring the changing demography and growing seroprevalence rates, a new challenge faces the country—HIV/AIDS in rural communities. Increasingly, HIV infection and AIDS are affecting areas outside of metropolitan cities (CDC, 1992; Rutherford et al., 1993; Tucker et al., 1991). This is especially true in the southeast where HIV seroconversion rates have escalated disproportionately (CDC, 1992). In fact, numerous investigators have found that rates of high-risk sexual behaviors in rural locales are much higher than rates in most urban AIDS epicenters (Fleming et al., 1987; Jones et al., 1987; St. Lawrence et al.,

1988). Clearly, health educators who hope to impact the pandemic must respond with prevention and education efforts inclusive of rural areas and sensitive to rural residents. In recent years, a recognized need for collaborative educational models that cover large rural geographic areas has emerged (Chang-Yit, et al., 1992). The importance, however, of responding in an effective way demands that educational efforts examine the challenges, as well as the strategies to overcome these challenges, when considering rural HIV/AIDS education.

In 1992, the Emory HIV/AIDS Mental Health Training Project (Emory Project), funded through the Center for Mental Health Services of the Substance Abuse and Mental Health Services Administration emerged to meet the need of enhancing the knowledge and skills of traditional and non-traditional mental health care providers about HIV/AIDS throughout Georgia. The Centers for Disease Control and Prevention reported that Georgia had the eighth highest cumulative number of AIDS cases reported among the 50 states, compared to its ranking as eleventh largest in population (CDC, 1994). The project currently serves the entire state of Georgia, including both urban and rural settings. As the percentage of the state's AIDS cases diagnosed in small towns and rural areas has increased from 18.2 % in 1989 to 36% in 1994 (CDC, 1994), the project staff have had many opportunities to explore the challenges faced when providing urban versus rural HIV/AIDS trainings. Utilizing this knowledge base as well as the collaborative expertise of the Southeast AIDS Training and Education Center in Georgia, strategies have been implemented to meet the challenges that health educators have found in Georgia's rural communities. This chapter draws from the experience of the Emory Project in defining the challenges, developing strategies for meeting these challenges, and implementing effective training methods to provide comprehensive AIDS education in rural settings in Georgia and the southeastern United States.

Unique Challenges of Rural Communities

Educators who provide HIV/AIDS education in rural areas in the United States are faced with unique challenges (see Table I). For example, many rural communities often retain traditional values, are less diverse and maintain church or family as having a central role in daily life. Fewer residents may have the formal education of urban residents, and geographic distance and limited resources may result in increased reliance on other community members. Social support is often channeled through informal social networking rather than the formal structures of larger cities. Therefore, new scientific ideas or alternative lifestyles made more public by the AIDS pandemic may not be easily tolerated in some rural communities which rely heavily upon conformity (Nelson, 1993).

Because community response to HIV/AIDS is significantly different in rural areas, educational interventions must be sensitive to these differences. For example, in rural communities traditional roles based on heterosexual relationships are usually the norm, resulting in increased stigma and fear of homosexuality. HIV status is often hidden and undisclosed due to fear of isolation and rejection from the community. This denial is evidenced by the rural community's attitude portraying HIV/AIDS as an urban or outside issue. HIV seropositive members of these communities are often invisible and remain isolated from support systems. Individuals may be fearful of seeking testing, treatment, or support services in rural areas for fear of public exposure; this fear may then prompt mistrust of local agencies' abilities to maintain confidentiality leading to underuse of available HIV-related services.

Given a history of low seroprevalence rates in these communities, rural regions have only recently been confronted with the complex psychosocial realities which accompany HIV/AIDS. Perhaps the foremost barrier to effectively integrating HIV/AIDS education is the fear and stigma that individuals and even whole communities experience when people disclose their HIV status. Historically, many rural communities first experienced AIDS when a gay man with AIDS, who grew up in the community and later moved to a more urban area, returns to be near his family as his HIV disease progresses. In many cases, the gay individual and his family not only face a community that is afraid of AIDS, but one that is also intolerant of homosexuals. Unlike most urban areas, these families have no gay community to buffer the hostility in the region and to offer support. This phenomenon is not unique to rural areas; however, given the lack of confidentiality and homogeneous nature of most rural communities, these attitudes are much more pronounced and their impact more strongly felt. Moreover, because rural individuals have limited exposure to persons who are different from themselves, they have less access to people modeling diverse ways of coping (Kinkel, 1986).

Because HIV/AIDS was identified historically as a disease of gay men or injection drug users, despite current epidemiology to the contrary, urban HIV/AIDS educational efforts initially experienced significant barriers of denial like those now confronting rural regions. This denial in some communities has facilitated a corresponding lack of ownership of HIV/AIDS as a public health threat. Given earlier low rural seroprevalence rates, many rural communities have comfortably maintained a level of denial that has now become a barrier to HIV/AIDS education. Therefore, the development of any educational outreach targeted to facilitate a rural response to HIV/AIDS must focus on efforts to decrease fear and stigma while increasing a sense of community ownership of the pandemic.

Such educational efforts must be sensitive to the unique cultural differences of rural individuals. In the southeast, an understanding of social support and social identity within the African American community is essential. For example, the African American community has historically held negative attitudes about homosexuality, stemming in part from conservative religious upbringing and the strong place of religion in African American culture (Icard, 1985). Educating persons about the spread of HIV infection among African American gay men must include an understanding that African American gay men may lack social support and social identity within the African American community, but many also may be viewed as outsiders in the larger gay community (Bell, 1991). HIV/AIDS education in the rural southeast, then, must acknowledge this history which will impact community perceptions of others, including African American women and children who test positive for HIV. Further, understanding the central role of religion as a primary social support for many rural and African American communities, will ensure the incorporation of religion into effective educational interventions.

Further complicating HIV/AIDS education in less urban locales is the lack of resources, both in terms of finances and staff, available for such education. Because most rural areas cover large geographic regions, concentrated educational efforts, such as those organized by community based AIDS organizations, often do not exist. Therefore, identifying ways to collaborate with existing organizations to provide rural education may be an important and perhaps essential tool. Such a model for rural collaboration of AIDS education exists in Minnesota where efforts have focused on the sharing of resources such as community educational programs, audio-visual and educational resources, and communication networks to ultimately foster a coordinated regional response to AIDS issues (Lippert et al., 1992). This has continually proven to be an effective method to address the problem of limited resources.

A lack of local leadership may also be a problem in rural areas in need of AIDS education. While usually not an impediment in urban areas, local leaders in rural communities may not provide adequate support for HIV/AIDS educational efforts. Because persons frequently seek the advice of friends concerning steps needed to reduce risk for HIV/AIDS, opinion leaders may give much needed support to a community's response to HIV and AIDS (Kelly et al., 1991). In fact, Kelly and colleagues (1991) have demonstrated that interventions that employ peer leaders to endorse change may produce or accelerate population behavior changes to lessen risk for HIV infection in the rural southeast. Therefore, the key to successfully mobilizing rural areas may lie in recruiting key community leaders as supporters of AIDS education.

Table I
Delivering HIV/AIDS Education in Rural Communities: Challenges

- **Community denial**
- **Cultural sensitivity**
- **Fear, stigma, isolation**
- **Gaining community trust and confidence**
- **Geographic distance**
- **Increasing rate of seroconversion**
- **Informal social support networks**
- **Lack of information about rural risk behavior patterns**
- **Lack of local leadership**
- **Lack of ownership of issue**
- **Lack of resources**
- **Less tolerance of alternative lifestyles**
- **Literacy**
- **Role of religion as a primary coping strategy**

Educational Strategies for Rural Communities

In its three years of operation, the Emory Project has trained over 5,000 participants, over one-third in rural areas, and has grown to appreciate key factors to successful trainings. Perhaps the most useful lesson learned has been the importance of teaming with local agencies who may also have a vested interest in bringing AIDS education to their region. Important agencies which have provided networking opportunities in rural Georgia have included rural community-based AIDS organizations, HIV-related health care facilities funded through the Ryan White Comprehensive AIDS Resources Emergency (CARE) Act of 1990, churches, business groups, palliative care agencies, hospitals, state AIDS committees, health departments, and professional medical organizations.

Overall, educational strategies for fostering positive attitudes and a supportive rural environment should focus on HIV/AIDS as a rural community issue rather than an urban issue. The objective of education is to help participants frame the issue in a way that will result in positive community responses. Trainings must include not only basic information about AIDS, but also must challenge individuals to examine and confront their fears and biases to reduce community hysteria and discriminatory acts toward PWAs and their families. The positive outcome of such educational outreach generally includes more community HIV/AIDS ownership.

To be effective, AIDS education must be delivered in a manner that is respectful of cultural differences inherent in rural settings. Developments in the last 10 years clearly indicate that the cultural beliefs of a community influence health attitudes, practices, and responses to the health delivery system (Foster et al., 1993). Educators must be prepared for negative misinformation, especially misinformation about the sexuality of women, gay men, African Americans, and Latinos (Crochet et al., 1993). Similarly, individuals may hold a variety of group-specific misconceptions about HIV and AIDS such as beliefs that the AIDS pandemic is a genocide attempt by a dominant culture, the idea that the disease is exclusively a white gay male disease, and misinformation about how the AIDS virus is transmitted (Crocteau et al., 1993). To address this misinformation appropriately, the educational AIDS message must be delivered in a culturally competent manner that makes effective use of skills, resources, and knowledge that are pertinent and responsive to the cultural values and norms, strengths, needs, and self- determined goals of the audience.

Rural Training Strategies of the Emory Project

The Emory Project has utilized a number of well-established strategies to overcome many of the challenges faced by AIDS educators in rural communities. Specific strategies that the Emory Project has integrated include a training approach that addresses each of the following areas of successful AIDS education: establishment of a collaborative training network; pre-training research and preparation; culturally sensitive execution of trainings targeted to audience needs; evaluation of delivered trainings; and maintenance of funding for training events. Table II provides an overview of general training strategies for rural communities.

Table II DELIVERING HIV/AIDS EDUCATION IN RURAL COMMUNITIES: STRATEGIES

- **ESTABLISH A TRAINING NETWORK THROUGH COLLABORATION**
  - —ALLY WITH COMMUNITY LEADERS
  - —UTILIZE EXISTING LOCAL AGENCIES
  - —ESTABLISH COMMUNITY STEERING COMMITTEE
  - —NETWORK WITH LOCAL COMMUNITY LEADERS

- **DELIVER EDUCATION THAT IS CULTURALLY SENSITIVE/AFFIRMING**
  - —PREPARE FOR NEGATIVE MISINFORMATION
  - —MAKE EFFECTIVE USE OF COMMUNITY SKILLS, RESOURCES, AND KNOWLEDGE
  - —RESPECT CULTURAL VALUES AND NORMS
  - —REINFORCE STRENGTHS AND SELF-DETERMINED GOALS OF THE COMMUNITY
  - —APPRECIATE UNIQUE, CULTURALLY RELEVANT NEEDS OF THE COMMUNITY

- **DEVELOP EDUCATIONAL PROGRAMS THAT FOSTER POSITIVE ATTITUDES**
  - —FRAME THE MESSAGE IN WAYS RESPECTFUL OF THE COMMUNITY
  - —INCLUDE BASIC INFORMATION ON HIV/AIDS
  - —UTILIZE TECHNIQUES THAT COMFORTABLY CHAL LENGE FEARS AND BIASES

- **PRE-TRAINING RESEARCH AND PREPARATION**
  - —ASCERTAIN AUDIENCE EDUCATIONAL NEEDS
  - —IDENTIFY WHO WILL COMPOSE THE TRAINING AUDENCE
  - —APPRECIATE LITERACY LEVEL OF PROPOSED TRAIN ING PARTICIPANTS
  - —FIND OUT THE TRAINING BACKGROUND OF THE TAR GET AUDIENCE

- **EXECUTION OF TRAININGS**
  - —DETERMINE TRAINING FORMAT (DIDACTIC, EXPERIENTIAL, PANEL DISCUSSION,ETC.)
  - —DETERMINE THE LENGTH OF TRAINING
  - —INCORPORATE LOCAL LEADERS AND/OR PERSONS AFFECTED BY AIDS INTO THE TRAINING AS SPEAKERS
  - —ENCOURAGE AUDIENCE PARTICIPATION

- **EVALUATION OF TRAININGS**
  - —UTILIZE PRE-TRAINING AND/OR POST-TRAINING EVALUATION FORMAT
  - —DETERMINE TRAINING PARTICIPANTS' SATISFACTION
  - —EVALUATE TRAINING PARTICIPANTS' KNOWLEDGE AND ATTITUDES
  - —CONSIDER LONGITUDINAL EVALUATIONS FOR ASSESSING BEHAVIORAL CHANGES

- **FUNDING**
  - —COLLABORATE WITH LOCAL AGENCIES TO SHARE RESOURCES
  - —UTILIZE STATE AGENCIES FUNDED TO PROVIDE CONTINUING EDUCATION
  - —UTILIZE VOLUNTEERS TO DECREASE STAFFING COSTS
  - —RESEARCH FOR GRANT SUPPORT

As outlined earlier, an effective training network consists of many components which may reflect a diverse range of local, regional, and state organizations. The key ingredient is choosing agencies and individuals that are visible, active and exhibit respect and power in the community. The Emory Project is guided by a Community Steering Committee representing the diversity of HIV infection within Georgia, including PWAs from both urban and rural communities. Many AIDS educators believe such steering committees or task forces are the most vital component of any training network (Rounds, 1988). Another important component of Emory's network has been the development of a formal linkage and partnership with a rural community based AIDS service organization in southern Georgia, Rainbow Partners, Inc., to facilitate reaching rural audiences. In addition to this organization being composed of local residents including community leaders, it also offers the opportunity to utilize local PWAs in trainings, an intervention that has been shown to be effective in many rural areas (Nelson, 1993; Lippert et al., 1992). Utilizing existing agencies is also a way to use more effectively the limited resources previously noted to be a problem in rural communities.

Pre-training preparation is an essential part of meeting training objectives. The first and most important step in the process is the identification of an audience's training needs. These needs may be ascertained through communication with a local organizer; however, the most effective means of establishing training needs allows for the participation of the intended audience. This process not only identifies training needs, but also identifies who will make up the audience. The Emory Project generally utilizes either pre-training focus groups when possible, or written needs assessments which can be returned by mail prior to a training. One obstacle in using such a written assessment in some rural communities may be the literacy level of some participants; therefore, it is important to phrase the assessment clearly and simply. For many audiences, the pre-training needs assessment or focus group can assist in identifying sexual norms and level of conservatism in the audience.

Once the audience needs have been ascertained, an educational program targeted to their unique training needs can be developed. One additional question that has proven helpful to include in the pre-training process is why the audience wants the training. One Emory training which had a particularly silent audience ended with the trainer discovering that a well-liked supervisor at the training site had recently died from AIDS, but had never disclosed his illness to his colleagues. While the pre-training needs assessment provided important information about the audience's knowledge base, the issue of why the training was requested was never asked. A follow-up training specifically included an experiential exercise which provided a comfortable environment for important communication and grieving.

The execution of the actual training event incorporates a variety of educational strategies aimed at meeting identified training needs. Generally, the Emory Project will request half-day to full-day commitments of audiences in order to ensure ample opportunity for sharing information and encouraging audience participation. Incorporating a local speaker, even if the local resident simply serves as the host and introduces the event to the audience, can greatly improve the effectiveness of the training. A typical training format utilizes a combination of a didactic presentation, an experiential exercise such as small group role playing, a speakers' panel composed of local PWAs or persons affected by AIDS, and an information sharing segment where the audience is given important information about local and regional HIV-related services available. Throughout the program, audience participation is encouraged. Dividing the audience into smaller groups for part of the program generally allows for more active participation and provides more effective training (Rounds, 1988; Nelson, 1993).

Post-training evaluation is a vital component for agencies such as the Emory Project which carefully monitor the effectiveness of individual trainings. The evaluation can be as simple as asking the audience participants to rate their level of satisfaction with the speaker(s), program format, handouts, meeting facility, etc. For more in-depth programs, the Emory Project utilizes a pre-training and a post-training evaluation assessing knowledge and attitudes as well as participant satisfaction. For selected trainings, these evaluations are re-administered over time, such as at three or six month intervals, to ascertain how well audience participants, such as health care providers, are able to incorporate these knowledge and attitude changes into behavior changes in their work settings. Obviously, these types of evaluation require staff who can longitudinally follow audience participants; therefore, extensive post-training evaluation may not be possible for smaller agencies. Nonetheless, the qualitative information obtained from participant satisfaction reports can be invaluable in ensuring that training objectives are met in a culturally sensitive and affirming manner.

Finally, maintaining funding for continued training events is an integral component to the Emory Project. Although funded through the federal Center for Mental Health Services, the Emory Project must stretch its resources to encompass training events throughout the state, some of which require extensive traveling. A key to cost-effective training and continued success for the Emory Project has been collaborating with local agencies, who often-times provide meetings facilities and manage local advertisement. Similarly, state agencies, hospitals, and other organizations may have specified funds available for financing continuing education. These collaborative efforts not only reduce project expenses, but also nurture local interest and participation. Finally, researching for specific requests for grant applications for AIDS education from such federal agencies as the Center for Mental Health Services of the Substance Abuse and Mental Health Services Administration, the Centers for Disease Control and Prevention, and the Health Resources and Services Administration may be key in maintaining larger statewide networks such as the Emory Project.

In conclusion, AIDS education remains a vital component of the national comprehensive outreach of HIV-related prevention and service delivery. The changing demography of the pandemic calls attention to the need to include rural regions in the outreach plan, especially education targeted to rural communities. Although the obstacles in effectively reaching rural audiences with AIDS education are significant, this chapter has outlined general strategies which have proven effective for the Emory Project in meeting the challenge of delivering rural AIDS education. Such education, delivered in a culturally sensitive manner, is essential to the task of changing common misconceptions and myths about HIV and AIDS which remain prevalent in many rural communities today.

References

Bell, N.A. (1991). Social/sexual Norms and AIDS in the South. *AIDS Education and Prevention*, 3(2), 164-180.

Centers for Disease Control and Prevention. (1994). *HIV/AIDS Surveillance Report*, 6(2), 1-39.

Centers for Disease Control and Prevention. (1992). HIV Infection and AIDS Georgia, 1991. *Morbidity and Mortality Weekly Report*, 41(46), 876-8.

Chang-Yit, L., Lippert, M. and Thielges, I. (1992). Model for Rural Collaboration for AIDS Education: A Case Study. *Family and Community Health*, 15(3), 62-69.

Crocteau, J.M., Nero, C.I., Prosser, D.J. (1993). Social and Cultural Sensitivity in Group-specific HIV and AIDS Programming. *Journal of Counseling and Development*, 71, 290-296.

Ellerbrock, T.V., Bush, T.J., and Chamberland, M.E. (1991). Epidemiology of Women With AIDS in the United States, 1981 Through 1990. *Journal of the American Medical Association*, 265, 2971-2975.

Fleming, D.W., Coch, S.L., Steele, R.S. et al. (1987). Acquired Immunodefeciency Syndrome in Low-incidence Areas: How Safe is Unsafe Sex? *Journal of the American Medical Association*, 258, 785-787.

Foster, P.M., Phillips, F.P., Belgrave, F.Z., Randolph, S.M., Braithewaite, N. (1993). An Africentric Model for AIDS Education, Prevention, and Psychological Services Within the African American Community. *Journal of Black Psychology*, 19(2), 123-141.

Icard, L. (1985). Black Gay Men and Conflicting Social Identities: Sexual Orientation Versus Racial Identity. *Journal of Social Work and Human Sexuality*, 4(1-2), 83-93.

Jones, C.C., Waskin, H., Gesety, B. (1987). Persistence of High Risk Sexual Activity Among Homosexual Men In An Area of Low Incidence of Acquired Immunodeficiency Syndrome. *Sexually Transmitted Disease*, 14, 79-82.

Kinkel, M.B. (1986). Stress-Coping-Support in Rural Communities: A Model for Primary Prevention. *American Journal of Community Psychology*, 14, 463.

Nelson, C.C. (1993). AIDS Prevention Programs In a Smaller Community. *Canadian Journal of Public Health* - Supplement 1, S39-S41.

Rounds, K.A. (1988). Responding to AIDS: Rural Community Strategies. *Journal of Contemporary Social Work*, 360-364.

Rutherford, G.W., Araba-Owoyele, L.A., Hughes, M.J., Singleton, J.A. (1993, June). HIV Infection and AIDS in Rural California: Is HIV Becoming Ruralized? *International Conference on AIDS*, 9(2), 664. (abstract no. PO-C05-2682).

St. Lawrence, J.S., Hood, H.V., Brasfield, T.L., Kelly, J.A. (1989). Risk Knowledge and Risk Behavior Among Gay Men in High- Versus Low-AIDS Prevalence Areas. *Public Health Reporter*, 104, 391-395.

Tucker, R., Pace, B., and Soth, I. (1991, June). AIDS and HIV Infection in Rural Washington State. *International Conference on AIDS*, 7(1), 356. (abstract no. M.C.3232)

Protocol 076: A New Look at Women and Children With AIDS

Nora Kizer Bell

The country's attention is finally focused on HIV/AIDS as it affects women, children and adolescents. During the 1990s, the World Health Organization (WHO) estimates an additional 3 million or more women and children will die from AIDS (Weekly Epidemiology Record, 1994). In major cities of the Americas, Western Europe, and sub-Saharan Africa, AIDS is becoming the leading cause of death for women aged 25-44. In New York City, it is already the leading cause of death among women aged 25 to 29 (Bacon, 1987). Ironically, it is the disease's effects on their children, not on women themselves, that has motivated this new focus on women in the AIDS epidemic.

HIV Infection Trends in Women and Children

In August of 1988, there were 5,840 cases of AIDS reported in women in the United States. At that time, the US Public Health Service projected that, by 1992, there would be between 29,000 and 36,000 women with AIDS (Bell, 1989,5). Data from the National Survey of Childbearing Women now indicate that in 1992, the estimated prevalence of HIV infection among childbearing women was 1.7 per 1000. In 1987, Surgeon General Koop predicted that, by 1991, 3000 children would be afflicted with AIDS. Yet, during the years 1989-1992, approximately 7,000 HIV-infected women gave birth each year (Davis, Gwinn et al., 1993), and an estimated 1000-2000 HIV-infected infants were born *annually* during those years in the United States (CDC Draft Recommendations, Feb. 1995).

The accumulating data indicate rapid increases in the numbers of women reported to have AIDS/HIV (Davis, Gwinn et al., 1993; Elias, 1995). In 1993, HIV infection was the fourth leading cause of death nationally among women 25-44 years of age (National Center for Health Statistics, 42(13) 1994) and the seventh leading cause of death among children one to four years of age in the United States. (National Center, 43(6S) 1994).

Through June of 1994, the US Centers for Disease Control and Prevention (CDC) had received reports of more than 53,000 AIDS cases among adult and adolescent women and more than 5,000 cases among children who acquired HIV infection perinatally (CDC Draft Recommendations, Feb. 1995). In 1994, 18% of the AIDS cases in the United States were female, almost three times the rate ten years ago. The 14,081 women reported with AIDS in 1994 represented nearly one-fourth (24%) of the total number of AIDS cases reported to date among women (CDC Training Bulletin, #123 1995).

Of great concern is the continued, steady rise of heterosexually transmitted cases of HIV (Wiley and Samuel, 1989). As the numbers of these cases have grown, heterosexual contact with an HIV-infected male has become the most rapidly increasing transmission mode among women (Fumento, 1989). Nearly two-fifths (38%) of all cases among women have been attributed to heterosexual contact; slightly more than two-fifths (41%) of all cases among women are thought to occur through injecting drug use (CDC Training Bulletin, #123 1995). Although black and Hispanic women constitute only 21% of all U.S. women, more than three-fourths (77%) of AIDS cases reported among women in 1994 occurred among blacks and Hispanics (CDC Training Bulletin, #123 1995). Almost 90 percent of cumulative AIDS cases reported in children, and virtually all new HIV infections among children, are attributed to perinatal transmission of HIV (CDC Draft Recommendations, Feb. 1995; PHS Guidelines, July 1995).

HIV infection can be passed from a mother to her fetus or newborn in three ways: during pregnancy, to the fetus *in utero* through fetal-maternal circulation; to the infant during labor and delivery, and to the newborn during the postpartum period, through breastfeeding (Freidland and Klein 1987, 1130; Piot, Plummer, et al. 1988, 575; Dunn, Newell et al. 1992, 585). From 15 to 40 percent of infants born to infected mothers become infected themselves (Connor, Sperling et al. 1994, 1173). While researchers know that HIV can be transmitted to the fetus as early as 8 weeks gestation, the preponderance of the evidence indicates that most transmission occurs late in pregnancy or during the time of labor and delivery (Mofenson and Wolinsky 1994; Connor, Sperling et al., 1994). Trends in women with AIDS are clearly ominous predictors of trends in pediatric AIDS cases.

Treatment of Pediatric AIDS

While much of the HIV/AIDS research over the past decade has focused on biomedical and behavioral interventions to prevent HIV transmission and infection, advances in treatment options over the last several years have improved survival rates and quality of life for HIV-infected persons. Despite these advances, however, pediatric HIV infection remains almost uniformly fatal. Reduction and/or prevention of pediatric HIV infection has consequently become the disquieting focus of recent research and policy recommendations.

Among children with perinatally acquired HIV infection, pneumocystis carinii pneumonia (PCP) remains the most common and devastating of their opportunistic infections. PCP in children under 12 months of age usually presents acutely and has a very poor outcome (MMWR 43(RR-11) 1994). Unfortunately, ongoing AIDS surveillance has detected no substantial decrease in PCP incidence among HIV-infected infants. In fact, the incidence remained relatively unchanged between the years 1989 and 1992 (MMWR 44(RR-4) 1995). Of the 7080 children born to HIV-positive mothers in 1992, 2.4 percent developed PCP. More significantly from the perspective of those recommending public health policy, a total of 199 of the 300 children diagnosed with PCP between 1991 and 1993 had never received prophylaxis (Simons, Lindegren, Thomas et al. 1995, 786).

This study and others suggest that the above continued incidence is associated both with a failure to identify HIV-infected infants before they develop PCP as well as with limitations in the current guidelines for identification of children at risk for PCP. For many, the failure to identify infants at risk is arguably linked to the failure to identify and evaluate pregnant women with HIV infection (PHS Guidelines, July 1995).

Against these data have now been juxtaposed the remarkable findings of the US AIDS Clinical Trials Group (ACTG), a team of clinical researchers headed by Dr. Edward M. O'Connor of the New Jersey Medical School in Newark. In a multicenter randomized placebo-controlled study (ACTG 076) involving 477 women known to be infected with HIV, half were given zidovudine (AZT) during the study and the other half (and their newborn children) were given placebo. The test group received AZT orally five times a day during the latter stages of pregnancy and intravenously during delivery. Newborns in this group were also treated with AZT for approximately six weeks following delivery.

Forty infected infants were born to the women who received placebo, representing a 25.5% rate of infection. By contrast, among the women who received AZT only 13 infants (8.3%) were born infected — a stunning 67.5% reduction in the incidence of transmission. Reported side-effects in mother and child were similar in both groups except for lower hemoglobin concentrations in the treated infants. Hemoglobin levels returned to normal when AZT administration was terminated. The results were considered impressive enough to halt the study, and patients in the control group were offered AZT treatment. The results of that study were released in February in the *New England Journal of Medicine* (Connor, Sperling et al. 1994).

The success of this trial, now known as Protocol 076, prompted researchers and clinicians to conclude that the use of antiretroviral therapy in the treatment of HIV-infected women and their newborns significantly reduces the risk of perinatal transmission of HIV. News of the success of the perinatal AZT treatment has met with mixed response from health care providers and those in health policy alike.

On one hand, the potential of AZT therapy for preventing transmission from mother to child, as well as AZT's potential for preventing infection in newborns, underscores the importance of detecting HIV infection during pregnancy. All children identified as HIV-exposed, either prenatally or postpartum, are recommended for diagnostic testing, monitoring and treatment (El Sadr, Oleske et al., 1994). Because perinatally infected children develop PCP most commonly between the ages of three and six months (Simonds, Oxtoby et al., 1993), effective treatment requires that children at risk for HIV infection because of maternal infection be identified early, *preferably prenatally*, and that prophylaxis begin as early as the second month of life. If HIV infection risks can be determined prenatally, the results of Protocol 076 suggest that we can expect significant reductions in pediatric AIDS.

On the other hand, because perinatal identification of HIV infection risks for newborns includes identification of maternal HIV, some have recommended that testing should only occur on newborns. Studies suggest, however, that only 35-55% of children with HIV infection risks are identified as newborns (Simons, Lindegren et al., 1995). Those infants not identified are, clearly, more likely to develop HIV infection and more susceptible to potentially fatal PCP during their first few months of life (CDC Training Bulletin, #140 1995). These considerations have led to a variety of recommendations for stepped-up, even mandatory, HIV testing of pregnant women. Understandably, talk of mandatory testing generates considerable medical and ethical controversy.

Framing the Debate

Women and children have always been among those who have AIDS. Nonetheless, there was little focus on women in earlier years of the epidemic, and CDC defining criteria for the diagnosis of AIDS did not even include conditions unique to women until January of 1993. In fact, a news report on National Public Radio on November 30, 1990, proclaimed that over half of the women who died of AIDS had never been diagnosed.

Historically, medical research has paid scant attention to women's health issues, except as they affect child health, and women have routinely been evaluated for health care intervention and treatment based on extrapolations from results obtained from studies conducted exclusively on men. In fact, numerical projections and statistics on AIDS/HIV were based, for many years, on data pertaining to transmission between males. Yet, as Kathy Anastos and Carola Marte point out in their article, "Women: The Missing Persons in the AIDS Epidemic," the problem of the "missing women" in the AIDS epidemic goes well beyond the epidemiology and case definition of AIDS or HIV. Societal attitudes toward women led to a pervasive inclination early in the epidemic to view women as "vectors" of HIV transmission to men and infants, rather than to focus on women's own risk of becoming infected and sick (Anastos and Marte, 1989). Women were not educated about their own risk factors, much less about the possible risks to a developing fetus. Women were, and still are, largely ignored by mainstream media in their (now dwindling) coverage of HIV/AIDS.

Although women are now included in clinical trials, they were eclipsed by much of the early HIV research leading many to suggest that there are still fundamental questions about disease progression in women that remain unanswered. Indeed, there are still fundamental questions about the long-term risks associated with AZT intervention, such as that used in Protocol 076.

In heralding the results of the ACTG 076 study, for example, little attention has been given to the clinical questions that remain unanswered — all questions of enormous importance to women. What are the long-term effects of this level of zidovudine exposure/treatment on mother and child? Could administration of lower levels of AZT be equally beneficial? If AZT were only administered late in pregnancy, could we expect the same results? Will treated infants develop AZT resistance, precluding the use of zidovudine later in the course of their illness? Is the effect of AZT sustained in infants? Is it in the best interest of mother or child to proceed on the basis of the results of a relatively small trial that has not been fully peer-reviewed?

Racism, unfortunately, is also implicated in the neglect of issues affecting women. Compared with men who have AIDS or are HIV-infected, women with HIV or AIDS are more likely to be ethnic minorities, drug users or sexual partners of drug users, and poor (CDC National HIV Seroprevalence summary, 1994). Factors potentially associated with the increased risk among racial/ethnic minorities include limited access to HIV prevention services and higher rates of sexually transmitted diseases (MMWR, 44(21) 1995). Researchers report further that while 78% of the reported cases of AIDS in children younger than six years old are in children of color, children of color constitute only 21% of the nation's population in that age group (Osterholm and MacDonald, 1987).

The disparities in the risk of HIV among blacks and Hispanics must be examined in the context of the social fabric in which HIV infection occurs, and at the core of that fabric one finds the problems of poverty, drug abuse, teen pregnancy, lack of education, inadequate health care and social support services, prostitution, and child and spouse abuse. For example, as Osterholm and MacDonald note, the rate of black, never married women aged 15 to 19 who are sexually active is 35% higher than that of white women (Osterholm and MacDonald, 1987). For many women, their address alone places them at risk. Anastos and Marte note, for example, that in New York City, the most socially and economically devastated inner-city areas are those with the highest incidence of HIV disease — often twice as many cases per 100,000 in those neighborhoods as in wealthier neighborhoods. Because the social and economic realities for women of childbearing age in the inner cities are not easily remedied, the great weight of female and pediatric HIV infection will continue to fall on communities of color, particularly in these urban settings.

Allegations of racism and class politics cannot be ignored in attempting to evaluate proposals for HIV prevention strategies that involve wider or mandatory screening. Women with HIV represent the least advantaged groups in American society. Already disenfranchised, these women lack the means to command the public's attention to their plight. These women are not the idealized "victim" woman.

HIV-infected women are more likely to be unemployed, intermittently employed, or employed in positions where they are particularly vulnerable to firings or layoffs. Many of these women have few personal or financial resources or lack the skills necessary for negotiating the fragmented American health care system. They are more likely than men to be crisis-oriented in seeking health care, and more likely to seek access to care through public health services (Moore, Smith et al., 1993).

Because many women are the sole caregivers and the heads of household in their homes, household and family responsibilities, including transportation needs and child care, often lead them to focus on children's and partners' or parents' needs before their own health care needs. Many of them find that the demands of work, coupled with the above responsibilities, leave little time to deal with bureaucratic social service agencies.

The dimension of power within her social and sexual relationships also defines the HIV/AIDS context for many women. The relationship to a male partner takes priority over everything else — in some cases because the woman is economically dependent on her partner. Dependence on a male partner is typically accompanied, especially among younger and poorer women, by the woman's clearly subordinate role in all aspects of the relationship. A heterosexual woman in a dependent relationship is also not an equal partner in the bedroom. If her partner does not want to use a condom, even if the woman feels she might be at significant risk of infection, she is unlikely to prevail in her requests that he use a condom or forego sex altogether. Indeed, because of women's great vulnerability to personal violence, many women feel more threatened by the possibility of beatings and abuse than they do by the risk of HIV infection (Nation's Health, 25(4) 1995). Hence, many women never ask for this element of control in their sexual relationships (National Hispanic Education, 1995; Cancer Epidemiology Studies, 1995).

A final disturbing factor is that almost one-half of infected women in various studies denied having knowledge of having engaged in any high risk behavior. Among women under 25 years of age, fully 68% claimed no knowledge of exposure to any risk factor associated with HIV transmission (Quinn, Glasser et al., 1988; Nation's Health, 25(3) 1995). Regrettably, large numbers of women learn of their HIV infection only after giving birth to an HIV-infected child.

Articulating the Ethical Concerns

As noted above, the demonstrated effectiveness of zidovudine in lowering the rate of perinatal HIV transmission is said to emphasize the importance of identifying pregnant women with HIV as early as possible. Since many women with HIV do not know they are infected, various recommendations have been made for increased testing and counseling of all pregnant women. Among these recommendations have been several that HIV testing of pregnant women be mandatory (Caplan, 1994; Caplan, 1995; Kolata, 1994; Purnick, 1995).

Such recommendations raise a number of ethical concerns that require more careful examination: issues of privacy and confidentiality, our "duty to warn" others of danger they may face, our duty to protect a child's best interest, and the conflict of rights that could occur between a mother's best interest and what could be said to be in the best interest of her unborn child.

Are There Ethical Limits to Privacy and Confidentiality?

Legislative and judicial law have long recognized a principle articulated by John Stuart Mill and typically identified as the "harm principle": one is free to do as one chooses so long as those actions harm no one else. This principle has often been used to justify paternalistic interventions designed to prevent harm to others. Rights of privacy, for example, are often compromised in favor of the public's health, as they are in public health laws that compel the reporting of otherwise personal or confidential information — such as one's infection with a contagious, infectious or sexually transmitted disease. The harm principle can also be said to justify contact tracing or partner notification, particularly when such diseases are relatively easily treated.

Following the *Tarasoff* case there is a growing acknowledgment in the law that provider/patient relationships also may carry duties to third parties who could be endangered by the patient. Disclosure of confidential or seemingly private information is sometimes deemed essential to warn a third party of both the source and nature of a danger to her or to alert public health officials of a threat to the public's health and safety. The protective duty to others is said to be exercised justifiably by allowing disclosure of such potentially harmful medical information when it is perceived that the third party is at serious risk. Indeed, the court in the *Tarasoff* case summarized this principle by observing that "[t]he protective privilege ends where the public peril begins" (*Tarasoff v. Regents*, 1976). However, only disclosure of necessary information is protected, and most courts insist that the information be given only to those with a clear need to know.

Compounding the ethical dilemma in the case of maternal-fetal HIV is the virtually universal agreement that when decisions are made on behalf of infants and young children, those children's "best interest" has incontrovertible moral and legal force. Medical evidence seems to indicate that we are in a situation where the medical interests of children with HIV are best served when their HIV status is known very early — preferably prenatally. This suggests that the mother's right to privacy with respect to her own HIV status is justifiably compromised in favor of the unborn infant's need to know. If we accept this reasoning, the interests of a newborn or an unborn child are placed in a necessarily adversarial posture with the mother's right to privacy.

Clearly the more difficult questions in this category of concern have to do with the rights of women as over and against fetal rights. For example, there have been suggestions that charges could be brought by or on behalf of a child infected with HIV *in utero*. Such charges could take the form of "wrongful birth" or "wrongful life" claims against mother, father and/or health care providers.

Essentially, a wrongful life or wrongful birth claim rests on the premise that, where infection is avoidable, the child should not have been born or should have been treated preventively before being born. Although few jurisdictions recognize wrongful life actions (Bell and Loewer, 1985), wrongful birth actions could lead some women to elect abortion. Hence, though many might argue that the outcomes of Protocol 076 recommend routine testing of all pregnant women as well as all women of reproductive age, others counter that such testing could generate new controversy over many of the reproductive choices articulated in *Roe v. Wade.*

And, while many might argue that the outcomes of Protocol 076 recommend routine testing of all pregnant women as well as all women of reproductive age, still others counter that the medical or clinical findings do not yet offer sufficient warrant for such an invasion of privacy. Based on public discussion of these issues in the past, it seems clear that American society will have great difficulty in agreeing on the morally responsible choice.

Mandatory Testing

Indeed, the recent policy discussions following publication of the ACTG 076 findings have suggested, among other things, that we reappraise strategies to screen individuals for HIV and to follow up on those whose test results are positive. Critics of the voluntarist approach to screening have charged that these earlier approaches to screening have been largely ineffective and more "politically correct" than sound public health policy. They urge the use of strategies analogous to those employed for combating TB and syphilis (Caplan, 1995; Kolata, 1995). HIV, they suggest, should be treated like any other infectious disease — those who carry infection should be identified, those who have been exposed should be notified, and those whom we can treat should be treated.

Currently, the CDC and state health departments use a variety of systems to monitor HIV and AIDS among childbearing women and their children. In addition to actual case reporting and contact notification, 45 states have conducted anonymous testing of blood samples routinely collected from newborns for metabolic tests in order to track HIV seroprevalence and epidemiological traits of HIV in mothers. Every mother whose newborn tests HIV-positive is positive. Through the newborn, health departments learned seroprevalence rates by testing the mothers, even though identifiers were removed so that test results could not be linked to a specific infant or its mother. These tests were recently halted when controversy erupted over whether all mothers should be informed of the results of the tests (What's News, 1995). One mother, Michele Faust, argued that if mandatory testing, disclosure or informed consent had been in place, her son would have been treated at birth, possibly preventing transmission of HIV to him. Faust only learned of her son's infection when he nearly died of PCP at two months of age (Washington Times, 1995).

That there might be strong moral and clinical reasons for preventing further spread of AIDS to newborns and for preventing pregnancy in infected women does not imply, however, that policy be *mandated* for accomplishing that end. For many women, mandatory testing carries with it the specter of forced celibacy, forced treatment, prohibitions against procreation (accompanied by the possibility of sanctions against violators), and even the threat of forced abortion (Lee, 1995).

In spite of the benefits suggested by Protocol 076, concerns have been raised about the possible negative effects of mandating testing and counseling in prenatal and other settings. Questions have also been raised about the moral, legal and practical consequences of enforcing mandatory testing.

A hidden assumption in some of the proposals for mandating testing during pregnancy is that women would not be permitted to refuse care for themselves, hence, their unborn fetuses. A positive test result would lead to mandated treatment. Many would argue that calls for mandatory testing are thereby flawed, because the principle of informed consent generally implies that competent adults have the right to refuse care, even where such a choice is self-destructive. Given the uncertainties about the long-term effects of AZT treatment for both mother and newborn, the importance of informed consent assumes heightened moral significance. Bayer argues, for example, that the proposal is also unjustified at this time because therapeutic interventions cannot yet substantially extend the lives of infected children. If they could, mandatory unblinded screening could be morally required because treatment of infected children, whether or not the parent(s) agreed, would be imperative. "By contrast, the mandatory screening of pregnant women is objectionable because mandatory treatment of competent adults is virtually never acceptable" (Bayer 1994, 1224).

Apart from evidence that suggests that mandatory testing in other populations would have had the effect of driving underground those most in need of testing and counseling, it is unclear what gains could be expected from forced testing perinatally. Many women in populations identified as "at risk" often cannot afford prenatal care and use midwives rather than physicians at delivery. There is the additional question of determining how such mandates might be enforced or sanctioned. By imprisonment? By steep fines? By intervention of child protective services? By termination of parental rights? Under such circumstances, if testing were mandated, the end hoped for still might not be realized. Testing not clearly perceived as voluntary could be a deterrent to the use of prenatal care services. Indeed, Nolan argues that mandatory screening policies would make it highly likely that we would see even more "marked decreases in the number of disadvantaged women who seek prenatal care" (Childress 1991, 66).

There are also economic issues inherent in proposals for mandatory testing. A single HIV test costs $25. About 4 million women give birth in the United States each year; testing each one of them for HIV would cost $100 million (Washington Post, 1995). Some place the cost of treating a single infected newborn at approximately $350,000 over his or her lifetime (Caplan, 1995), hence, argue that testing is both prevention-oriented and a more cost-effective way of managing the costs of pediatric HIV. Others are quick to point out that nothing in the results of ACTG 076 suggest that mandatory testing will completely eliminate pediatric HIV infection or obviate the need for budgeting treatment costs for children infected perinatally.

There is a final important argument to examine, one that will be more familiar to those who have a longstanding interest in issues affecting women: A woman must be allowed to weigh for herself the risks inherent in undergoing AZT treatment during pregnancy if she is found to be seropositive. Only she can evaluate the moral validity of her options. As James Childress concludes, "the most defensible policy, because the most respectful of pregnant women's autonomy and also the most productive of desirable consequences, is to offer pregnant women, in high seroprevalence areas or with risk factors, prenatal testing for HIV with adequate information so that they can make their own decisions, with appropriate pretest and posttest counseling and services" (Childress 1991, 66). Moral and practical difficulties in compelling women to follow a prescribed regimen of treatment and care argue instead for the importance of enlisting the woman's voluntary cooperation.

Future Policy Deliberations

Advocacy of voluntary approaches stems not from ideology but from the facts of the case: since private behavior is at issue, the most effective policies will be those that enlist the cooperation of those at greatest risk, thus optimizing both human rights and the health of the public (Osborn, 1988). Clearly, development of public health policy rests on assumptions about what prevention measures or any HIV intervention should accomplish. These assumptions obviously shape recommendations for new public health policy. It is important to ask, therefore, what should count as a measure of any successful public health strategy.

It seems clear from policy discussions and deliberation that for many in HIV/AIDS prevention, the bottom line — the public health goal — is elimination of disease, zero transmission, 100 percent risk reduction. Short of that, public health efforts are said to have failed.

These goals seem to reflect an impoverished understanding of where we are relative to a disease like HIV/AIDS. Serious public health and social consequences can flow from a failure to appreciate how likely it is in a democratic society that we will ever bring about 100% risk reduction or complete behavior change. Equally serious consequences can flow from an expectation that they would.

Even if we were to agree that completely eliminating risky behaviors is desirable in combating HIV, our commitment to the kind of education we champion in a democratic society will not allow us to realize that end (Bell, 1991). A democratic society places a high value on pluralism; hence, the principle of respect for persons has important moral force. Respecting persons requires a presumption in favor of individual responsibility, just as it leads us to embrace certain values, such as mutual respect among persons. Placing a high value on individual responsibility requires not only that we accept all persons as equally possessing moral status, but also that we treat them with such respect — that we affirm their moral right to be treated equitably and that we affirm their right to be different.

The criteria for successful public health policy in such a context will be very different from those criteria implicit in policies that mandate certain behaviors or outcomes. Under public health policy conceived as voluntarist, strategies for reducing transmission of HIV must rely heavily on moral persuasion, rational deliberation, persons' respect and concern for others, and hence, on the availability of current and accurate information on HIV transmission and prevention.

Under such a conception of public health policy, success is achieved if persons can be participants in their own learning and if they can differentiate and accept responsibility for moral choices. Such a conception of public health policy carries with it certain risks, however — namely, that some people will learn and understand but will not change their behaviors, that they will forget, that they will make mistakes, that HIV will not be entirely eliminated. In fact, a voluntarist approach to HIV prevention strategies may make some persons more willing to take risks with themselves and others than they were before; it may even make some people less responsible citizens than they were before. And, not surprisingly, those are risks that some who would determine public health policy are unwilling to accept.

The issues involved in developing a successful program of HIV prevention should not be conflated with issues involved in effecting behavior change. Only if we think that successful prevention programs must eventuate in specific behaviors (or absence of those behaviors) are we pushed to think that prevention is equivalent to coercion. So, for example, while we might agree that HIV/AIDS prevention requires telling people what their responsibilities are to others (including their offspring), it is a very different project to force them to act responsibly or to determine what will happen to those who fail to do so. In fact, history teaches us that coercion and "magic bullets" have only short-lived success in combating sexually transmitted diseases.

Not all resistance to mandatory HIV testing of pregnant women is generated by social or political considerations. Many institutions and organizations *in principle* oppose mandatory screening or testing, except for blood and blood products or organs and tissues being considered for organ transplantation. Many others want to see clear evidence that the efficacy of the regimen is as high in women with advanced disease as it was in the women in the trial — a group of women exhibiting mild to moderate immunosuppression. Still others believe that the focus should be on continuing efforts to develop a range of strategies for preventing perinatal transmission of HIV, including better educational and outreach programs, vaginal cleansing with antiretroviral agents, and caesarian delivery (Rogers and Jaffe 1994, 1222).

Unfortunately, discussions such as the above point to the fact that the moral and social context within which we must evaluate policy dimensions of HIV have remained relatively unchanged over the past decade. In August of 1994, the Center for Strategic and International Studies released a report that emphasized once again the fact that the main barriers to effective strategies against the epidemic are stigmatization and discrimination. The report argued for refitting prevention strategies to address the special needs of women (Global HIV/AIDS, 1994).

One of the great tragedies of the epidemic is that AIDS is affecting populations that have historically been disadvantaged. Sadly, what seems to emerge from the foregoing discussion is that we may really have fewer options for averting the disastrous consequences to women than we would like to admit.

References

076 Fact Sheet. (1995). CDC Public Health Service guidelines for HIV Counseling and Voluntary Testing for Pregnant Women. July 7.

AIDS Testing. (May 16, 1995). *Washington Times*, A6.

AIDS Testing for Pregnant Women Urged. (February 23, 1995). *Washington Post*, A5.

Anastasio, C., McMahan, T., Daniels, A. et al. (1995). Self-care Burden in Women With HIV. *Journal of the Association of Nurses in AIDS Care*, 6 (3): 31.

Anastos, K. and Marte, C. (Winter, 1989). Women: The Missing Persons in the AIDS Epidemic. *Health/PAC Bulletin*, 19(4), 6.

Bacon, Lisa. (1987). Lessons of AIDS: Racism, Homophobia Are the Real Epidemic. *Listen Real Loud*, 8(2), 5-6.

Bayer, Ronald. (May 26, 1995). It's Not 'Tuskegee Revisited. *Washington Post*, A27.

Bayer, Ronald. (1994). Ethical Challenges Posed by Zidovudine Treatment to Reduce Vertical Transmission of HIV. *New England Journal of Medicine*, 331(18), 1223-25.

Bell, Nora. (1991). Ethical issues in AIDS education. In F. G. Reamer (Ed.), *AIDS and ethics*. New York: Columbia University Press.

Bell, N. and Loewer, B. (1985). What is Wrong With 'Wrongful Life Cases? *Journal of Medicine and Philosophy*, 10(2), 127-145.

Bell, Nora K. (1989). Women and AIDS: Too Little, Too Late? *Hypatia*, 4(3), 1-22.

CDC. (1994). Recommendation of the US PHS Task Force on the Use of Zidovudine to Reduce Perinatal Transmission of HIV. *MMWR*, 43: (RR-11).

CDC. (1994). National HIV Seroprevalance Summary: Results Through 1992. Vol. 3—US Dept. of HHS.

CDC. (1995). Update—trends in AIDS Among Men Who Have Sex With Men: US, 1989-94. *MMWR*, 44(21).

CDC. (March 10, 1995). HIV Counseling and Testing—US 1993. *MMWR*, 44(9).

CDC National AIDS Hotline Training Bulletin. (February 9, 1995). #123.

CDC National AIDS Hotline Training Bulletin. (February 24, 1995). #129.

CDC National AIDS Hotline Training Bulletin. (May 1, 1995). #140.

CDC National AIDS Hotline Training Bulletin. (March 24, 1995). #133.

CDC press release. (May 22, 1995). Talking Points on the Survey of Childbearing Women.

Can Women Demand Condom Use? Gender and Power in Safe Sex. (1995). Cancer Epidemiology Studies. San Francisco, CA.

Caplan, Art. (March 15, 1995). Women Who Are Pregnant Should be Routinely Tested. *Philadelphia Enquirer*, A13.

Caplan, Art. (November 15, 1994). Make this AIDS Test Mandatory. Albany, New York newspaper. Viewpoint.

Childress, J.F. (1991). Mandatory HIV Screening and Testing. In F. G. Reamer (Ed.), *AIDS and Ethics*. New York: Columbia University Press.

Connor, E., Sperling, R., Gelber, R., Pavel K., et al. (1994). Reduction of Maternal-Infant Transmission of Human Immuodeficiency Virus Type I with Zidovudone Treatment. *New England Journal of Medicine*. 331(18), 1173-1180.

Culture and Sexual Behavior. (1995). National Hispanic Education and Communications Projects. Washington, DC.

Davis, S., Gwinn, M., Wasser, S., Fleming, P., Karou, J. (December 12-16, 1983). *HIV Prevalence Among U. S. Childbearing Women*, 1989-1992. Abstract. Presented at First National Conference on Human Retroviruses and Related Infections.

Washington, DC.

Dunn, D., Newell, M., Ades, A., Peckham, C.(1992). Risk of Human Immunodeficiency Virus Type I Transmission Through Breastfeeding. *Lancet* 340, 585-88.

El Sadr, W., Oleske, J., Agins, B. et al. (1994). Evaluation and Management of Early HIV Infection. Clinical Practice Guidelines. AHCPR Publication no. 94-0572. Rockville, MD: Agency for Health Care Policy and Research. US Dept. of HHS. Public Health Service.

Elias, M. (March 24, 1995). AIDS Rate Increasing Faster Among Women Than Men, Study Shows. *USA Today*, 7A.

Fact Sheet—Children, Adolescents, Young Adults. (1995). National Pediatric HIV Resource Center. Washington, DC.

Friedland, G. and Klein, R. (1987). Transmission of Human Immunodeficiency Virus. *New England Journal of Medicine*, 317(18), 1125-1135.

Fumento, M. (1989). *The Myth of Heterosexual AIDS*. New York: New Republic Books.

Global HIV/AIDS: A Strategy for U. S. Leadership. (1994). *Health Affairs*, 13 (5), 256.

Harrigan, P. (1995). Routine Testing of HIV Status of Babies? *Lancet* 345 (8957), 1102.

Hinman, A. (1991). Strategies to Prevent HIV Infection in the U.S. *American Journal of Public Health*, 81, 1557-9.

Kolata, G. (November 3, 1994). Discovery That AIDS Can be Prevented in Babies Raises Debate on Mandatory Testing. *New York Times*.

Lee, F. (May 9, 1995). For Women With AIDS, Anguish of Having Babies. *New York Times*. A1.

Macklin, R. (September, 1989). *HIV Infection In Children: Some Ethical Conflicts*. Technical Report on Developmental Disabilities and HIV Infection. Silver Springs, MD: American Association of University Affiliated Programs. Report #3.

Mofenson, L. and Wolinsky, S. (1994). Current Insights Regarding Vertical Transmission. In P. Pizzo & C. Wilfert (Eds.), *Pediatric AIDS: The Challenge of HIV Infection in Infants, Children and Adolescents* (pp. 179-203). Baltimore: Williams & Wilkins.

Monthly vital statistic report. (1994). 43(65), Hyattsville, MD: PHS

Moore, J., Smith, D., Solomon, L., et al. (1993). *Quality of Life Measures in HIV-Infected and At-risk Women*. Presented at IXth International Conference on AIDS. Berlin. June 6-11.

National Center for Health Statistics. (1994). Advanced Report of Final Mortality Statistics: US, 1992.

National Center for Health Statistics. (1994). *Annual Summary of Births, Marriages, Divorces and Deaths*: US, 1993. Monthly Vital Statistics Report 42 (13): Hyattsville, MD: PHS.

National Commission on AIDS. (December, 1992). *The Challenge of HIV/AIDS in Communities of Color*. Washington, DC: National Commission on AIDS.

New AIDS Estimates Show Demographic Changes. (1995). *AIDS Alert* 10 (6), 83.

Osborn, J. (1988). AIDS, Politics and Science. *New England Journal of Medicine*, 381, 444-447.

Osterholm, M. and MacDonald, K. (1987). Facing the Complex Issues of Pediatric AIDS: A Public Health Perspective. *Journal of the American Medical*

Association, 258(19), 2736-2737.

Piot, P., Plummer, F., Mhalu, F., Lambaray, J., Chin, J., Mann, J. (1988). AIDS: An International Perspective. *Science*, 239, 573-579.

Purnick, Joyce. (May 18, 1995). When AIDS Testing Collides with Confidentiality. *New York Times*, B4.

Quinn, T., Glasser, D., Cannon, R., Matuszak, D., Dunning, R., Kline, R., Campbell, C., Irace, E., Fauci, A., and Hook, E. (1988). Human Immunodeficiency Virus Infection Among Patients Attending Clinics for Sexually Transmitted Diseases. *New England Journal of Medicine*, 318(4), 197-203.

Revised Guidelines for Prophylaxis Against Pneumocystis Carinii Pneumonia for Children Infected With or Perinatally Exposed to Human Immunodeficiency Virus. (1995). CDC/US HHS Publication (CDC) 95-8017. *MMWR*, 44 (RR-4). April 28.

Rogers, M. and Jaffe, H. (1994). Reducing the Risk of Maternal-infant Transmission of HIV: A Door is Opened. *New England Journal of Medicine*, 331(18), 1222-23

STD Education Initiative Seeks to Stem Large Number of Cases in US. (March, 1995). *Nation's Health*, 25(3), 9.

Simonds, R., Lindegren, M.L., Thomas, P., et al.(1995). Prophylaxis Against Pneumocystis Carinii Pneumonia Among Children With Perinatally Acquired Human Immunodeficiency Virus Infection in the United States. *New England Journal of Medicine*, 332(12), 786.

Simonds, R., Oxtoby, M., Caldwell, M., Gwinn, M., Rogers, M.(1993). Pneumocystis Carinii Pneumonia Among U. S. Children With Perinatally Acquired HIV Infection. *Journal of the American Medical Association*, 270, 470-3.

Study links HIV, STD Infection Risk With Rape for Poor, Urban Women. (1995). *Nation's Health*, 25(4), 11.

Tarasoff v. Regents of the University of California. (1976). 551 P.2d 347.

The Current Global Situation of the HIV/AIDS Pandemic. (1994). *Weekly Epidemiology Record*, 69, 191-92.

US Public Health Service Recommendations for HIV Counseling and Testing for Pregnant Women. (February 23, 1995). DRAFT guidelines.

Voelker, R. (1995). Foes of Mandatory Maternal HIV Testing Fear Guidelines Will Lead to Reprisals. *Journal of the American Medical Association*, 273 (13), 977.

What's News: US Officials. (May 12, 1995). *Wall Street Journal*, A1.

Wiley, J. and Samuel, M.(1989). Prevalence of HIV Infection in the U. S. A. *AIDS* (suppl), 571-578.

We Are A Part of All That We Have Met: Women and AIDS

Lynn Morrison and Sepali Guruge

"I am a part of all that I have met"
— Alfred, Lord Tennyson

Introduction

Reproductive and sexual health in women is determined not only by biological factors but by a complex interplay of social, cultural, economic, and political factors each of which is steeped in a historical context. At no time has this become more evident than during the HIV epidemic. Women, largely ignored in the past, are now being diagnosed at an ever-increasing rate. Some researchers estimate that by the year 2000, 38-110 million people worldwide may become infected with HIV (Mann et al., 1992). Approximately 75% of HIV transmission is through heterosexual intercourse (Mann et al., 1992), a statistic that will likely continue to increase. Women are at a greater risk for HIV infection than men both physiologically and socially (de Bruyn 1992; Carovano 1991; O'Malley & Ridley, 1993; Pizzi, 1992; Whipple 1992). As of 1992, it was estimated that nearly five million women were either infected, ill, or already dead because of HIV (Reid, 1992). Yet, women are still misdiagnosed, under-represented, and denied the medical attention and social support they deserve and have the right to expect.

The escalating rate of HIV among women is a particularly dramatic example of the historical neglect women's health issues have received from the medical, behavioral, and social sciences. This long legacy has had tragic consequences. An examination of historical sources shows that the stigma attached to women as carriers of sexually transmitted diseases is not unprecedented; women have had to bear this burden in decades and centuries past. Indeed, not only are we a part of all that we have met as individuals, but also as a gender. We must learn from our collective histories, act in the present and plan for the future.

WOMEN, SEX AND HISTORY

One cannot ignore the many similarities between AIDS today and sexually transmitted diseases (STDs) in the past.[1] Before the advent of antibiotics, syphilis was the most dreaded, and, if left untreated, fatal sexually transmitted disease (Fee, 1988). Syphilis, like AIDS, precipitated deep-rooted fears surrounding sexuality and disease (Brandt, 1988). The societal conception of syphilis was equated with fear, immorality, and "scapegoatism," defined here as the act of discriminating against and blaming other individuals or groups for the spread of HIV. AIDS has evoked similar responses including the unfounded condemnation of already marginalized groups such as prostitutes, homosexuals, IV drug users, and people from different ethnic backgrounds or countries.[2] Not only is a dichotomy created between the "ill" and the "well" (McCullum, 1992), but that dichotomy is socially reconstructed as the "bad" and the "good."[3] Those judged by the masses to have contracted HIV through no "moral" fault of their own i.e., individuals who had "few" sexual partners or contracted the virus through a blood transfusion, are lumped with the "good" while those who acquired it via "promiscuous" sex or injection drug use, are lumped with the "bad."

A society's attitudes and beliefs towards many issues including sexual behaviour (Morton, 1990a) and disease are often reflected through artistic media. Although stylistically images differ over time, themes are recurrent and can be transposed from one century to the next. Women have long been depicted as the source of contamination, completely denying and obfuscating men's role in sexual relationships or networks. Figure 1 illustrates the strong sentiment felt towards women with syphilis as the head of a syphilitic prostitute is brought in on a platter as an offering of blame. As early as the 18th and 19th centuries, women were portrayed as the "deceivers," hoodwinking "innocent" men into sexual play (see Figure 2).[4] Interestingly, the same theme recurs in a poster produced some 200 years later regarding HIV/AIDS (see Figure 3). Not only are women grievously portrayed as the transmitters of a

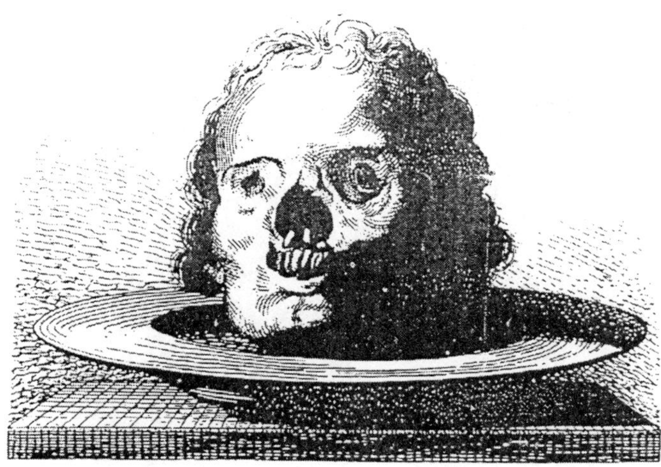

Figure 1. *AIDS and Syphilis: The Iconography of Disease* by Sander L/ Gilman. From "AIDS: Cultural Analysis/Cultural Activism" by D. Crimp (ed.), 1988, Cambridge, MA: MIT Press, p.96.

disease, but in their skeletal manifestations, they are portrayed as death itself. More importantly, these images illustrate how stunted progress has been in dealing with sexuality, disease, and what is often misplaced morality.

By the 1860s, blaming women went beyond social censure to legal censure. Discriminatory measures such as the Contagious Diseases Act of 1864 were introduced in England as a preventive measure which allowed for the arrest, physical examination and detention of women thought to spread syphilis and gonorrhea (Amstey, 1994; Littlewood & Mahood, 1991; Morton, 1990b). Similar acts were also being enacted in the rest of Europe and generally did not apply to men. McLaren (1991) states, "...the legislation clearly infringed on individual rights and unabashedly sustained the sexual double-standard; women were examined, men were not." This attitude was in keeping with the Victorian view of prostitutes as greedy and vain women suffering from personal "character flaws" rather than a social problem steeped in poverty and lack of education (Littlewood & Mahood, 1991).

In a further contradiction of sensibilities, the chaste Victorian woman was kept on a pedestal of piety and respectability by the men in her society (Nead, 1988). This view, however, was in contrast to how women were actually treated as Figure 4 illustrates. Woman may have been the "...queen of humanity..." but she nevertheless had to be subservient to the man in her life. Those very same men who wanted chaste wives also frequented prostitutes but still gave themselves licensure to stand in moral judgement of women giving further accreditation to the double-standard. Women were thus put on a pedestal of virtuosity empowered to control men's libidos in sharp contrast to the subservient role

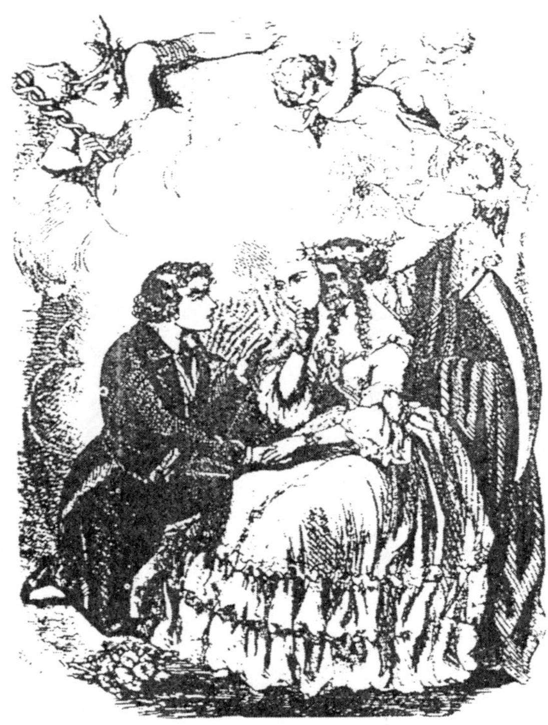

Figure 2. *AIDS and Syphilis: The Iconography of Disease* by Sander L/ Gilman. From "AIDS: Cultural Analysis/Cultural Activism" by D. Crimp (ed.), 1988, Cambridge, MA: MIT Press, p.97.

they actually held. One could argue that the very same notion persists today.

The attitude which dichotomizes women into "good" and "bad" denies society's responsibility for the demand that exists for prostitutes and the lack of many other options these women face regardless of the century they live in. Not only do they bear the brunt of society's neglect but are often made responsible for the occupational hazards they must face. These hazards include an increased exposure to STDs, exploitation, violence, assault, and rape.

The category of prostitution was and still is very ill-defined (Littlewood & Mahood, 1991).[5] We can begin to appreciate the difficulty in talking about women and sexuality without incorporating prostitution into the discourse. There does not seem to be a very clear distinction between women and prostitutes since a woman's membership into one group or the other is often mutually exclusive and largely based on the moral scrutiny of that particular time period. A woman who passes the moral test remains (just) a woman, but one who does not pass the various imposed social standards of that time period or culture becomes a "fallen" woman, or a "prostitute," and is rarely referred to again as a "woman." Her primary label is that of prostitute.

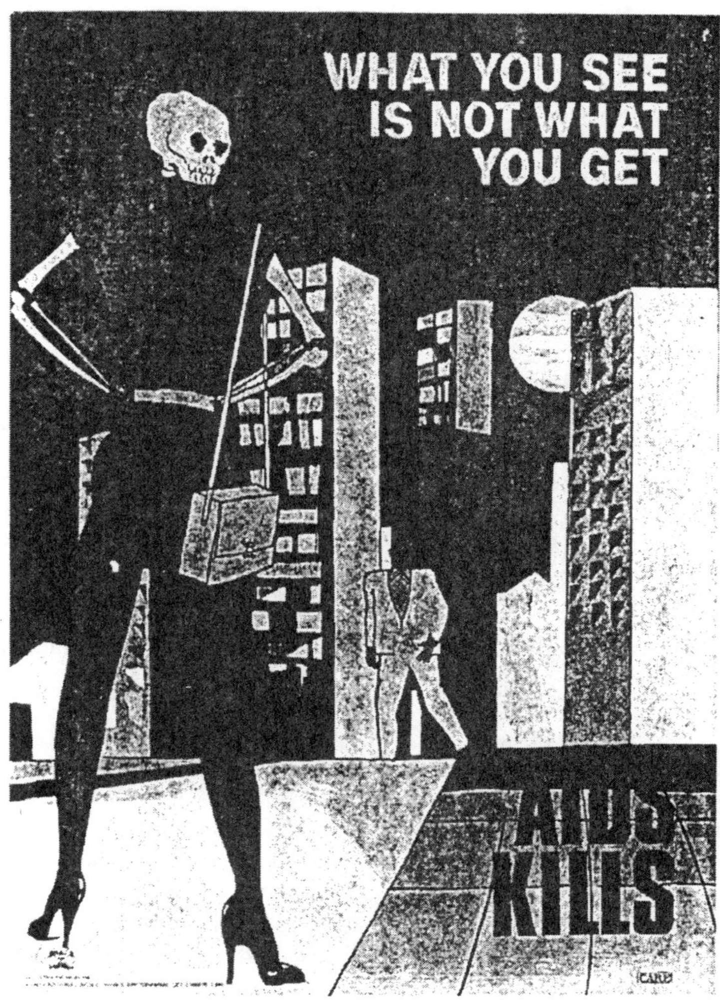

Figure 3. From *"Women and HIV/AIDS"* by Marge Berer and Sunanda Ray (eds.), 1993 London: Pandora Press, p.41.

Early Twentieth Century

The social construction of morality regarding STDs continued throughout the 1900s and was particularly evident during World War I. Soldiers afflicted with syphilis were regarded as the innocent victims while prostitutes were blamed for their defilement. (Brandt, 1988; Thibierge, 1918). Barmaids, waitresses, and laundresses are indentified as ". . . sources of contagion . . . " who " . . . give themselves up to clandestine prostitution . . ." (Thibierge, 1918, p. 11). By 1915, 28.7 percent of men in the Canadian forces had an STD (Cassel, 1987). Women were again regarded as a source of temptation/infection to be "eliminated" for the protection of the men.

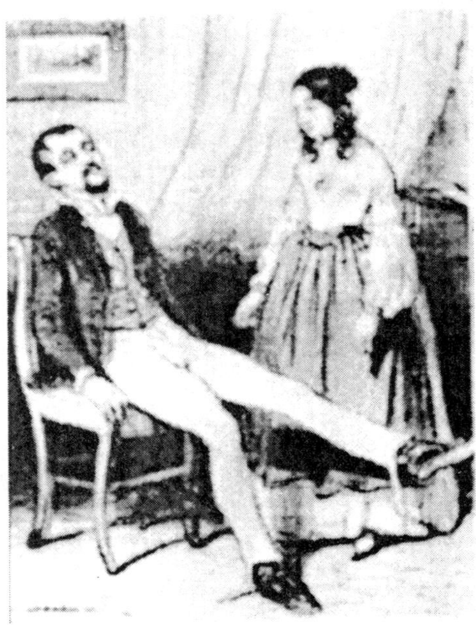

Figure 4. "Oh, woman! Masterpiece of creation, queen of humanity, mother of the human race...Take my boots off!" by Reay Tannahill, 1992, NY: Stein and Day/Publishers, p.391.

Reminiscent of the Contagious Diseases Act of the 1860s, these staggering statistics once again prompted the institutionalization of infected women (Sanger, 1939). In fact, the stringent measures the United States took in controlling sexually transmitted diseases which included denying women their civil rights, having them quarantined, and publicly identifying them with a placard on their door denouncing their diseased status was applauded (Amstey, 1994). The underlying assumption was that women would purposely continue to infect men but that the reverse did not or would not occur; that men would not knowingly infect women or put them at risk for infection. Sanger (1939), writing on the history of prostitution, states "The summit of ambition with [women] is to keep their liberty; so long as they can earn enough to provide themselves shelter, and feed their ravenous appetite for intoxicating liquor, they are content to submit to the pains and ravages of syphilis, alike heedless of their own sufferings and the injuries they inflict on others" (p.646). This attitude denies men's responsibility in the transmission of STDs.

Numerous medical discoveries made in the last few decades before World War II placed an even greater emphasis on hygiene and sanitation which was relegated to the woman's domain. Figure 5 reveals the extent to which the societal expectation regarding women, dirt, and cleanliness permeated. Although not directly related to STDS, this image illustrates the social con-

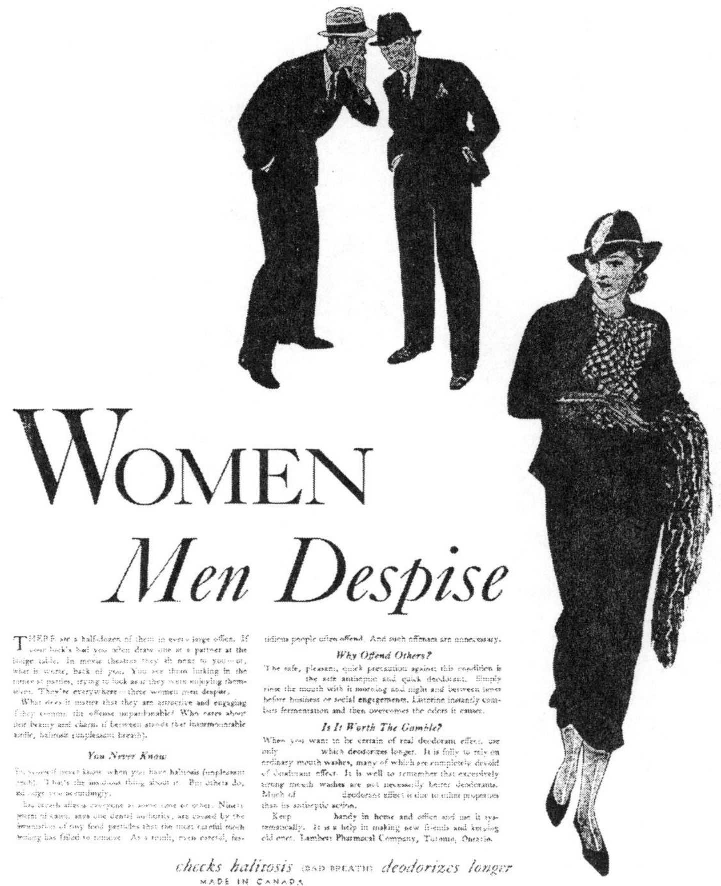

Figure 5. From "Chatelaine" June 1935, p.1 (In agreement with the present-day manufacturer, the product name was deleted.)

text within which women found themselves. Similarly, Chatelaine published a Lysol advertisement in 1928 entitled "It's *worry* - not *work* that ages a woman." The advertisement continues:

> Worry and nerves, in so many cases, are a woman's own faults.
>
> Neglect of the proper care of herself, or misunderstanding of the facts about personal hygiene, often lead to listlessness, premature old age, needlessly unhappy marriage.
>
> Don't experiment in this critical, vital matter. Use "Lysol" Disinfectant.

If men could "despise" women for having bad breath or poor hygiene, for being "unclean," what chance did women have in such a judgmental society in escaping the blame for spreading STDs? What disinfectant could be applied to those women and why were men not held accountable for their bad breath, unhappy marriages, or their responsibility in transmitting STDs? The social construction of cleanliness penetrated deeply and women were allowed very few transgressions. The indelible link between women and cleanliness was used to further subordinate women by adding more stigma to an already heavy burden.

By the 1940s, the "dirt" could still not be removed. Public health campaigns mounted to combat STDs even alluded to the "all-American girl" being the all-American deceiver out to get those otherwise righteously clean young men (see figure 6), again denying men's culpability. During both the syphilis and the AIDS epidemic, chastity and virtuosity were and have been espoused by the public and religious sectors not only as a means of protection but as a reason to blame those infected. In essence, those who chose not to have chaste lives deserved what they got.

Late Twentieth Century to the Present

It is the historical construction of sexuality, disease, blame, and "scapegoatism" that has resulted in women being so deeply affected by HIV. History does indeed repeat itself with dire consequences. Although current research shows that women are at greater risk for contracting HIV than men, they are still largely regarded only in their role as transmitters or "vectors" of the virus (de Bruyn, 1992; Carovano, 1991; Overall, 1991; Smeltzer, 1992).

The term vector, which appears in the medical and behavioral literature regarding women and HIV, is inappropriately used as it is a term reserved for the various arthropods which act as transmitters of parasitic diseases. Most notable are the malaria and yellow fever parasites which are transmitted by mosquitos. In these cases, the "vectors" are often not affected by the disease making the analogy of women as vectors of HIV that much more damning.

The "spread to heterosexuals" seems to imply the spread to heterosexual men, not heterosexual women (Overall, 1991) even though in Canada, 59.4% of HIV+ women acquired the virus heterosexually (Quarterly surveillance update, 1995). When women are depicted it is often because of their connection to men and children (Carovano, 1991; Krieger & Margo 1991; Overall, 1991). The concern is not so much for the women themselves, but for their child-bearing capabilities and their sexual interactions with men. Too many AIDS prevention programs for women have targeted pre-natal women or women in the sex industry. AIDS prevention efforts for mothers and prostitutes are really aimed at the protection of men and children (de Bruyn, 1992; Carovano, 1991). Krieger and Margo (1991) succinctly state, "Utterly ignored, if not deliberately negated, is the possibility that women might be autonomous, sexually active beings whose right and need to be pro-

SHE MAY LOOK CLEAN—BUT
PICK-UPS
"GOOD TIME" GIRLS
PROSTITUTES
SPREAD SYPHILIS AND GONORRHEA

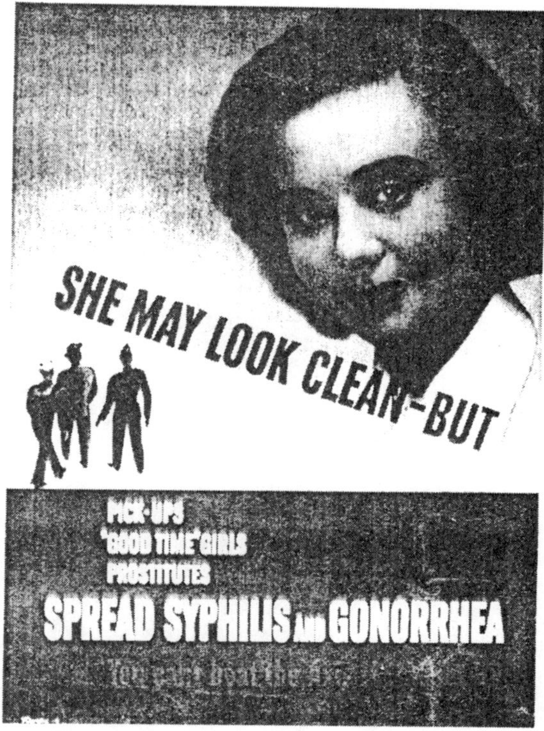

Figure 6. From "History of Syphilis" by Claude Quetel, translated by J. Braddock and B. Pike, 1990, Cambridge: Polity Press, p.190.

tected from HIV infection is as legitimate and necessary as that of children and men" (p.128).

WOMEN AND THEIR MANY SPHERES

At the crux of the matter is not only *how* women are depicted but *why* they are depicted merely as "vectors." Fundamental to the problem of women's negative, or at best, inconsequential, portrayal are issues of disempowerment and inequity which affect women worldwide and are present, in varying degrees, in many societies, cultures, and households. Women who are at most risk for HIV/AIDS are those women who are likely to have the least control over their bodies and lives (Carovano, 1991). As in earlier decades and centuries, many women are socially, educationally, and economically disadvantaged. This has impacted on the many spheres of women's lives including lack of diagnostic criteria for women and AIDS (Allen and Marte, 1992; Denenberg, 1991; Hitt, 1991; Smeltzer, 1992), moral and legal censure of a woman's ability to reproduce (Hunter, 1995; Overall, 1991), and general lack of control and autonomy of her life on a daily basis.

Biological Sphere

Only as of 1993 did Canada and the United States add cervical cancer and bacterial pneumonia, opportunistic infections specific to women, to the official case definition for AIDS. Until that time the case definition was largely based on opportunistic infections seen mostly in men. There still exists a wide range of gynecological manifestations not yet accurately represented or given proper diagnostic recognition resulting in poor overall health-care management of HIV+ women (Allen & Marte, 1992; Brettle & Leen, 1991). Moreover, many health-care professionals do not recognize tell-tale gynecological problems as manifestations of HIV. Women have been dying of AIDS without fitting the case definition which means they received inadequate medical care,may not have had access to medication such as AZT, or could not participate in drug trials (Hunter, 1995; Overall, 1991).

Reproductive Sphere

As in the past, when women were blamed for transmitting syphilis to their infants, there exists today the social condemnation of women who inadvertently transmit HIV to their unborn children. This has resulted in pressure put on present-day women for screening, counselling, and mandatory actions such as termination of pregnancy or use of medications such as AZT to reduce risk of perinatal transmission (Denenberg 1991; Hunter, 1995; Smeltzer, 1992). Some states in the United States have suggested or are considering legislation that would require pregnant women to be tested for HIV infection in an effort to decrease the incidence of pediatric AIDS (Hunter 1995; Smeltzer, 1992). The unspoken presumption of such considerations is that once pregnant and determined to be HIV+, there are no options to absolutely ensure decreasing the risk of HIV transmission to the infant except to abort. A basic infringement on women's rights, this completely neglects the value women, and cultures as a whole, place on fertility.

The medical and legal establishments are dealing with the end product — a fetus — while ignoring why women want to get pregnant. The ability and desire to conceive is not simply part of women's physical evolution but is deeply ingrained in our cultural evolution. In many women's lives, motherhood is equated with status, security, self-esteem, and validation (Campbell, 1990; Carovano, 1991; Williams, 1990). The problem with current AIDS prevention strategies which include using condoms, having non-penetrative sex, or not having sex at all also means no conception. Society has not provided a valid role for women that does not include childbearing (Carovano, 1991). Until we broaden our understanding of the high value placed on fertility, telling women to use condoms is not realistic and may well be regarded as paternalistic.

Social and Economic Spheres

Socioeconomic precursors such as patriarchal societies, racism, and poverty place women at high risk for HIV (Shroff, 1992). For many women, sex is associated with coercion, violence, disease, employment, power, or procreation. As Ward (1991) eloquently states, "Sex often means prostitution, sexual bargaining, sexual marketing and exploitation before it means poetry, orgasm, or personal fulfilment" (p.298). Therefore, to tell women, either explicitly or implicitly, to practice safer sex completely disregards the context within which women live and their world-view. Women face a much greater problem than simply convincing the men in their lives to wear condoms. They face a deeply-ingrained and societally supported inequity between the sexes that has evolved over millennia.

Given the high incidence of sex-related violence against women, women's perceived risks to their social and economic survival impact on their decision to introduce safer sex (Worth, 1989). For many women who are not in an egalitarian relationship, survival is based on short term needs such as obtaining household money for food, securing her living arrangements, protecting her children, and avoiding violent outbursts (Worth, 1989). In some instances, the *immediate* repercussions of introducing safer sex with a partner may very well outweigh the benefits of protecting herself from a *possible* future cost of HIV illness. Telling women to practice safer sex does not necessarily empower them to do so and may even exacerbate situations in which men react violently (Overall, 1991; Worth, 1991). Holloway (1994), a staff writer for *Scientific American,* emphasizes "Improving women's health means overhauling attitudes towards sex and addressing hidden epidemics, such as domestic violence" (p.77).

AIDS is a human rights issue as it regards not only unequal access to education, employment, and health care between men and women but also between rich and poor, and majority and minority groups on a global scale. Although women in developed countries are sometimes perceived as having greater equality, the sexual sphere still remains a frontier to be conquered from male dominion. Individual control and autonomy over one's life is highly dependent upon that individual's circumstances. It does not appear that AIDS education has been any more or less successful in one country or another based on its level of development. Further, many developed countries have large immigrant populations who are in the midst of transition and are experiencing the inevitable difficulties in adjusting to a new and unfamiliar country. The issues of disempowerment may be exacerbated in a foreign country where familial support is lacking leaving some women to rely on their husbands to an even greater extent. The lack of power and autonomy are part of an ever-changing continuum which transcends temporal, cultural, and familial boundaries.

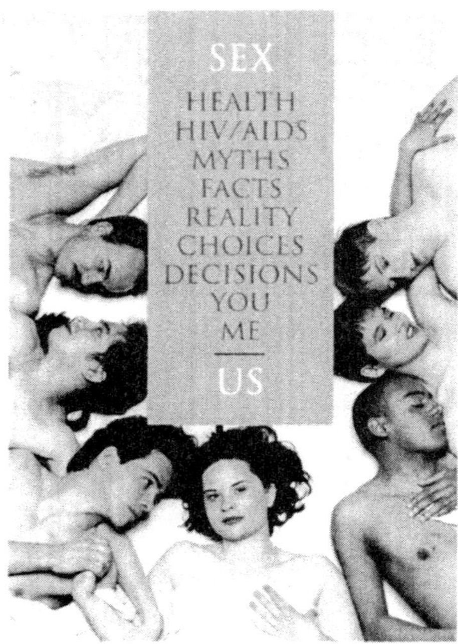

Figure 7. Poster and pamphlet produced by the Ryerson AIDS Education Project, Ryerson Polytechnic University, August 1994.

Plans for the Future

In order to challenge this long legacy towards women's health issues, research and education must address the empowerment of women, their perceptions of sexuality, and the impact men have on their lives. We can begin to appreciate that the various spheres of women's health and HIV are inextricably linked.

Research

Even when women acknowledge themselves as being at risk, they experience difficulty in using barriers to prevent HIV transmission (Bury, 1992). Holloway (1994) encapsulates this pervasive dilemma in the following statement:

> Social customs, health policies and a largely male medical community have tended to treat women as wives or wombs and little else. Consequently, as chronicled in report after report, aspects of women's health have received minimal attention or funding. Upgrading women's health entails, in large part, reexamining sexuality and cultural mores; it entails improving male and adolescent sexual health; it entails involving men. Put simply, securing women's health means social transformation. (p.77)

Somebody else in your picture?
GET IT ON
EVERYBODY
EVERYTIME

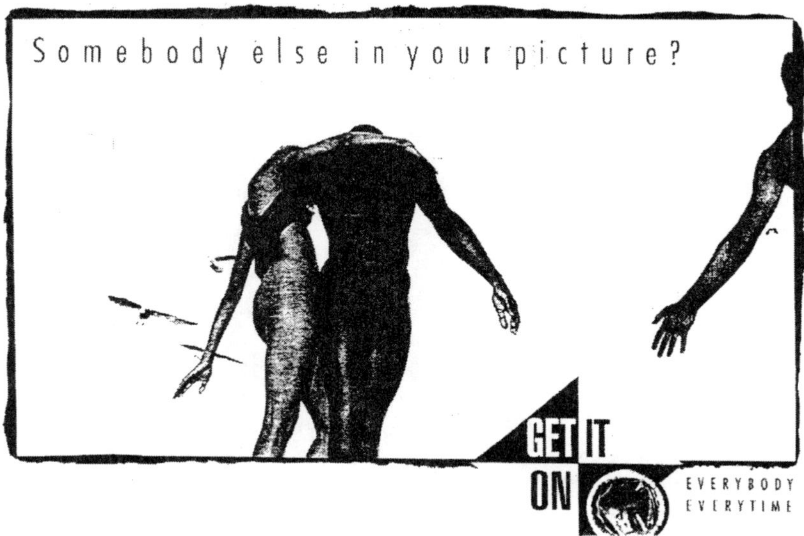

Figure 8. Poster produced by the Black Coalition for AIDS Prevention, the AIDS Committee of Toronto, and the Black Gay and Lesbian Discussion. reprinted with permission from BlackCAP.

Research must investigate sexual decision-making, sexual exchanges, and the social and cultural norms that support these. Women's attitudes towards their own sexuality and the ambivalence some women feel about the role they play within a sexual encounter may be the most important factor in AIDS prevention (Bury, 1992).

It is time to go a step beyond education towards empowerment in an attempt to foster healthy sexuality among women and between genders. Education, as a preventative strategy, has been saturated. Giving people the information does not elicit behavioral change. Messages bearing the words "have safer sex" do not address the issues of why people do not or cannot have safer sex (Morrison, 1994). Researchers need to look at a comprehensive approach to the political economy of health to find the underlying causes of the AIDS epidemic in all cultures. Specifically, what can we learn about women's lives and the context within which they live to empower them to change their behavior and maintain a healthier sexuality? What do we know about men that will also change their perceptions of women and their outlook and behavior regarding sexuality? What do we know of their influence over women, their sexuality, sexual decision-making, and sexual practices including safer sex? Under what conditions and circumstances will men and women practice safer sex and what motivates them to do so? Relationships are dyadic and change will not be affected if we focus on just one gender (Morrison, 1994). The focus should be on people's sexual behavior in its totality.

MORE WOMEN ARE BUYING MENSWEAR. It's not taboo. It's smart.
More women are buying condoms because they can prevent the spread of HIV – the virus that causes AIDS. But we don't want this to be a case of 'all action and no talk'. Because a large part of the population is unaware of the risk.
So talk. To your partner, your family, and your friends. If word spreads quickly, the virus won't.

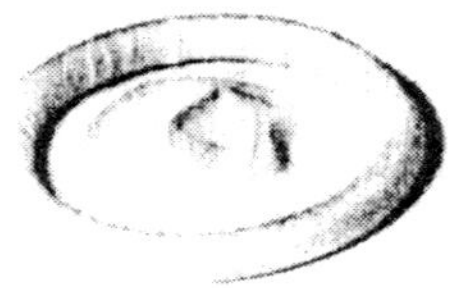

Figure 9. Reprint with permission of the Canadian Public Health Association and Alberta Health's HIV/AIDS Prevention Program for Young Adults.

To talk about sexuality and safer sex openly, to empower both women and men to engage in healthier sex and to respect each other's choices is not a moral issue; it is a human right that would go a long way in bridging the gap between men and women. Wright and Mackereth (1993), writing from a nursing perspective, state "The stress placed on `family values' and `moral behavior' at the expense of giving facts about how to make having sex and injecting drugs safer is a refusal to wake up to the reality of what some people do with their bodies. If clean needles, free condoms and information on safer sex are not available, then more people and their partners risk becoming infected." (p.33).

Women around the world are affected by AIDS.
We are caregivers. We are women living with AIDS.
We are mothers and sisters.
We are friends and lovers.

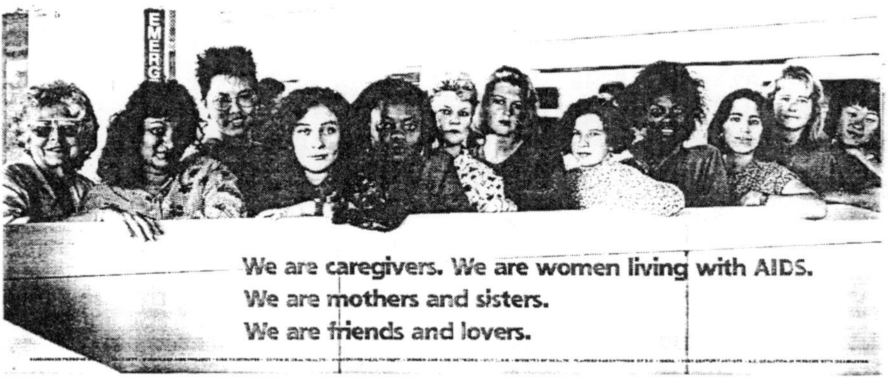

Figure 10. Poster produced by numerous governmental agencies in British Columbia. Reprinted with permission from Pacific AIDS Resources Centre.

Education

Policy-makers and AIDS activists also need to be aware of the different cultures that exist within their societies. For example, the City of Toronto gives multilateral funding to approximately 50 agencies and community organizations that target various groups who receive AIDS education, prevention, and counselling in their own language and in a way that was developed specifically for them. These highly community-oriented projects take into account cultural, religious, and medical beliefs as well as the priority AIDS prevention may have in the lives of new immigrants relative to the numerous other problems they may be encountering.

A major factor that inhibits HIV/AIDS prevention is people's lack of perception of themselves as being at risk (Stockdale et al., 1989). Added to this is the fact that there is a continuing tendency to refer to "high risk groups" and to attribute blame which allow people to believe AIDS as a disease that other people get. It is the responsibility of AIDS educators, policy-makers, and funders to make safer sex everybody's issue. People must take responsibility for their own health and their partner's health. Visual images must be all-inclusive to represent the multi-cultural and multi-sexual societies we live in (see Figures 7 and 8). Some campaigns have already contributed to the elimination of old stereotypes (see Figures 9 and 10) and are instrumental in paving the way for a more progressive approach to AIDS education and prevention that is not dependent on blame, stereotypes, and the kind of "scapegoatism" we have seen in the past.

Conclusion

As we have seen in the past, women being held responsible for not only their own sexuality, which is often out of their control, but also for men's sexuality is not a novel situation. What has been occurring with women and AIDS in the last 15 years is a mirror-image of how women, sexuality, and disease have been portrayed in past decades and centuries. Not only are women blamed for the transmission of STDs but a deliberate intent to do so is implicit in many of the graphic depictions.

This historical legacy has resulted in the neglect of health, medical, and social/cultural issues for women in the current HIV/AIDS epidemic. It is the reason why stereotypes dichotomizing women into `good' and `bad' have evolved and persisted; why women's symptoms were not included in the case definition until 1993; and why AIDS education and prevention, in its simplicity, neglected the deeply imbedded and intertwined spheres of women's lives. HIV infection in women is a serious and unrelenting problem. Women who are at risk for HIV come from all walks of life and therefore, their issues cross all economic, religious, geographical, and cultural boundaries.

Although we may be a part of all that we have met, the ingenuity, creativity, and resourcefulness exists within all cultures and age groups to change the direction of this long historical legacy. Women and men must stand up, speak out, and work together because we are fighting for a much deeper issue than just HIV/AIDS. Women are struggling to be counted as fully autonomous human beings in all the spheres of their lives be they medical, political, economic, or social. Whether the multiple labels women wear include mother, wife, girlfriend, care-taker, nurse, secretary, laborer, commercial sex-worker, or executive-director, we can pass on a much more positive legacy to future generations.

Notes

1. Many of the early accounts refer to sexually transmitted diseases as venereal diseases or VD. For the sake of uniformity, all references to venereal diseases will be regarded as sexually transmitted disease.
2. The judgement passed upon Haitians as a "risk group" is a particularly poignant example. See Farmer's exposé in *AIDS and Accusation: Haiti and the Geography of Blame.* Los Angeles, Ca.: University of California Press.
3. See Carovano 1991 and Schneider and Jenness 1995 for a more in-depth discussion of the "good girl/bad girl" complex.
4. Gilman (1988) uses figures 1 and 2 in his chapter "AIDS and Syphilis: The Iconography of Disease" to trace the social construction of syphilis and its similarities to AIDS. The author gives particular attention to those afflicted by either disease and how society portrays them.
5. The social construction of prostitution and the problems associated with using the term broadly transcend temporal and geographical boundaries. At one extreme a prostitute may be someone who sells sex for money as his/her primary

profession. At the other extreme, it may refer to a person who exchanges/barters sex for something that is essential to that person's survival whether it be on a short-term or long-term basis.

References

Allen, M.H. and Marte C. (March 15, 1992). Presentations and Protocols. *Hospital Practice,* 155-162.

Amstey, M.S. (1994). The Political History of Syphilis and its Application to the AIDS Epidemic. *Women's Health Issues,* (1), 16-19.

Berer, M. with Ray, S. (1993). *Woman and HIV/AIDS.* London: Pandora Press.

Brettle, R.P. and Leen L. S. (1991). The Natural History of HIV in Women. *AIDS, 5,* 1283-1292.

de Bruyn, M. (1992). Women and AIDS in Developing Countries. *Soc.Sci. Med, 34*(3), 249-262.

Brandt, A.M. (1988). AIDS from Social History to Social Policy. In E. Fee & D.M. Fox (Eds.), *AIDS: The Burdens of History.* California: University of California Press.

Bury, J. (1992). Education and the Prevention of HIV Infection. In J. Bury, E. Morrison, and S. McLachlan (Eds.), *Working with Women and AIDS* (pp.99-109). NY: Tavistock/Routledge.

Campbell, C. A. (1990). Women and AIDS. *Soc. Sci. Med.,* 30(4), 407-415.

Carovano, K. (1991). More Than Mothers and Whores: Redefining the AIDS Prevention Needs of Women. *International Journal of Health Services, 21*(1),131-142.

Cassel, J. (1987). *The Secret Plague: Venereal Disease in Canada 1838-1939.* Toronto: University of Toronto.

Denenberg, R. (1991). Pregnancy and HIV. *Treatment Issues, 5*(6), 6-10.

Fee, E. (1988). Sin Versus Science: Venereal Disease in Twentieth-century Baltimore. In E. Fee & D.M. Fox (Eds.), *AIDS: The Burdens of History* (pp.121-146). California: University of California Press.

Gilman, S. L. (1988). AIDS and Syphilis: The Iconography of Disease. In D. Crimp (Ed.), *AIDS: Cultural Analysis/cultural Activism* (pp.86-107). Cambridge, MA: The MIT Press.

Hitt, R.S. (Sept. 1991). Women and HIV: What do We Know?. *Being Alive 8 Newsletter.*

Holloway, M. (August 1994). Trends in Women's Health: A Global View. *Scientific American,* 76-83.

Hunter, N.D. (1995). Complications of Gender: Women, AIDS, and the Law. In B.E. Schneider and N.E.Stoller (Eds.), *Women Resisting AIDS: Feminist Strategies of Empowerment* (pp. 32-56). Philadelphia: Temple University Press.

Krieger, N. and Margo G. (1991). Women and AIDS: Introduction. *International Journal of Health Services, 21*(1), 127-130.

Littlewood, B. and Mayhood L. (1991). Prostitutes, Magdalenes and Wayward Girls: Dangerous Sexualities of Working Class Women in Victorian Scotland. *Gender and History, 3*(2), 160-175.

Mann, J., Tarantola, D. J. M. and Netter, T. W. (Eds.)(1992). A *Global Report: AIDS in the World.* Cambridge, MA: Harvard University Press.

McCullum, C. (1992). Disease and Dirt: Social Dimensions of Influenza, Cholera, and Syphilis. *The Pharos, 55*(1), 22-29.

McLaren, A. (1991). Book Reviews. Gender and History, 3, 224-227.

Morrison, L. (1994). *The Flipside: Anthropological Contributions to Women's Health Issues.* Paper presented at the Canadian Anthropology Society/Societe Canadienne d'Anthropologie, University of British Colombia, Vancouver, B.C.

Morton, R.S. (1990a). Syphilis in Art: An Entertainment in Four Parts. Part 1. *Genitourinary Medicine, 66*(1), 33-40.

Morton, R.S. (1990b). Syphilis in Art: An Entertainment in Four Parts. Part 4. *Genitourinary Medicine, 66*(4), 280-294.

Nead, L. (1988). *Myths of Sexuality, Representation of Women in Victorian Britain.* Oxford: Basil Blackwell Ltd.

O'Malley, K. and K. Ridley (1993). Women Living with AIDS. *The AIDS report.* Massachusetts: Harvard AIDS Institute.

Overall, C. (1991). AIDS and Women: The (Hetero)-sexual Politics of HIV Infection. In C.Overall and W.Zinn (Eds.) *Perspective on AIDS: Ethical and Social Issues* (pp. 27-42). Oxford University Press.

Pizzi, M. (1992). Women, HIV Infection and AIDS: Tapestries of Life, Death, and Empowerment. *The American Journal of Occupational Therapy, 46*(11), 1021-1027.

Quarterly Surveillance Update: AIDS in Canada (Jan. 1995). Division of HIV/AIDS Epidemiology. Bureau of Communicable Disease. Epidemiology Laboratory Centre for Disease Control Health Canada: Ottawa.

Quetel, C. (1990). *History of Syphilis.* Translated by J. Braddock and B. Pike. Cambridge: Polity Press.

Reid, E. (1992). Gender, Knowledge, and Responsibility. In J. Mann, D.J.M. Tarantola & T.W. Netter (Eds.), *AIDS in the World: A Global Report* (pp.657-667). Cambridge: Harvard University Press.

Sanger, W. W. (1939). *The History of Prostitution.* New York: Eugenic Publishing Co.

Schneider, B.E. and Jenness, V. (1995). Social Control, Civil Liberties, and Women's Sexuality. In B.E. Schneider and N.E. Stoller (Eds.), *Women Resisting AIDS: Feminist Strategies of Empowerment.* Philadelphia: Temple University Press.

Shroff, F.M. (1992). The Social Construction of AIDS, Heterosexism, Racism and Misogyny: The Challenges Facing Women of Color. *RFR/DRF, 20*(3/4), 115-122.

Smeltzer, S. C. (1992). Women and AIDS: Sociopolitical Issues. *Nursing Outlook, 40*(4), 152-157.

Stockdale, J.E., Dockrell, J.E. and Wells, A.J. (1989). The Self in Relation to Mass Media Representations of HIV and AIDS - Match or Mismatch? *Health Education Journal, 48*(3), 121-130.

Tannahill, R. (1992). *Sex in History.* NY: Stein and Day Publishers. P.390.

Thibierge, G. (1918). *Syphilis and the Army.* C.F. Marshall (Ed.). London: University of London Press Ltd. pp. 7-15.

Ward, M.C. (1991). Cupid's Touch: The Lessons of the Family Planning Movement for the AIDS Epidemic. *Journal of Sex Research, 28*(2), 289-305

Whipple, B.(1992). Issues Concerning Women and AIDS: Sexuality. *Nursing Outlook, 20*(5), 203-206

Williams, A. B. (1990). Reproductive Concerns of Women At Risk for HIV Infection. *Journal of Nurse-Midwifery, 35*(5),292-298

Worth, D. (1989). Sexual Decision-making and AIDS: Why Condom Promotion Among Vulnerable Women is Likely to Fail. *Studies In Family Planning, 20*(6), 297-307.

Wright, S. and P. Mackereth, P. (1993). Waking Up to Reality. *Nursing Times, 89*(26): 32-33.

Part Four

Education and Prevention

INTRODUCTION

At present, there is no cure or vaccine for HIV/AIDS. The effort to reduce the rate of HIV infection should be directed to education and prevention strategies to encourage changes of behavior. The articles in this section examine the cultural impediments to effective education in preventing HIV infection and suggests strategies that may enhance acceptance and the practice of positive health behavior for HIV prevention by specific populations.

In "Overcoming Barriers in HIV/AIDS Education for Asian Americans: Toward More Effective Cultural Communication," Gust A. Yep identifies and discusses some of the barriers associated with HIV/AIDS education for Asian Americans. He examines potential cultural, socio-cultural, psycho-cultural and communication barriers in HIV intervention. He also discusses ways of designing, implementing and evaluating culturally appropriate HIV/AIDS education programs for Asian Americans.

Gerjo Kok et al., in "Applying Social Psychology to HIV Prevention: Solving a Dilemma in the HIV Prevention Communication on Anal Sex as an Example," systematically applied different social psychological theories to HIV/AIDS prevention. They found that the application of the theories does not provide a simple solution to the dilemma but it focuses attention on the most relevant aspects of a possible solution. Their discussion focuses on the existence of high barriers to behavior change and the potential of continued improvement in intervention techniques. The authors suggest the need for tailored educational messages to overcome barriers to behavior changes.

Frank Machlica, in "HIV/AIDS Prevention Strategies Affecting Special Population," presents an overview of HIV/AIDS prevention and educational strategies that focus on special population groups in New York City. His discussion is directed to women of color, children, adolescents, the severely and persistently mentally ill, mentally ill chemical abusers, intravenous drug users, people with disabilities, immigrants and undocumented residents.

Janet L. Mitchell et al., in "AIDS in the Black/American Community: A Central Harlem Experience - 1989-1992," studied three groups of women targeted for enhanced delivery of health care services and education about

HIV transmission and prevention. The results indicate that women were more receptive to HIV/AIDS information when that information is integrated into the regular clinic activities and when their general health care needs are met. One-on-one risk reduction counseling may actually work most effectively with this population of high risk women. Data also show the need for increased provision of information about the availability and accessibility of free counseling and testing for HIV.

In "Relevant Measurement of HIV/AIDS Prevention Beliefs for African American Youth," Howard Stevenson and Helen Rupp studied beliefs about preventing AIDS among African American adolescents. The Beliefs About Preventing AIDS scale (Koopman et. al, 1990) was factor analyzed and a three factor solution best fit the data. The factors self-efficacy (SE), Self Control (SC), and Condom-Efficacy (CE) were used to differentiate between the sub-populations of the students. All three factors were positively correlated with AIDS knowledge. Religion was found to influence SE, and gender, sexual activity, and knowledge to influence social control (SC).

Ifeanyi Emenike, in "Sexual Abstinence: A Viable Option for Young Adolescents in HIV/AIDS Prevention," states that sexual abstinence is the best strategy for adolescents to adopt in preventing HIV transmission. He emphasizes that intervention to prevent associated negative health outcomes must address the very factors that influence the sexual behaviors of teenagers. These interventions should focus on increasing adolescents' competence in decision making, building social skills and social supports, and enhancing self-esteem. The development of these intervention strategies will enable adolescents to develop attitudes and abilities to withstand peer and social pressure toward sex.

Overcoming Barriers in HIV/AIDS Education for Asian-Americans: Toward More Effective Cultural Communication

Gust A. Yep

The HIV/AIDS epidemic is rapidly spreading in Asian American[1] communities in the United States (Aoki et al., 1989; Choi et al., 1995; Gock, 1994; Yep, 1993a, b, in press-a). In fact, Choi and associates (1995) observed that "the incidence of AIDS is increasing at a higher rate among Asian and Pacific Islanders than among whites" (p. 115). Such increase may be attributed to high-risk sexual behavior among Asian Americans reported in recent studies (e.g., Choi et al., 1995; Cochran et al., 1991; Fairbank et al., 1991). To motivate this population to engage in health protective behaviors, HIV/AIDS education programs have been developed and implemented (Aoki et al., 1989; Yep, 1993a, c). However, most of these programs have not addressed the cultural needs of Asian Americans (Choi et al., 1995; Yep, 1993a, in press-a).

Researchers and practitioners (e.g., Estrada, 1995; Jue, 1987; Michal-Johnson & Bowen, 1992; Weeks et al., 1995; Yep, 1993a, 1994a, in press-a) maintain that HIV/AIDS education is a cultural communication process. Michal-Johnson and Bowen (1992) succinctly captured the need to focus on culture: "HIV education and prevention efforts that take into account the cultural experiences of those who bear the disproportionate burden of AIDS have the best opportunity to offer believable messages and messengers in communities of color" (p. 147). In terms of Asian Americans, Choi and associates (1995) added, "any new education and risk-reduction efforts must effectively address ... [these] interconnected social and cultural issues" (p. 130).

Although some attempts have been made to provide guidelines for culturally appropriate HIV/AIDS education for Asian Americans (e.g., Yep, 1994a, b, in press-a), there appears to be no scientific literature that attempts to unify key cultural barriers and their implications for HIV education, prevention, and service delivery for this population. To partially fill this gap, this chapter attempts to identify some of the key cultural barriers by using Gudykunst and Kim's (1992) intercultural communication model as a unifying framework. More specifically, it: (a) examines potential cultural, sociocultural, psychocultural, and communication barriers in HIV interventions for Asian Americans, and (b) discusses ways of designing, implementing, and evaluating culturally appropriate HIV/AIDS education programs for this group. Finally, it explores potential avenues for future research.

Gudykunst and Kim's Intercultural Communication Model

As stated earlier, effective HIV/AIDS intervention programs for communities of color must take into account their cultural and social realities. Michal-Johnson and Bowen (1992) called HIV/AIDS education "a cultural communication process" (p.148) in which the health educator must carefully assess how cultural beliefs influence individual behavior and how cultural norms define gender roles, language use, and ways in which intimate partners talk and interact sexually and interpersonally. To understand this cultural communication process, Gudykunst and Kim (1992) proposed a unifying framework that isolates and identifies the factors influencing intercultural interaction. This widely adopted model posits that the creation and interpretation of messages is an interactive process influenced by conceptual filters including cultural, sociocultural, psychocultural, and communication factors.

The increase of HIV infection and AIDS-related infectious disease in Asian American communities remains largely unnoticed and untreated because of many cultural barriers preventing health education and action regarding HIV transmission, infection, prognosis, and treatment. In the following analysis, based on both review of the existing literature and findings from a forum examining cultural factors in HIV education for Asian Americans,[2] I will identify and discuss cultural, sociocultural, psychological, and communication barriers that inhibit awareness, education, and action for this group.

Cultural Barriers

These are obstacles to HIV/AIDS intervention that are associated with cultural values, norms, and assumptions. Three such factors were identified: (a) Individualism versus collectivism, (b) fatalism, and (c) shame.

The first is lack of individualism. Asian Americans come from more collectivistic cultures than their Euro-American counterparts (Aoki & Ja, 1987; Aoki et al., 1989; Choi et al., 1995; Jue, 1987; Lee & Fong, 1990; Reyes & Yep, in press-a; Yep, in press-b). In collectivistic cultural orientations, the social group such as the family or the community is more important than the individual person (Jue, 1987; Lee & Fong, 1990; Reyes & Yep, in press). Because individual thoughts and expression are of lesser importance than those of the larger social group, many Asian American individuals do not feel comfortable talking about personal issues including sexuality and HIV.

The second factor is fatalism. The perception that HIV infection is a matter of fate that cannot be controlled or prevented prevails among Asian Americans. According to anecdotal evidence, "If it is God's will" is quoted by many Asian Americans in relation to contracting the virus. Most Asian Americans do not discuss illness and death (Aoki et al., 1989; Jue, 1987). It is believed that if one talks about disease, it will become a self-fulfilling prophecy (Aoki & Ja, 1987). Thus, difficulty arises in conveying preventive education as people feel they have little control over their lives. By neglecting open discussions about disease, individuals impede progress in the prevention of HIV/AIDS through education.

The third cultural factor is shame (Carrier et al., 1992; Chan, 1989; Chang, 1993; Yep, in press-a). While Euro-Americans are often thought of being guilt-driven, it is often argued that Asian American cultures are more shame-regulated (Benedict, 1946/1989; Gagnon & Simon, 1973). Abramson (1986) noted that "while 'guilt' societies provide the opportunity for the atonement of one's sins... shame is a life long burden" (p. 4). This personal tendency or concern to act in such a way that one does not bring embarrassment or loss of face and honor to oneself and his/her social group can also be a major barrier in HIV/AIDS intervention (Chang, 1993). Many Asian American individuals are reluctant to discuss — not to mention disclose their serostatus — because of apprehension related to bringing shame to their own families (Aoki & Ja, 1987; Jue, 1987).

Sociocultural Barriers

The second category of barriers is sociocultural. These are obstacles associated with the individual's social relationships within a cultural environment. Four factors were identified: (a) family as a potential barrier, (b) sex, sexuality, and gender roles, (c) perceptions of sexuality, homosexuality, transgenderism/transsexuality, and HIV/AIDS-related stigma, and (d) denial of injecting drug use and sexual abuse.

The first potential sociocultural barrier is the family (Aoki et al., 1989; Choi et al., 1995; Jue, 1987; Morales, 1990; Reyes & Yep, in press; Yep, 1993a). Family ties are a strong social force in Asian American communities (Aoki & Ja, 1987; Reyes & Yep, in press). These ties can also be a barrier to HIV education. The traditional Asian American family is supposed to care for all family needs and the individual should not turn to outside sources for assistance. If one does, sensitive issues can be exposed and bring shame to a family especially when the individual is both gay and living with HIV infection. As stated earlier, the power dynamics of the Asian American family tend to de-emphasize individuality. Typically, the family is close and non-confrontational. It is assumed that the family will not abandon family members. Yet, individual needs and aspirations are secondary to the family. In addition, family care for a person living with AIDS (PLWA) is often conditional. Examples of conditional care by the family may include limiting contact with friends or not admitting contraction of the disease. The final outcome may be restriction of the individual's aspirations, needs, and feelings (Yep, 1993a).

The second sociocultural barrier is sex, sexuality, and gender roles within Asian American communities. Sexuality and gender roles are subjects not typically broached by many Asian Americans (Aoki et al., 1989; Yep, 1993a). It is assumed that individuals will automatically learn what sex is. Since sex itself is not discussed, the importance of safer sex and communication with one's partner are not talked about, especially by women. A power imbalance also exists between men and women in many traditional relationships. Women are typically viewed as either exotic or submissive, and may not have the personal resources to openly discuss sexuality with their partners. In addition, potentially high-risk activities involved in prostitution and massage parlors are silently accepted rather than openly discussed.

The third group of sociocultural barriers are perceptions of sexuality, homosexuality, transgenderism/transsexuality, and HIV/AIDS-related stigma. The reticence typically associated with discussion of sexuality among Asian Americans becomes more extreme with the subject of homosexuality, bisexuality, and transgenderism/transsexuality. Homosexuality is often denied in Asian American communities (Carrier et al., 1992; Chan, 1989; Chang, 1993; Choi et al., 1995; Lee & Fong, 1990; Reyes & Yep, in press; Wu & Pak, 1989; Yep, 1993a). Homosexual and bisexual behaviors are believed to be "Western phenomena" and outside the realm of Asian cultures (Jue, 1987; Lee & Fong, 1990). If people engage in homosexual behavior, they often do not identify themselves as "homosexual" or "bisexual" or have ambivalent and conflicted identities (Choi et al., 1995). This situation is further exacerbated for transgender and transsexual Asian Americans (Yep, 1994b). Denial of homosexuality and bisexuality hampers HIV and AIDS-related educational efforts because people engaging in potentially risky sexual behavior do not identify themselves as being at risk (Choi et al, 1995). Further, HIV/AIDS education in Asian American communities is difficult because of the relationship between "taboo subjects" and stigma attached to HIV/AIDS (Aoki et al., 1989; Chang, 1993; Yep, 1993c). For example, AIDS is seen as a "gay, white" (Lee & Fong, 1990, p. 18) disease; it can be literally translated from Chinese as a "white devil disease." The perception of AIDS as a Western epidemic gives Asian Americans the impression that the disease can be avoided by restricting contact with westerners (Jue, 1987; Lee & Fong, 1990). In addition, Asian American communities feel they have no ownership of the epidemic (Yep, 1994a). Because the virus is affiliated with taboo subjects such as homosexuality, death, and illness, it is very shameful to contract the disease. Not only does the shame affect the individual but also his or her family and communities. An infected individual is often made to feel responsible for contracting the virus and bringing shame to the family. This shameful burden places great stress on the infected individual (Aoki et al., 1987; Reece et al., 1993).

The final set of sociocultural barriers is denial of injecting drug use and sexual abuse (Chang, 1993). Injecting drug use provides another example of a high-risk behavior denied in Asian American communities. This may result in consequences similar to the denial of homosexuality, bisexuality, and transsexuality. Sexual abuse, incest, and ritual abuse are not openly discussed among Asian Americans. Sexual abuse relates to the gender and power imbalances between men and women. Abusive behavior can contribute to a decline in a woman's self-esteem and a reluctance to talk to her partner about safer sex and past sexual history. Besides the direct risk associated with sexual behaviors in abusive relationships; sexual abuse, incest, and ritual abuse can hamper communication between individuals making the enactment of health protective behaviors problematic, if not impossible.

Psychocultural Barriers

These are obstacles to HIV/AIDS intervention that are associated with the person's psychological orientation to the external world within a cultural context. Three such factors were identified in the context of HIV education for Asian Americans: (a) stereotyping, (b) eurocentrism, and (c) attitude toward utilization of health services.

The stereotype that Asian Americans are responsible, diligent, compliant, quiet, and less likely to contract HIV has been developed both within Asian American communities and between Euro-Americans and communities of color (Lee & Fong, 1990). Because "the public health establishment was slow to include Asians and Pacific Islanders in the AIDS epidemiological picture" (Choi et al., 1995, p. 126), HIV/AIDS has been largely invisible in Asian

American communities at all levels (Aoki et al., 1989), thus, little community ownership of the health threat exists (Yep, 1994a).

Closely related to stereotyping, eurocentric attitudes continue to persist in funding, education, and delivery of services to Asian American communities affected by HIV/AIDS. In terms of funding, Yep (1993a) noted:

> In the AIDS crisis, Asian and Pacific Islander communities are faced with a classic Catch-22: they receive limited, if any, funding for services or research because there are relatively few reported Asian AIDS cases, but no one can financially, socially, and ethically afford to wait for an explosion of HIV infection in these communities. (p. 294)

Additionally, as noted earlier, most HIV/AIDS education and research programs have traditionally targeted white gay men (e.g., Catania et al., 1990; Ekstrand & Coates, 1990; Jemmott & Jones, 1993; McKusick et al., 1990) and many of these programs reflect a eurocentric perspective that largely ignores social and cultural factors present in communities of color.

Asian Americans appear to display unfavorable attitudes toward utilization of HIV educational services because of feelings of embarrassment, shame, and loss of face, in addition to stigma associated with HIV and marginalized sexual behaviors (Choi et al., 1995; Yep, 1993a, c) and lack of adequate knowledge about the American health care system (Chang, 1993). Such attitudes may be manifested in terms of under-utilization of health services and educational programs that can empower them to engage in health enhancing behaviors (Choi et al., 1995; Murase, 1992; Yep, 1993a).

Communication Barriers

Communication barriers are those obstacles to HIV/AIDS intervention that are related to cultural styles of self expression, modes of interaction, and representations in the mass media. Such barriers encompass a wide array of factors including: (a) language diversity, (b) communication with health care providers, (c) cultural communication style — both verbal and nonverbal, (d) intimate communication, and (e) media representations of Asian Americans with respect to HIV/AIDS.

Language diversity is the first communication barrier. The diversity of Asian American communities throughout the United States makes it difficult for health educators to communicate with members of such communities (Chang, 1993; Choi et al., 1995; Gock, 1994; Lee & Fong, 1990). There is no single "Asian community"; in fact, there are over 40 Asian and Pacific Islander groups residing in this country (Yep, 1993a). Gock (1994) noted that in order to reach most Asian Americans, health education programs need to target at least 10 Asian Pacific subgroups that speak more than 15 languages and dialects. Levels of acculturation and communication differ between immigrants and U.S.-born Asian Americans. For example, AIDS education materials targeting immigrants need to be printed in their native language whereas this may not be necessary for native-born Asians. In Southern California, a substantial portion of the Asian American population is non-English speaking monolingual (Carrier et al., 1992) or multilingual (Yep, 1992, 1993d). Moreover, regional differences separate the distinct Asian Pacific ethnic groups. Groups isolate and separate themselves from others of the same ethnic origin based on native regional hometowns; for example, although Okinawans and mainland Japanese are of the same nationality, these two groups do not generally associate with one another. Differences between sexual identities sometimes divide a cultural group even further; for example, Carrier and associates (1992) found two groups of Vietnamese American men who have sex with men: (a) Vietnamese "gays" (those who are moderately acculturated and maintain a harmonious gay and ethnic identity), and (b) Vietnamese homosexual "outsiders" (those who are unacculturated or moderately to highly acculturated and without a clear sexual identity). At times these groups harbor prejudicial views toward each other which may hinder group educational efforts. Therefore, a health educator faces the daunting task of targeting different groups within the same Asian communities. Differences between urban and rural upbringings can also be a barrier to HIV/AIDS education. The level of basic education and cultural differences of the two areas can further inhibit intervention efforts.

The second barrier is communication with health care and service providers. HIV/AIDS education emphasizes the importance of safer sex activities and negotiation skills. Any educational program requires open communication between the person delivering the information and the person receiving it. Unfortunately, such openness may not exist between service providers and target groups within Asian American communities (Reece et al., 1993). In addition, communication barriers between health educators who are unaware of Asian cultural norms and beliefs present another major cultural hurdle in HIV/AIDS education and prevention programs (Chang, 1993).

The third barrier is derived from differences in styles of communication including both verbal and nonverbal aspects. Generally, Asian cultures do not directly speak about sensitive subjects but, rather, talk about subjects metaphorically (Aoki et al., 1989; Jue, 1987). For example, Asian languages do not have words for homosexuality, only representations of it. This method of indirect and context-based communication can lead to misunderstandings (Yep, in press-b). In addition, many Asian Americans tend to exhibit a nonconfrontational style of relating which may create additional challenges to situations requiring open and direct expression like talking about one's risk to a disease threat (Yep, in press-b). Further, in Asian American communities, open communication about feelings is not generally approved — one is not to speak of his/her feelings or expose his/her problems (Reece et al., 1993). For example, Asian Americans frequently hide and refuse to recognize feelings of anger (Reece et al., 1993). Anger and frustration surround life-threatening illnesses such as AIDS. When emotions get repressed because of intolerance, emotionally-ladden subjects such as sex, HIV, and AIDS remain undiscussed, thus, possibly further compromising immunological suppression.

The fourth barrier is intimate communication. As indicated earlier, discussions about sex and safer sex practices are considered taboo (Aoki et al., 1989; Yep, in press-b). If a person carries condoms and talks about safer sex, he or she may be viewed as sexually promiscuous. In more extreme cases, some people may even believe that expressing a desire to engage in safer sex indicates HIV infection. This paradox inhibits HIV/AIDS education.

Finally, the lack of HIV-positive Asian representation in the media paints a misleading picture of the incidence of the disease in Asian American communities (Yep, in press-a). Because of this, these communities do not think the disease affects them. Such lack of ownership continues to create denial, low perceptions of susceptibility to HIV infection, and a general lack of interest in learning about modes of transmission, HIV prevention, antibody testing, and early intervention.

Toward More Effective Cultural Communication

As stated earlier, HIV intervention efforts that incorporate cultural factors associated with their target population have greater likelihood of achieving their educational objectives. Based on both review of the existing literature and on the findings deriving from a forum of HIV-related experts in both research and service delivery areas, I have identified and discussed some important cultural, sociocultural, psychocultural, and communication barriers associated with HIV education for Asian Americans.

To increase the effectiveness of intervention programs for this population, HIV/AIDS education must overcome these identified obstacles. For example, conventional emphasis on individual self-protective behaviors (e.g., "protect yourself — use a condom") can be replaced with more collectivistic messages for Asian Americans (e.g., "protect your family — use a condom"). Similarly, HIV educational messages should come from Asian American faces — gay, bisexual, transsexual, transgender, heterosexual — to create visibility and representation that may increase perceptions of risk and susceptibility to HIV in these communities. Further, educational programs should be developed in consultation with those communities they are designed to target; for example, HIV educational programs targeting Asian American youth of a specific age and ethnic group should invite individuals from such groups to assist in the design, creation, implementation, and evaluation of the curriculum and intervention. Such approach enhances community ownership of the AIDS epidemic and promotes community empowerment.

HIV education programs for Asian Americans should also reflect the cultural and social realities of this population; in other words, they should be culturally appropriate. As such, these programs need to address the profound feelings of shame, isolation, rejection, oppression, racism, and heterosexism that many potential clients may experience. Some community members have suggested the need to broaden the definition of familial relationships in Asian American communities while others have recommended greater representation of Asian American diversity to fight against the racism, sexism, and heterosexism that are present in HIV intervention efforts (Reyes & Yep, in press). Cultural, linguistic, and socioeconomic heterogeneity in Asian American communities should also be considered. To accomplish this, Choi and associates (1995) suggested that HIV intervention programs should simultaneously "target each subgroup with interventions that are culturally and linguistically syntonic with its subculture... [and] identify cultural norms that are shared across subgroups within a target population to address the remaining diversity found in any risk group" (p. 131). Such programs also need to emphasize anonymity and confidentiality in the delivery of HIV-related services.

In addition to developing programs that cater to various segments in the diverse landscape of Asian American communities, such intervention efforts also need to target those individuals who are uninfected by HIV and those who are living with it (Yep, 1993a, in press-a). For example, Yep (1993a) suggested that prevention programs for Asian Americans should include messages that will increase: (a) awareness of the AIDS problem, (b) knowledge about HIV transmission, (c) perceived vulnerability to HIV infection, (d) feelings of efficacy associated with risk reduction behaviors and safer sex negotiation, and (e) competence in the performance of health protective actions. Similarly, education programs for Asian American living with HIV infection should provide: (a) information about early treatment and medical updates, and (b) psychosocial support services to help these community members face the challenges of living with HIV.

HIV education programs should also encourage the adaptation of innovative strategies that incorporate common Asian cultural beliefs and practices. For example, Yep (1994a) reported some innovative outreach strategies: The use of the Fortune Cookie and the Chinese Red Envelope concepts in face-to-face community education efforts. The Fortune Cookie, a symbol of Asian American food, has been used to include and disseminate safer sex as well as HIV antibody testing messages. Similarly, the Chinese Red Envelope, which Chinese and other Asian groups have traditionally used to give money in such packets to celebrate Chinese New Year, has been adopted to give the "gift of life" — the inclusion of safer sex kits (containing condoms and instructions on how to use them, dental dams, a list of sexual behaviors that are considered risky, possibly risky, and safe, and a number to call for further information) to preserve good health. Such face-to-face approaches have been generally well received as they are nonthreatening, face-preserving, and culturally accepted vehicles for HIV education for these groups.

The effectiveness of these suggested HIV intervention efforts remains to be evaluated. At the present time, little information is available regarding the effectiveness of current culturally-specific educational programs for Asian Americans (Choi et al., 1995; Gock, 1994; Yep, 1993a). The question of culturally appropriate evaluations must also be addressed (Yep, 1994a).

Because of the paucity of research focusing on HIV education targeting Asian Americans, future research faces many challenging tasks. At the theoretical level, researchers must ascertain how culture and behavioral models come together to produce health enhancing outcomes. At the service delivery level, health educators must be able to incorporate theoretically sound principles in their intervention efforts to produce successful, cost-effective, culturally-sensitive, and community-empowering programs to limit the growth of AIDS cases in Asian American communities in this country.

Notes

1. According to the U.S. Census Bureau, there are over 40 Asian and Pacific Islander groups from over 40 countries and territories, who speak more than 100 different languages. It is recognized that each group has a distinct culture and heritage. The term "Asian American" is a label of convenience used by government agencies including the Centers for Disease Control and Prevention (CDC) and the author does not intend to imply cultural and/or linguistic homogeneity.
2. A forum entitled "Cultural Factors in HIV/AIDS Education and Prevention for Asian and Pacific Islanders: A Multidisciplinary Exploration" brought together 14 health educators, community representatives, university researchers, and medical and social scientists who have extensive experience working with HIV-related issues in Asian American communities. One of their main objectives was to identify barriers in HIV/AIDS education, prevention, and delivery of services to these groups.

References

Abramson, P.R. (1986). The Cultural Context of Japanese Sexuality: An American Perspective. *Psychologia*, 29, 1-9.

Aoki, B., & Ja, D.Y. (1987, August). *AIDS and Asian Americans: Psychosocial Issues*. Paper presented at the Annual Meeting of the American Psychological Association, New York.

Aoki, B., Ngin, C.P., Mo, B., & Ja, D.Y. (1989). AIDS Prevention Models in Asian-American Communities. In V.M. Mays, G.W. Albee, & S.F. Schneider (Eds.), *Primary Prevention of AIDS: Psychological Approaches* (pp. 290-308). Newbury Park, CA: Sage.

Benedict, R. (1946/1989). *The Chrysanthemum and the Sword: Patterns of Japanese Culture*. Boston, MA: Houghton Mifflin.

Carrier, J., Nguyen, B., & Su, S. (1992). Vietnamese American Sexual Behaviors and HIV Infection. *Journal of Sex Research*, 29, 547-560.

Catania, J.A., Gibson, D.R., Chitwood, D.D., & Coates, T.J. (1990). Methodological

Problems in AIDS Behavioral Research: Influences on Measurement Error and Participation Bias in Studies of Sexual Behavior. *Psychological Bulletin*, 108, 339-362.

Chan, C.S. (1989). Issues of Identity Development Among Asian-American Lesbians and Gay Men. *Journal of Counseling and Development*, 68, 16-20.

Chang, R. (1993). *U.S. National Asian and Pacific Islander HIV/AIDS Agenda*. San Francisco, CA: Asian Pacific AIDS Coalition.

Choi, K., Salazar, N., Lew, S., & Coates, T.J. (1995). AIDS Risk, Dual Identity, and Community Response Among Gay Asian and Pacific Islander Men in San Francisco. In G.M. Herek & B. Greene (Eds.), *AIDS, Identity, and Community: The HIV Epidemic and Lesbians and Gay Men* (pp. 115-134). Thousand Oaks, CA: Sage.

Cochran, S.D., Mays, V.M., & Leung, L. (1991). Sexual Practices of Heterosexual Asian-American Young Adults: Implications for Risk of HIV Infection. *Archives of Sexual Behavior*, 20, 381-391.

Ekstrand, M.L., & Coates, T.J. (1990). Maintenance of Safer Sexual Behaviors and Predictors of Risky Sex: The San Francisco Men's Health Study. *American Journal of Public Health*, 80, 973-977.

Estrada, A.L. (1995). Deriving Culturally Competent HIV Prevention Models for Mexican American Injection Drug Users. In R.A. Brooks, B. Solis, & D.E. Hayes-Bautista (Eds.), *Defining the Path for Future Research: Proceedings of the National Latino HIV/AIDS Research Conference* (pp. 93-108). Los Angeles: Regents of the University of California.

Fairbank, Bregman, & Maullin, Inc. (1991). *A Survey of AIDS Knowledge, Attitudes and Behaviors in San Francisco's American-Indian, Filipino and Latino Gay and Bisexual Male Communities*. Santa Monica, CA: Author.

Gagnon, J.H., & Simon, W. (1973). *Sexual Conduct: The Social Sources of Human Sexuality*. Hawthorne, NY: Aldine.

Gock, T.S. (1994). Acquired Immunodeficiency Syndrome. In N.W.S. Zane, D.T. Takeuchi, & K.N.J. Young (Eds.), *Confronting Critical Health Issues of Asian and Pacific Islander Americans* (pp. 247-265). Thousand Oaks, CA: Sage.

Gudykunst, W.B., & Kim, Y.Y. (1992). *Communicating with Strangers: An Approach to Intercultural Communication*. New York: McGraw-Hill.

Jemmott, J.B., & Jones, J.M. (1993). Social Psychology and AIDS Among Ethnic Minority Individuals: Risk Behaviors and Strategies for Changing Them. In J.B. Pryor & G.D. Reeder (Eds.), *The Social Psychology of HIV Infection* (pp. 183-224). Hillsdale, NJ: Lawrence Erlbaum.

Jue, S. (1987). Identifying and Meeting the Needs of Minority Clients With AIDS. In C.G. Leukefeld & M. Fimbres (Eds.), *Responding to AIDS: Psychosocial Initiatives* (pp. 65-79). Silver Spring, MD: National Association of Social Workers.

Lee, D.A., & Fong, K. (1990). HIV/AIDS and the Asian and Pacific Islander Community. *SIECUS Report*, February/March, 16-22.

McKusick, L., Coates, T.J., Morin, S., Pollack, L., & Hoff, C. (1990). Longitudinal Predictors of Reductions in Unprotected Anal Intercourse Among Gay Men in San Francisco: The AIDS Behavioral Research Project. *American Journal of Public Health*, 80, 1-8.

Michal-Johnson, P., & Bowen, S.P. (1992). The Place of Culture in HIV Education. In T. Edgar, M.A. Fitzpatrick, & V.S. Freimuth (Eds.), *AIDS: A Communication Perspective* (pp.147-172). Hillsdale, NJ: Lawrence Erlbaum.

Morales, E.S. (1990). Ethnic Minority Families and Minority Gays and Lesbians. In F.W. Bozett & M.B. Sussman (Eds.), *Homosexuality and Family Relations* (pp. 217-239). New York: Haworth Press.

Murase, K. (1992). Models of Service Delivery in Asian American Communities. In S.M. Furuto, R. Biswas, D.K. Chung, K. Murase, & F. Ross-Sheriff (Eds.), *Social Work Practice With Asian Americans* (pp. 101-120). Newbury Park, CA: Sage.

Reece, S.T., Yep, G.A., & Negron, E.L. (1993, December). *Group Psychotherapy for Asians with HIV Infection: Emerging Issues*. Paper presented to the 12th Annual Meeting of the Japanese Clinical Psychology Association, Okinawa, Japan.

Reyes, E.E., & Yep, G.A. (in press). Challenging Complexities: Strategizing with Asian Americans in Southern California Against (Heterosex)isms. In J.T. Sears & W.L. Williams (Eds.), *Combating Heterosexism: Strategies That Work*. New York: Columbia University Press.

Weeks, M.R., Schensul, J.J., Williams, S.S., Singer, M., & Grier, M.(1995).AIDS Prevention for African-American and Latina Women: Building Culturally and Gender-appropriate Intervention. *AIDS Education and Prevention*, 7, 251-264.

Wu, S., & Pak, S. (1989). The Hidden Minority: Perspectives on Being Asian and Gay. *East Wind*, 2 (2), 22-25.

Yep, G. A. (1992). The Effects of Community-based HIV/AIDS Education and Prevention Messages on Knowledge, Attitudes and Behavioral Enactment Skills Among Asian Men. In *Proceedings of the Ninth International and Intercultural Communication Conference* (pp. 19-22). Miami, FL: University of Miami.

Yep, G.A. (1993a). HIV/AIDS in Asian and Pacific Islander Communities in the United States: A Review, Analysis, and Integration. *International Quarterly of Community Health Education*, 13, 293-315.

Yep, G.A. (1993b). HIV Prevention Among Asian-American College Students: Does the Health Belief Model Work? *Journal of American College Health*, 41 (5), 199- 205.

Yep, G.A. (1993c). First Asian/Pacific Island Men's HIV Conference, Los Angeles, California. *AIDS Education and Prevention*, 5, 87-88.

Yep, G.A. (1993d, November). *Attitude Toward Condoms and AIDS-phobia Among Gay/bisexual Asian Men: An Assessment of a Community-based HIV Education Program*. Paper presented to the 79th Annual Meeting of the Speech Communication Association, Miami, FL.

Yep, G.A. (1994a). HIV/AIDS Education and Prevention for Asian and Pacific Islander Communities: Toward the Development of General Guidelines. *AIDS Education and Prevention*, 6, 184-186.

Yep, G.A. (1994b). *Working with Transgender and Transsexual Asian Americans at Risk for HIV Infection.* Unpublished manuscript.

Yep, G.A. (in press-a). 'See No Evil, Hear No Evil, Speak No Evil:' Educating Asian Americans About HIV/AIDS Through Culture-specific Health Communication Campaigns. In L.K. Fuller (Ed.), *Media-Mediated AIDS*. Amherst, MA: Human Resource Development Press.

Yep, G.A. (in press-b). Safer Sex Negotiation in Cross-cultural Romantic Dyads: An Extension of Ting-Toomey's Face Negotiation Theory. In N. Roth & L.K. Fuller (Eds.), *Women's Ways of Acknowledging AIDS: Communication Perspectives*. Binghamton, NY: Haworth Press.

Applying Social Psychology to HIV Prevention: Solving a Dilemma in the HIV Prevention Communications on Anal Sex as an Example

Gerjo Kok, Harm J. Hospers & John B.F. de Wit

Health education interventions should be based on insights derived from the behavioral sciences, especially social psychology. In this paper we will describe a difficult decision that had to be made regarding a health education intervention, namely the possible revision of the Dutch HIV prevention communications about anal sex. In short, until recently, the Dutch preventive message focused on abstinence from anal sex. However, there were suggestions that this message had an unwanted side effect: men who continued to engage in anal sex would not (always) use condoms. Revision of the abstinence-message was debated, especially a double message was proposed. Since there were no empirical data on this specific issue and there was no time for adequate empirical research, the authors examined the problem by applying different social psychological theories. Based on the outcomes of these applications we formulated a solution that strongly influenced the final decision that was made by the responsible governmental agency.

Social psychologists are supposed to be trained to apply their theories, but given a complex problem it is sometimes difficult to find the optimal approach. A study of the available theoretical and empirical materials on social psychology did not provide easily applicable answers. However, it did facilitate the final decision making with regard to the dilemma.

The problem was whether the main HIV-prevention educational communications about anal sex needed to be changed. Until 1991, HIV prevention messages for gay men in the Netherlands strongly advised them to refrain from any form of anal sex; only in case people felt unable to practice abstinence was the use of special condoms advised. The focus on refraining from anal sex was primarily based on studies that showed substantial failure rates of condoms used during anal sex (between five and 15%). Furthermore, as we now realize, the decision to focus on abstinence underestimated how difficult refraining from anal sex was for many gay men. Because the messages did not say much about condom use, there was a lack of easily accessible information on correct condom use for anal sex.

Several years into the epidemic, cohort studies among gay men in Amsterdam showed dramatic changes in behavior: in 1984-85 11.5% refrained from anal sex vs. 37.5% in 1987-88 (Van Griensven et al., 1989). Within the group of men who had anal sex, one-third consistently used condoms but two-thirds did not use condoms or used condoms inconsistently. Men who still had anal sex were obviously aware of the risks of HIV-infection. For instance, the number of partners of these men had decreased dramatically since the outbreak of the epidemic, which can be seen as a means of reducing their risk.

Health educators responsible for HIV prevention expressed concern about the possible negative effects of the strong focus on refraining from anal sex. They argued that the abstinence message might be effective for one group, but might be countereffective for men who were not able or not willing to refrain from anal sex. As a result of the lack of attention to social and other skills related to condoms and also to easy accessibility to condoms, this latter group of men might use condoms inconsistently. Indeed, data from countries where the focus of HIV education for gay men was solely on condom use, showed that fewer men refrained from anal sex, but that the actual use of condoms was higher than in The Netherlands (Bochow, 1989; Pollak et al., 1989). Moreover, some gay men may intend to abstain from anal sex, but nevertheless get into a situation where they have anal sex, and should then also be able to adequately use condoms. In short, the issue was *whether the abstinence message needed to be revised, and if so, what the optimal educational message would be.* The decision would result in an immediate nationwide implementation (which excludes intervention-control groups' designs) and it needed to be taken fast. As a result, it was not possible to conduct specific research and the decision had to be made based on the available knowledge at that moment. In the discussion that followed, various arguments, including some that were ideological, were exchanged, ranging from an extreme position that only advice promoting 100% safety could be disseminated, to the accusation that the abstinence message was the result of moral intolerance and homophobia. In the analysis in this article we will restrict ourselves to the arguments that were derived from a social psychological analysis of this dilemma.

The dilemma of providing a message that is optimal from an epidemiological point of view but very difficult to perform, against a message that is more feasible but at the same time less optimal *and implicitly contradicts the first message* (a "double bind"), is not unique in health education (Stein, 1992). The dilemma is comparable to the choice between educating IV-drug users to use new needles through needle exchange programs (optimal and difficult), or giving the message to clean used needles with bleach (less optimal but more feasible). The same kind of dilemma is present in programs that suggest total abstinence in case one has to drive a car (optimal) or to rest a number of hours after drinking (feasible). A final example is not smoking at all for baby protection or only smoke when the baby is not present (Strecher, 1989). Within these kinds of dilemmas, there are, of course, combinations of the two messages, but in practice there is a tendency to choose for one to avoid double and confusing messages. There is no conclusive research on these dilemmas, in particular not with respect to HIV prevention (Stein, 1992).

A Further Analysis of the Problem

The availability of safer condoms for anal intercourse would largely solve the current dilemma in the sense that educational messages could then concentrate on skills for adequate condom use. However, recent studies still show a substantial failure rate in condoms for anal sex (Chan-Chee et al., 1991; De Wit et al., 1993; Golombok et al., 1990; Richters et al., 1988; Ross, 1987; Valdiserri et al., 1988; Van Griensven et al., 1988, Voeller et al., 1989; Wigersma & Oud, 1987). At this moment we do not know what part of failure is related to the quality of condoms and what part is related to improper use (e.g. inappropriate lubricant; De Wit et al., 1993). As a consequence we may not yet assume that the main reason for failure is a lack of skills. It seems possible to improve the safety rate of anal condoms, although at present manufacturers do not see economic incentives to do so.

Assuming that the failure rate of anal condoms is 10%, refraining from anal sex is preferable to condom use in a population where there are a number of seropositives. However, if we assume that a substantial part of the population will continue to have anal sex, the consistent use of condoms is preferable to inconsistent use or non-use. Hypothetically, a situation where 100% of the population use condoms is safer with 90% protection than the situation where 25% do not use condoms, even if the other 75% refrain from anal sex (75% protection). If, hypothetically, all the men within the population who have anal sex consistently use condoms, the protection rate will improve when more men begin to refrain from anal sex. Thus, from an epidemiological perspective, the objective for health education is not only to get the target group to refrain from anal sex but also to get them to use condoms in case they cannot or will not refrain from anal sex. The question is what kind of message can achieve this complex goal. We will first review available data on determinants of having anal sex, to get more insight into reasons why men are not able or willing to refrain from anal sex. Then we will identify concepts and theories that are possibly relevant to a solution.

Determinants of (Unprotected) Anal Sex

What are the reasons for anal sex by men? Most recent studies on determinants focus on unsafe sex as the dependent variable, often operationalized as having unprotected anal sex (see for a review Hospers & Kok, 1995). Our interest here is also in men who use condoms for anal sex. However, specific data are difficult to derive from studies that defined condom use as safe. Moreover, most studies report on convenience samples which limits the generalizability of the results. Several studies document higher risk taking among gay men who are younger (Ekstrand & Coates, 1990), who live in low AIDS prevalence areas (Kelly et al., 1990c), and who have a steady partner (which may actually be safe; Bochow, 1990). Alcohol and drug use seem to be related to unsafe sex, although a direct causal path is questionable (Gold et al., 1991). Knowledge about HIV-infection is very high among gay men but recent studies show that that knowledge is unrelated to preventive behavior (e.g. Kelly et al., 1990b). Risk perception is often adequate but only weakly related to risk behavior (Joseph et al., 1987). However, men who have protected anal sex tend to see themselves as completely safe instead of just safer. For a substantial proportion of gay men, anal sex is a very important part of their life style, being physically satisfying, emotionally satisfying (Connell & Kippax, 1990), and an essential part of their own gay identities (Prieur, 1990). Men at higher risk (unprotected anal sex) are relatively more loosely related to a gay social network, lonelier, more isolated and more closeted (Connell et al., 1990). These men often indicate that their partners insist on unprotected anal sex. Self-efficacy, that is the gay man's estimation of being able to avoid unprotected anal intercourse including the ability to negotiate safer sex with potential partners, is strongly related to actual preventive behavior (Bandura, 1989). To summarize: beliefs about the importance of anal sex, lack of social support and low self-efficacy expectations are strongly related to more risk taking. Focusing specifically on the distinction between men who refrain from anal sex vs. men who have protected and/or unprotected anal sex, the special importance of having anal sex seems an essential determinant for that latter group. If we focus on the group of men who have anal sex and specifically on the difference between having protected vs. unprotected anal sex, then negative attitudes toward condoms, lack of support and low self-efficacy expectations appear to predict high risk taking.

Relevant Concepts

Given the further analysis of the problem, "should we revise the message and if so, how?" and the available empirical data, what are relevant concepts in this dilemma that may help identify useful theories and effective solutions? In our approach we tried not to limit ourselves to some well-known theories, but to look at the problem from as many different viewpoints as possible and to search for different concepts that could be related to the theories. All authors are (social) psychologists with research and practice experience in HIV prevention and health education.

At first, brainstorming, free association and free generation of ideas suggested two major possible reasons for the insufficient effectiveness of the abstinence message: the educational message may have been inadequately developed and implemented, or the message may have targeted an unrealistic goal. The first reason suggests that the message should be improved, whereas the second reason suggests that condom use should be promoted.

Perhaps the original message on HIV prevention failed to reach the target group successfully, was confusing, or failed to convince people. Here, the relevant concepts that are related to social psychological theories are the diffusion of innovations, comprehension and change and risk perception. Another possibility is that the abstinence-message does indeed aim for a behavioral change that is too difficult to realize, at least for part of the population. Theoretical concepts related to this are discrepancy between message and receiver, goal setting and self-efficacy. We will analyze the problem further by applying theories that are related to the concepts that were suggested, In addition, we will try to indicate whether these theories support improvement of the educational intervention or if they suggest changing the message into the promotion of condoms.

As we will see, a further theoretical analysis of these two issues suggests the possibility of a third major reason: one overall message for the whole population of gay men may have been inappropriate because of large individual differences among the target population. This suggests that tailored education might be a solution to the problem.

Applying Theories

For each of the relevant concepts mentioned we will describe the theory that is linked to that concept and suggest possible solutions for our dilemma. Where possible, we will distinguish between an improved intervention on refraining from anal sex vs. changing to a message promoting consistent condom use, as that distinction is most relevant to our dilemma.

Diffusion of Innovations

E. M. Rogers (1983) has described the adoption of innovations in a population as an S-shaped cumulative normal distribution. Early adopters' decisions are based on direct information about characteristics of the innovation: e.g. compatibility (with life style and values), relative advantage, observability, and the possibility for trying out. However, the majority of people base their adoption decisions on information received through interaction with other members of the community. Rogers stresses the impact of communication in the social network and the importance of opinion leaders in the community. As a consequence, the diffusion of taboo issues about which people do not communicate easily, is very slow. Rogers also indicates that an innovation may be rejected if it is incompatible or does not provide (relative) advantages. Sometimes the target group will re-invent and adopt the innovation in a different, better fitting form.

Applying Rogers' theory to our problem, we recognize the likelihood of non-adoption in men who are loosely related to the gay social network: e.g. young gays and closeted gays. Health education activities should try to get these men more involved in the gay community (Fisher, 1988), using techniques from community development (Bracht, 1990). Even in these marginal groups, there are patterns of interaction that we can try to use for our preventive messages. For instance, the gay community started to organize HIV prevention outreach activities directed at younger gays and gays involved in anonymous sex. Men who may serve as reference persons and who successfully refrained from anal sex can be used as a model for other gay men ("modeling," Bandura, 1986; "social comparison," Suls & Wills, 1991).

For part of the target group, the compatibility and relative advantage of refraining from anal sex will be lower when compared to consistent condom use. This group may never adopt the proposed abstinence or may try to re-invent the abstinence-message as a more acceptable message, e.g. condom use or even a reduction in the number of sexual partners. However, compared to other health-related behaviors (e.g. smoking) the adoption rate of the abstinence-message is actually rather high. We may even be able to stimulate faster adoption, especially when the issue is repeatedly the object of communication in the gay community, opinion leaders support the message and experiences with refraining from anal sex result in positive feedback, e.g. in terms of safety or responsibility. Overall, it follows from the diffusion approach that educational efforts should continue with improved strategies.

Comprehension and Change

McGuire (1985) explained in his communication-persuasion matrix why so many relationships between communication variables and change are curvilinear, a reversed U-curve. The same variable may have different influences in the subsequent steps of the change process: attention, comprehension, attitude change, behavior change, and maintenance. For instance, a complex message can be difficult to understand but at the same time it can be very convincing when understood. The model also indicates that changing a message may undermine its credibility. However, when receivers subsequently find out that the message is incorrect, its impact will diminish, and the source will be discredited. Petty & Cacioppo (1986) stress the importance of elaboration: only changes that are based on extensive processing of information will be maintained. Elaboration can be stimulated by active learning (Bandura, 1986), although it will be biased if people have strong initial opinions.

Applying McGuire's ideas to our problem, we recognize the potential difficulty in understanding the original, twofold, message. However, changing the educational message into a strong plea for condoms has the risk of being seen as over-simplified and therefore unconvincing. It may, moreover, be countereffective for those men who did successfully refrain from anal sex. In accordance with Petty & Cacioppo, we could promote refraining from anal sex by stimulating the active processing of information on the risk of condom use in anal sex (without lowering peoples' self-efficacy, see Self-Efficacy Improvement) by using techniques such as role playing or creative assignments. On the other hand, when people decide to have protected anal sex, skills for adequate negotiation about, and correct use of condoms also deserve optimal educational strategies.

This approach supports the intervention improvement solution by implying that the desired behavior changes are indeed possible. Subsequently, McGuire stresses the importance of tailored messages for different subgroups within the population. The target group should be involved in the development of messages to improve the attention value, understandability, and compatibility with existing values and norms. In general, pretesting educational materials on a representative sample of the target population is an essential part of intervention development (Romano, 1984).

Risk Perception

Several theories, the Health Belief Model (Janz & Becker, 1984), Protection Motivation Theory (R.W.Rogers, 1983), and Precaution Adoption Theory (Weinstein, 1988), assume that awareness of risk (fear, threat) motivates action. However, the actual form action takes depends on outcome expectations of the advised behavior, in combination with self-efficacy expectations about performing that behavior. A high level of fear combined with low outcome expectations and/or low self-efficacy results in dysfunctional behavior such as denial of one's own susceptibility and scape- goating of risk groups.

It is certain that our population is aware of the risks of anal sex. However, we lack sufficient information on how aware they are of the risks of condom use. Data from cohort studies on the dramatic reduction of partners for anal sex, suggest that the target men recognize risks of anal sex, even when they use protection. There is evidence that some of the men who have unprotected anal sex do not believe that condoms are safe (Valdiserri et al., 1988). Most gay men however, are convinced that condoms can prevent HIV infection. The main determinants of unsafe sex are probably feelings of low self-efficacy and many perceived barriers among gay men to refraining from anal sex as well as to consistent condom use. In general, the risk perception approach is not optimistic about possibilities for improved interventions: interventions that focus strongly on high risk may be counterproductive if people do see many barriers to effective action. Some of these barriers are real and difficult to overcome. Getting men to consistently use condoms may even be too difficult an objective. Educational messages should focus on skills training and self-efficacy (see Self-Efficacy Improvement).

Discrepancy, Ego-Involvement and Change

Fishbein & Ajzen (1975, p. 451-509) summarized the empirical data and theoretical ideas about the effect of message-receiver discrepancy on attitude change as follows: the relation is a reversed U-curve, with most change at intermediate levels of discrepancy. The reason for this curvilinear relation is that discrepancy is positively related to potential change but negatively related to acceptance (McGuire, 1985). Discrepancies that are too large may even become countereffective. As high ego-involvement (personal commitment) is also negatively related to acceptance, discrepant messages will be ineffective or countereffective with highly involved people. On the other hand, high source credibility, social support and high response-involvement promote change. Therefore, with increasing discrepancy between the message/source and the receiver, attitude change will increase up to a certain point. After that point, attitude change will decrease as the discrepancy increases further. The position of that point, at the top of the reversed U-curve, depends on ego-involvement and on the credibility of the source and response-involvement. The higher the receiver's ego-involvement, the earlier the curve starts to decline; the higher the source credibility and response-involvement, the later the curve starts to decline.

Getting gay men to use condoms consistently will require discrepant behavior with regard to their initial position; getting them to refrain from anal sex altogether requires even more discrepant behavior. The theory predicts that for men with high ego-involvement this discrepancy will often be too great, leading to a rejection of the message. Ego-involvement is strongly anchored in values, other beliefs, social environment and (past) behavior. For many gay men anal sex is part of their identity and will be an issue of high ego-involvement. Consistently using condoms may be acceptable, but refraining from anal sex will probably fall within the "latitude of rejection" (McGuire, 1985). McGuire's approach is more supportive for messages that would promote condom use instead of an abstinence message. However, getting gay men to refrain from anal sex may be possible by using highly credible sources, strong social support and persuasive messages stressing the importance of abstinence (response-involvement).

Goal Setting and Feedback

Locke & Latham (1991) have posited that setting a challenging goal will result in higher achievements than setting an easy goal or no goal, given the conditions of task-relevant abilities and self-efficacy, goal commitment and acceptance, and feedback. Acceptance of challenging goals is promoted by participation of the target person, high self-efficacy and social support. Setting a challenging goal is supposed to improve achievements through increased effort, persistence and concentration, and, with complex tasks, through strategy development.

Completely refraining from anal sex will be a more difficult goal for many gay men than consistently using condoms. However, individual differences may be large; for some people consistent condom use may be too difficult while refraining is totally impossible. This theory suggests that we can promote the acceptance of a challenging goal by letting people participate in goal setting, improving their skills, promoting the use of effective strategies and self-efficacy, giving social support, and organizing feedback and reinforcement (e.g. from the community). On the one hand this approach is supportive for the improved intervention solution and suggests adopting the most challenging goal; on the other hand, it recognizes individual differences, suggesting that tailored messages are needed.

Self-Efficacy Improvement

Self-efficacy is the estimation of the person about his/her ability to perform a specific behavior (Bandura, 1985). Den Boer et al. (1991) summarized the psychological strategies to improve self-efficacy through attributional retraining (Försterling, 1988; Weiner, 1986) and relapse prevention (Marlatt & Gordon, 1985). Low self-efficacy (or learned helplessness) is seen as the result of multiple failures and the interpretation of these failures as caused by stable, internal and uncontrollable factors. People can learn that they are indeed able to change their behavior by acquiring skills and investing more effort. Skills training involves observational learning and enactive learning (learning from the consequences of behavior; Bandura, 1986). Relapse prevention theory adds that people also have to be taught coping skills for high-risk situations that might occur. In general, this approach implies that failure to consistently behave in the desired way is a normal phenomenon that requires improved educational techniques.

Self-efficacy is an essential concept in our dilemma. Because refraining from anal sex will be seen by most gay men as more difficult than consistent condom use, their self-efficacy for refraining will be lower. Even self-efficacy for consistently using condoms may be low for many men. Theory suggests however, that self-efficacy can be improved through understanding the importance of skills and effort, observing other people's successes, recognizing high-risk situations, and developing adequate coping responses. Hospers & Kok (1992) reviewed studies on promising relapse prevention approaches for HIV prevention with gay men (e.g. Kelly et al., 1989; 1990a). Basically, the relapse prevention approach would suggest that it is possible to achieve the objective of getting gay men to refrain from anal sex, but also that that is probably more difficult than getting them to consistently use condoms. Educational techniques are, in this case, mostly directed at individuals through counseling or small groups, but in other areas of health education, self-help manuals have also been shown to be effective.

In addition to message failure or goal difficulty, most of the theoretical applications so far suggest a third reason for our problem, namely the existence of major individual differences among members of the target population. Relevant to this are concepts such as communication channels and tailored messages for people in different stages of change.

Interpersonal vs. Mass Media Communication Channels

McGuire's (1985) summary of the potential effects of mass media vs. interpersonal communication implies that mass communication will have a greater impact on the first steps in the change process: attention, comprehension, and — sometimes — attitude change because of its potential to reach a larger group of people. It is however, assumed that interpersonal communication is needed for behavior change and maintenance, because of its potential to adapt to individuals' values and barriers. There are exceptions. When people are motivated to change but lack knowledge about simple adequate behavioral responses, mass media may improve behavior change and maintenance. In general however, it is very difficult, though not impossible to target mass communication at individual differences.

Our dilemma is concerned with public education messages on HIV prevention. These are by definition part of mass communication, even when directed at a specific "risk group." However, public educational activities are combined with more intensive interpersonal strategies: telephone hotlines, counseling, small group interventions, and other out-reach activities. It is possible that the main HIV prevention mass media message can be general and challenging, while individuals in small group or counseling situations derive their own personal subgoals from their individual strategies. For this purpose, the accessibility of tailored communication services should be improved.

Tailoring of HIV Prevention Messages According to Stage of Change

The Transtheoretical Model of Stages of Change (Prochaska & DiClemente, 1984) has strongly influenced health education by stressing the importance of individual differences among people depending on their stage of change: precontemplation, contemplation, action, maintenance. The model does not suggest new techniques, but it focuses on the linkage between educational techniques and the stage people are in. In practice this implies the use of different strategies and materials for people in different stages, often in the context of individual or small group counseling. For example, contemplators need interventions that improve their motivation for action; actors need interventions that prevent relapse. It is also possible for people to categorize themselves and then work through specific self-help manuals that are developed per stage. Abstaining from anal sex as well as consistently using condoms can both be described in terms of stages of change. In fact, an individual can be identified as being in a stage for both behaviors; for instance, a consistent condom user (maintainer) may be a contemplator for abstinence. The stages of change approach is comparable to relapse prevention and in the same way optimistic about possibilities for change: people need time and skills to pass through all the stages, and better, more tailored, health education strategies can promote preventive behavior. The abstinence message may need more time and effort to really be effective.

Theory-Based Suggestions for Solutions:

Our application of theories does not provide a simple solution to our dilemma: a safe but possibly unrealistic message promoting abstinence from anal sex, or a more feasible but also less safe message about condom use. It does however, focus attention on the most relevant aspects of a possible solution: the existence of high barriers for behavior change, the potential of continued improvement of intervention techniques, and the need for tailored educational messages.

Arguments for a Condom Use Message: High Barriers

A substantial group in the gay population perceives high barriers for refraining from anal sex. Anal sex is a highly ego-involving issue for these gay men: it is meaningfully related to important values. An abstinence message may not be compatible with the person's current life-style. While many men recognize the risks of HIV infection, a number of them report low self-efficacy for refraining from anal sex. Even consistently using condoms may be too difficult for some of the men. It is clear that education on condom use needs to be improved: we need to apply our knowledge on effective health education in an optimal way.

Arguments for an Abstinence Message: Continued Improvement of Intervention Techniques

Decision makers in HIV prevention who are not trained in health education, often have unrealistic expectations about major short-term effects of HIV education. Changing people's behavior through health education is a slow and time-consuming process. Changes in the community are indirect and follow diffusion patterns. Compared to the public education messages on smoking, HIV education in the gay community has been extremely successful.

A consistent plea to refrain from anal sex is justified for epidemiological reasons, moreover, the resistance against this message is in itself not a sufficient argument to choose a message that is less safe. The abstinence message is certainly feasible from the viewpoint of theories about diffusion of innovations, persuasion-communication, goal setting, relapse prevention, and stages of change. In fact, a number of educational techniques such as relapse prevention methods, that are very effective in other areas, have not yet, or only very superficially have been applied to HIV education on anal sex. The abstinence message can certainly be improved.

Arguments for a Combined Message: Tailored Educational Messages

Our analyses until now suggest two messages for the entire target group: one advising abstinence from anal sex, and one promoting correct use of anal condoms. Focussing on only one of these two messages may have serious disadvantages: relatively less consistent condom use may occur as a result of an abstinence-only educational message, whereas a relative underestimation of the risks of condom use may occur as a result of a condoms-only message. Thus, one conclusion is that we should combine the two messages. Moreover, most theories stress the importance of individual differences and the need to tailor health education messages. The mass media educational message should be combined with different types of interpersonal communication with individuals and subgroups of the gay population.

Theories such as the stages of change model and goal setting theory suggest that we see the two objectives as sequential: people with a low general self-efficacy for HIV-preventive behavior can first try to learn how to use condoms consistently. After they have mastered that, they can gradually learn how to refrain from anal sex. This stepwise approach requires that messages be tailored to the target person, using techniques to improve self-efficacy in different domains subsequently. Theories about involvement and diffusion of innovations, however, suggest that there may be a group that will never adopt the abstinence message. For this group the focus should be on the promotion of condom use. Both theories may be right, implying that the group of men who are currently unsafe can partially be convinced to abstain from anal sex while being encouraged to consistently use condoms.

Intervention Development

Our social-psychological analyses of the problem lead to a solution that is rather complex:

1. The public message should contain *both objectives in a position of equality*: "refrain from anal sex or consistently use a condom; never have unprotected anal sex." Equality here means getting equal attention; the message is not that using condoms is as safe as refraining from anal sex. Moreover, the message should facilitate a choice between those two alternatives, and not cause inaction (unprotected anal sex) as a result of the inability to choose (Romis, et al., 1989).
2. The public message needs to be supported by easy access to resources for *tailored messages*: e.g. personal, group, and anonymous counseling.
3. Available theoretical and empirical knowledge on the effectiveness of health education should be applied *to both parts of the message and to the combination* (Green & Kreuter, 1991; Glanz et al., 1990; Zimbardo & Leippe, 1991). Special attention is needed for: pretesting of messages with the target group (especially to avoid confusion and low self-efficacy), tailoring messages to different subgroups, promoting community development and community communication, active information processing and social support, anchoring the objectives in existing values and goals, skills training by observational and enactive learning, improving self-efficacy by attributional re-training and relapse prevention techniques. Continual *pretesting, monitoring and evaluation* is essential for the development and improvement of interventions and for the identification of unwanted effects.
4. Finally, a completely different kind of solution (but perhaps the best) is the development of *safe(r) condoms* for anal sex, combined with skills training for optimal use. Health educators should stimulate policy makers and manufacturers to promote this development. Health education messages could then solely focus on skills for adequate condom use.

Epilogue

As we have seen, the application of social psychological theories to real-life problems is not without difficulties. Theories are often too general for specific predictions or too conditional for generalizations to other situations. Given a problem, we have to find relevant concepts that guide us to appropriate theories. In this case the problem was extremely complex and the different theories suggested different solutions.

We started by recognizing two positions in the debate: first, the message may have failed and could be improved. Secondly, the message could have been unrealistic and should be changed to promote condom use. Different theories that were suggested by concepts derived from the two positions actually partly supported, as well as partly undermined, both positions, making it clear that simple solutions were not available. Moreover, the theoretical analyses brought forward a new concept of individual differences that had to be taken into account. Finally, the integrated solution which emerged was rather complex, but certainly feasible. A selective focus on only one theory would probably have resulted in a one-sided and ineffective, or even countereffective, solution.

Afterwards, some of the parties involved in the decision making concluded that social psychologists provide answers that other people can infer much faster from common sense and practical experience. As we had documented the diverse and often extreme positions in this debate, this accusation was certainly not an adequate perception. A more correct observation is that the official new Dutch policy on the HIV preventive message about anal sex was strongly influenced by the social-psychological analysis of the problem and as a result resembles the solution proposed here very closely: "Refrain from anal sex or consistently use a condom."

References

Bandura, A. (1986). *Social Foundations of Thought and Action*. Englewood Cliffs, NJ: Prentice-Hall.

Bandura, A. (1989). Perceived Self-efficacy in the Exercise of Control over AIDS Infection. In V.M.Mays, G.W.Albee, & S.F.Schneider (Eds.), *Primary Prevention of AIDS; Psychological Approaches* (pp. 128-141). Newbury Park, CA: Sage.

Bochow, M. (1989). Wie leben schwule Männer heute? *Deutsche AIDS Hilfe*, X, 27-32.

Bochow, M. (1990). AIDS and Gay Men: Individual Strategies and Collective Coping. *European Sociological Review, 6*, 181-188.

Bracht, N. (Ed.) (1990). *Health Promotion at the Community Level*. Newbury Park, CA: Sage.

Chan-Chee, C., De Vincenzi, I., Sole-Pla, M.A., Ancelle-Park, R., & Brunet, J.B. (1991). Use and Misuse of Condoms. *Genitourinary Medicine, 67*, 173-175.

Connell, R.W., & Kippax, S. (1990). Sexuality in the AIDS Crisis: Patterns of Sexual Practice and Pleasure in a Sample of Australian Gay and Bisexual Men. *The Journal of Sex Research, 27*, 167-198.

Connell, R.W., Crawford, J., Dowsett, G.W., Kippax, S., Sinnott, V., Rodden, P., Berg, R., Baxter, D., & Watson, L. (1990). Danger and Context: Unsafe Anal Sexual Practice Among Homosexual and Bisexual Men in the AIDS Crisis. *Australian and New Zealand Journal of Sociology, 26*, 187-208.

Den Boer, D.J., Kok, G., Hospers, H.J., Gerards, F.M., & Strecher, V.J. (1991). Health

Education Strategies for Attributional Retraining and Self-efficacy Improvement. *Health Education Research, 6*, 239-248.

De Wit, J.B.F., Sandfort, T.G.M., De Vroome, E.M.M., Van Griensven, G.J.P. & Kok, G.J. (1993). The Effectiveness of Condoms Use Among Homosexual Men. *AIDS, 7*, 751-752.

Ekstrand, M.L., & Coates, T.J. (1990). Maintenance of Safer Sexual Behaviors and Predictors of Risky Sex: The San Francisco Men's Health Study. *American Journal of Public Health, 80*, 973-977.

Fishbein, M., & Ajzen, I. (1975). *Belief, Attitude, Intention and Behavior*. Reading, MA: Addison-Wesley.

Fisher, J.D. (1988). Possible Effects of Reference Group-based Social Influence on AIDS Risk Behavior and AIDS Prevention. *American Psychologist, 43*, 914-920.

Försterling, F. (1988). *Attribution Theory in Clinical Psychology*. New York: Wiley.

Glanz, K., Lewis, F.M., & Rimer, B. (1990). *Health Behavior and Health Education*. San Francisco: Jossey-Bass.

Gold, R.S., Skinner, M.J., Grant, P.J., & Plummer, D.C. (1991). Situational Factors and Thought Processes Associated With Unprotected Intercourse in Gay Men. *Psychology and Health*, 5, 259-278.

Golombok, S., Sketchley, J., & Rust, J. (1990). Condom Failure Among Homosexual Men. *Journal of AIDS, 2*, 404-409.

Green, L.W., & Kreuter, M.W. (1991). *Health Promotion Planning: An Educational and Environmental Approach*. Mountain View, CA: Mayfield.

Hospers, H.J., & Kok, G. (1992). *AIDS Prevention for Gay Men and Relapse Prevention Approaches*. Paper presented at the Second European Conference on Homosexuality and HIV, Amsterdam, February 14-16, 1992. *Workshop D*, p. 1.

Hospers, H.J., & Kok, G. (1995). Determinants of Safe and Unsafe Sexual Behavior Among Gay Men: A review. *AIDS Education and Prevention*, 7, 74–96.

Janz, N.K., & Becker, M.H. (1984). The Health Belief Model: A Decade Later. *Health Education Quarterly, 11*, 1-47.

Joseph, J.G., Montgomery, S.B., Emmons, C-A., Kessler, R.C., Ostrow, D.G., Wortman, C.B., O'Brien, K., Eller, M., & Eshleman, S. (1987). Perceived Risk of AIDS: Assessing the Behavior Consequences in a Cohort of Gay Men. *Journal of Applied Social Psychology, 17*, 231-250.

Kelly, J.A., St Lawrence, J.S., Hood, H.V., & Brasfield, T.L. (1989). Behavioral Intervention to Reduce AIDS Risk Activities. *Journal of Consulting and Clinical Psychology, 57*, 60-67.

Kelly, J.A., St Lawrence, J.S., Betts, R., Brasfield, T.L., & Hood, H.V. (1990a). A Skills Training Group Intervention Model to Assist Persons in Reducing Risk Behaviors for HIV Infection. *AIDS Education and Prevention, 2*, 24-35.

Kelly, J.A., St Lawrence, J.S., Brasfield, T.L., Lemke, A., Amidei, T., Roffman, R.E., Hood, H.V., Smith, J.E., Kilgore, H., & McNeill, C. (1990b). Psychological Factors that Predict AIDS High-risk Versus AIDS Precautionary Behavior. *Journal of Consulting and Clinical Psychology, 58*, 117-120.

Kelly, J.A., St Lawrence, J.S., Brasfield, T.L., Stevenson, Y., Diaz, Y.E., & Hauth, A.C. (1990c). AIDS Risk Behavior Patterns Among Gay Men in Small Southern Cities. *American Journal of Public Health, 80*, 416-418.

Locke, E.A., & Latham, G.P. (1991). *A Theory of Goal Setting and Task Performance*. Englewood Cliffs, NJ: Prentice Hall.

Marlatt, G.A., & Gordon, J.R. (1985). *Relapse Prevention: Maintenance Strategies in*

the Treatment of Addictive Behaviors. New York: Guilford.
McGuire, W.J. (1985). Attitudes and Attitude Change. In G.Lindsay & E.Aronson (Eds.), *The Handbook of Social Psychology, Volume 2* (pp. 233-346). New York: Random House.
Petty, R.E., & Cacioppo, R.T. (1986). The Elaboration Likelihood Model of Persuasion. In L.Berkowitz (Ed.), *Advances in Experimental Social Psychology, Volume 19* (pp. 123-205). New York: Academic Press.
Pollak, M., Dubois-Arben, F., & Bochow, M. (1989). La Modification des Pratique Sexuelles. *La Recherche*, 20, 1100-1111.
Prieur, A. (1990). Norwegian Gay Men: Reasons for Continued Practice of Unsafe Sex. *AIDS Education and Prevention, 2*, 109-115.
Prochaska, J.O., & DiClemente, C.C. (1984). *The Transtheoretical Approach: Crossing Traditional Boundaries of Therapy*. Illinois: Dow Jones-Irwin Homewood.
Richters, J., Donovan, B., Gerofi, J., & Watson, L. (1988). Low Condoms Breaking Rate in Commercial Sex. *The Lancet,1988ii*, 1488.
Rogers, E.M. (1983). *Diffusion of Innovations*. New York: The Free Press.
Rogers, R.W. (1983). Cognitive and Physiological Processes in Fear Appeals and Attitude Change: A Revised Theory of Protection Motivation. In J.T.Cacioppo & R.E.Petty (Eds.), *Social Psychophysiology; A Source Book* (pp. 153-176). New York: Guilford.
Romano, R. (1984). *Pre-testing in Health Communications*. Bethesda, MD: National Cancer Institute.
Romis, D.L., Yates, J.F., & Kirscht, J.P. (1989). Attitudes, Decisions, and Habits as Determinants of Repeated Behavior. In A.R.Pratkanis, S.J.Brecker & A.G.Greenwald (Eds.), *Attitude Structure and Function* (pp. 213-239). Hillsdale, NJ: Lawrence Erlbaum.
Ross, M.W. (1987). Problems Associated with Condom Use in Homosexual Men. *American Journal of Public Health, 77*, 877.
Stein, Z.A. (1992). Editorial: The Double Bind in Science Policy and the Protection of Women from HIV Infection. *American Journal of Public Health, 82*, 1471-1472.
Strecher, V.J., Bauman, K.E., Boat, B., Fowler, M.G., Greenberg, R.A., & Stedman, H. (1989). The Development and Formative Evaluation of a Home-based Intervention to Reduce Passive Smoking by Infants. *Health Education Research, 4*, 225-232.
Suls, J., & Wills, T.A. (1991). *Social Comparison, Contemporary Theory and Research*. Hillsdale, NJ: Lawrence Erlbaum.
Valdiserri, R.O., Lyter, D., Levitan, L.C., Callahan, C.M., Kingsley, L.A., & Riwalde, C.R. (1988). Variables Influencing Condom Use in a Cohort of Gay and Bisexual Men. *American Journal of Public Health, 78*, 801-805.
Van Griensven, G.J.P., De Vroome, E.M.M., Tielman, R.A.P., & Coutinho, R.A. (1988). Failure Rate of Condoms During Anogenital Intercourse in Homosexual Men. *Genitourinary Medicine, 64*, 344-346.
Van Griensven, G.J.P., De Vroome, E.M.M., Tielman, R.A., Goudsmit, J., De Wolf, F., Van der Noorda, J. & Coutinho, R.A., 1989. Effects of Human Immunodeficiency Virus (HIV) Antibody Knowledge on High-risk Sexual Behavior with Steady and Nonsteady Sexual Partners Among Homosexual Men. *American Journal of Epidemiology*, 129, 596-603.
Voeller, B., Coulson, A.H., Bernstein, G.S., & Nakamura, R.M. (1989). Mineral Oil Lubricants Cause Rapid Deterioration of Latex Condoms. *Contraception, 39*, 95-102.

Weiner, B. (1986). *An Attributional Theory of Motivation and Emotion.* New York: Springer.

Weinstein, N.D. (1989). Effects of Personal Experience on Self-protective Behavior. *Psychological Bulletin, 105*, 31-50.

Wigersma, L., & Oud, R. (1987). Safety and Acceptability of Condoms for Use by Homosexual Men as a Prophylactic Against Transmission of HIV During Anogenital Sexual Intercourse. *British Medical Journal, 295*, 94.

Zimbardo, Ph.G., & Leippe, M.R. (1991). *The Psychology of Attitude Change and Social Influence*. Philadelphia: Temple University Press.

HIV/AIDS Prevention Strategies Affecting Special Population Groups

Frank Machlica

Historically, the AIDS pandemic has entered its second decade and is certain to be a lifelong issue for many individuals. Since there is currently no cure, no effective treatment, and no vaccine available to prevent HIV infection, the only realistic way of controlling the spread of AIDS is through prevention and education. Several research initiatives currently focus on HIV/AIDS prevention and education for special population groups.

The AIDS pandemic is different from previous ones, which were spread randomly through air or water, because HIV can only be spread through a limited number of biological pathways and thus has a strong behavioral component. The traditional epidemiological approaches to prevention lack mechanisms which account for individual behavioral changes in response to a disease, and the impact of information on behavior. Therefore, since most AIDS interventions are based on epidemiological models that involve either gathering or disseminating information, but cannot account for the effects of information, AIDS program planners and administrators have no method of evaluating the effects of their programs on the spread of HIV/AIDS (Philipson, et al., 1994).

Another difficulty with HIV prevention/education programs has been the inappropriate focus on individuals or populations ("gay men") instead of specific behaviors. Thus, men who have sex with men and who don't identify themselves as being "gay" have not considered themselves at risk. Furthermore, sexual behaviors identified with gay men (unprotected anal intercourse) have been considered higher risk than unprotected vaginal intercourse when in fact, 75% of the AIDS cases worldwide are attributed to heterosexual transmission (Ungvarski, 1994). In addition, "the number of cases of heterosexually-transmitted AIDS has been increasing steadily and more rapidly than cases in any of the other transmission categories" (Greenspan, et al., 1990, pg.1).

In addition, HIV prevention efforts have concentrated on HIV negative people. The false assumption was that if the two groups did not interact, there would not be an epidemic. However, in reality, both HIV positive and HIV negative individuals do not exist in a vacuum and therefore both groups must be addressed in prevention programs.

For AIDS prevention and education programs to be successful, they must demonstrate an understanding of the various levels of risk and the dynamics involved in changing human behavior, as well as an awareness of the unique cultural factors of the region where the behavior change is to be conducted (Livingston, 1992). AIDS education programs usually describe what AIDS is and how it can be transmitted. Information dissemination alone is not enough. Education strategies must address issues such as attitudes and motivation which influence behavioral change over long periods of time. AIDS researchers need to accurately communicate the level of risk and allow individuals to respond to AIDS in proportion to the risk that they face personally (Odets, 1994). "Innovative health education messages, perhaps via film, folklore, or popular music, should go beyond the avoidance of risky sexual behaviors and include additional messages regarding HIV transmission to the entire family and community... More specifically, messages should tell of and provide ways to discourage social practices that may also weaken the immune system or increase risk of HIV infection, such as drug abuse, excessive alcohol consumption, untreated sexually transmitted diseases (STDs), and unsanitary home environments" (Livingston, 1992, pg.11).

Additionally, interpersonal methods of communicating (including testimonials of people living with AIDS) may be more effective than mass media campaigns for educating and influencing the behavior of select groups within the community (Livingston, 1992).

Prevention strategies must address cultural factors, including norms, values and beliefs, which influence the past, present and future behaviors of individuals. Two aspects of cultural factors are significant: 1) the conceptualization held by the target group of the variables being studied (sexual behaviors and drug use); and 2) their belief systems about disease, sickness, and death and how these relate to AIDS. People with low incomes generally experience a higher incidence of illness and a lower survival rate than the general population. Poor people of color usually are less likely to obtain early treatment for

HIV infection, likely to have been less healthy when they contracted the virus, and likely to have more advanced symptoms when they first seek treatment. In addition, tuberculosis also links race, poverty and disease because transmission often occurs in crowded environments with inadequate ventilation such as housing shelters and prisons which are disproportionately shared by persons of color (National Commission on AIDS, 1993).

AIDS has directly impacted special populations such as men who are sexually involved with men, women — especially women of color, children and adolescents, the severely and persistently mentally ill, mentally ill chemical abusers, intravenous drug users, middle-aged and older individuals, people with disabilities, and immigrants and undocumented residents who may have language and cultural barriers and be less likely to receive information, or act on information once it is received.

Men Who Are Sexually Involved With Men

"The difficulty of compliance with condom use... should make us pause and think about crusades for the supremacy of the condom in preventing the transmission of HIV. People need choices in reducing their risk of infection, but each method requires demonstration of its effectiveness" (Johnson, 1994, pg. 392).

In early 1992, AIDS educators publicly acknowledged that gay men were having unprotected sex (Odets, 1994). It has been estimated that between 31-53% of gay and bisexual men nationwide are having unprotected anal intercourse (Odets, 1994; Signorile, 1994). Forty-three percent (43%) of 17-19 year old gay males in San Francisco reported having unprotected sex. Fifty-two percent (52%) of African-American young gay men in San Francisco reported having unprotected sex (Signorile, 1994). Thirty percent (30%) of 20 year olds in San Francisco will be infected or dead of AIDS by age 30 and the majority will become HIV infected at some time during their lifetimes. The life expectancy of a gay male in San Francisco between the ages of 16-24 is about 45 (Odets, 1994). There is a 50% overall infection rate of gay men nationwide with 10-40% infection rates among young gay males and 70% among older gay males (Odets, 1994). Thirty-three percent (33%) of all currently uninfected 20 year old gay and bisexual men in Baltimore, Chicago, Los Angeles and Pittsburgh, will seroconvert by age 30 (Signorile, 1994).

These statistics translate into depression, loss, grief, isolation, hopelessness, guilt and despair. AIDS prevention can no longer focus only on simplistic behavior changes and ignore the role of emotions in dealing with the complexity of this life-long epidemic, particularly issues of intimacy, sex and death.

Mental Hygiene Issues

Mental hygiene issues must be incorporated into prevention/education strategies, in order for them to become effective. In order to help individuals get in touch with their thoughts and feelings about sex, intimacy, alcohol and other drug use, death and AIDS, they must be encouraged to talk about these "taboo" subjects.

The practice of unprotected sex usually leads to shame and guilt. Individuals "often feel they have crossed into forbidden territory from which there is no return... Gay men must be allowed to know their conflicted feelings about protected/unprotected sex are shared by many, and the transgression of 'community standards' neither excommunicates them from the gay community nor makes their lives irretrievable" (Odets, 1994, pg. 6).

"Terms like 'unsafe sex' and 'risky behavior' are value judgements that imply certain acts are 'bad' and 'dangerous' in themselves, despite our knowledge that they may be dangerous in the presence of HIV...In pursuit of making thoughts and feelings accessible, we must speak about 'protected' and 'unprotected sex'" (Odets, 1994, pg. 6).

Odets (1994) suggests that several psychological issues should be incorporated into AIDS prevention and education programs:

"The sense of inevitability that so many men feel about contracting HIV."

This is expressed in depression, hopelessness, helplessness, anxiety, the false belief that one has HIV, the careless exposure to HIV, the abandonment of any effort to protect oneself from HIV, and the deliberate pursuit of HIV infection. This is the result of a profound identification with AIDS, with those dead of AIDS, or those who are HIV positive.

"The variety of human meanings of sex."

AIDS education has identified "the exchange of body fluids" as the primary mode of HIV transmission, without acknowledging that this has been a significant expression of intimacy for many men. Future approaches to education should consider that oral sex without condoms might be a minimum (.0003%) risk alternative for men for whom semen exchange is a meaningful part of intimacy. "Is a .0003% risk over 5 years a universally acceptable reason to preclude an important expression of intimacy?"

"Trait behaviors."

People are less likely to repeat undesired behaviors if they attribute them to a *state* rather than to a *trait*. State-determined behavior (feeling in love, being influenced by a partner, being under the influence of alcohol/drugs) is due to "temporary" external or internal influences. Trait-determined behavior is the expression of "permanent" character traits.

The danger in AIDS educators connecting behavior to character traits (having common sense), can encourage occasional behaviors to become continuous ones "because for those compelled to practice unprotected sex for reasons they do not understand, character-based education colludes with the rationalization, "I guess it's just in my nature."

New approaches to education must acknowledge the complexity of feelings about sex and that many men occasionally engage in sexual behaviors that they wish they had not. This will lead to an understanding of the reasons of these behaviors.

"Off line/on line."

People exist in different states of consciousness when they are being educated and when they are having sex. These states of consciousness need to be addressed in the context of AIDS education which must also affirm the importance of erotic life by showing it realistically integrated into other aspects of life (intimacy, friendship, love, communication).

Substance Use/Abuse.

There is a strong correlation between substance use/abuse and sexual behaviors that increase the risk of HIV infection. Substance use typically lowers inhibitions and impairs judgement. It has been found that HIV sexual risk behaviors increases as substance use advances from alcohol and cigarettes to marijuana, cocaine and other illicit drugs (Lowry, et al., 1994).
Consequently, mental hygiene issues must be addressed in HIV/AIDS prevention programs targeting men who have sex with men. Strategies need to be developed to increase self esteem to combat racism, sexism, homophobia, and poverty. For example, before working with low income women of color who abuse drugs, or gay teenagers, mental health and social service providers must first help clients become aware of and discuss how they feel about themselves, because feelings of low self esteem will probably not result in safer sex behaviors. In other words, if an individual is not permitted to think about why s/he may *not* feel like surviving the pandemic, then s/he cannot think about why s/he might feel like surviving it.

Women, Including Women of Color

Nationwide, women represent the fastest growing group of people with AIDS (Osborn, 1990; Lerner, 1994). In New York City, women, especially Black and Hispanic women, comprise 19% of the reported AIDS cases. Poor Black and Latina women are at high risk for HIV because of poverty, lack of resources and lack of opportunities which prevent them from leaving areas of high HIV seroprevalence (Alexander, 1990). Women of color often have limited access to medical, legal and social support systems and thus have had few opportunities to learn about HIV disease. Many do not have health insurance and seek medical care only for emergencies. In New York City, 40% of Latinas have late or no prenatal care (Maldonado, 1990). Additionally, many women of color often do not identify themselves as members of "high risk populations" (Perez, 1990).

The many issues related to pregnancy need to be addressed by prevention programs. HIV infected pregnant women can infect their infants in utero, during delivery, and through breast-feeding. About 30% of babies born to HIV positive mothers will be born and remain seropositive (Perez, 1990). Providing counseling to HIV positive women during pregnancy has become more complex in light of recent developments related to the use of AZT during pregnancy and childbirth. Treating mothers with Zidovudine during the second and third trimesters and during labor and delivery has been shown to reduce HIV transmission to infants by two-thirds (Saag, 1994). Medical, ethical and confidentiality issues will surge to the forefront over the next few years as guidelines are developed for practitioners on how to counsel HIV infected women who are pregnant or considering having children. Medical information will need to be presented to women, including those who are pregnant, and/or HIV positive (whether infected before or during pregnancy) in an objective, non-judgmental manner to allow them to make informed decisions regarding HIV testing, and taking AZT during pregnancy.

Due to the high rate of women becoming HIV-infected through drug use, women need increased access to drug treatment services, particularly with child care components, and these programs must address the link between drug use and HIV transmission. In addition, existing community programs such as STD clinics, prenatal care programs, family planning programs, substance abuse programs, and primary care clinics should be expanded to include HIV prevention, screening, and treatment for women and families. There should be an integration of multiple, interrelated services: health, mental health, substance abuse, nutrition, case management, etc. (Perez, 1990).

Current prevention efforts regarding the sexual transmission of HIV infection have focused on abstinence and safer sex. More work needs to be done in the development and marketing of microbicides, chemicals that can be used intravaginally to kill HIV infection and other sexually transmitted diseases, but not damage the reproductive tracts of either partner. Women need a method to use when they suspect their partner may have an STD or HIV infection and they can't convince their male partners to use condoms. "Microbicides should be seen as an additional HIV prevention option, one that complements rather than supplants the others" (Lerner, 1994, pg. 13). Just as the FDA has accelerated the route for testing AIDS therapies, it needs to expedite the review process to result in the labeling of a vaginal microbicide against HIV infection (Potts, 1994). The potential of microbicidal products to slow the spread of HIV infection should provide motivation for the development of these products and their future availability to women in need of more HIV prevention methods (Lerner, 1994).

Children and Adolescents

"Adolescents' perceptions of invincibility may inflate their risk of HIV transmission, especially when combined with their misconceptions and misinformation about AIDS" (Livingston, 1992, pg. 10). AIDS is the sixth leading cause of death among youth and is being increasingly spread via heterosexual transmission in urban minority areas in the United States. Thus, there is a need for AIDS education programs that target children and adolescents, particularly those of color, living in high risk environments (Romer, et al., 1994). Most HIV prevention approaches focus on health-related attitudes and behavioral skills of the individual. Youth need help in obtaining the skills (how to negotiate safer sex) and access to the resources needed for lower risk behaviors (how to purchase condoms and other STD prevention supplies). "Although these factors are important in initiating safe behavior, they may not be sufficient to maintain this behavior when social environments continue to encourage risk... Knowledge about the hazards of unprotected sex is not sufficient to overcome the host of other influences that increase risky sexual behavior... Even changing individual attitudes and skills may not undo the influence of peer norms" (Romer, et al., 1994, pgs. 977, 984).

Interventions should target not only the knowledge, attitudes and beliefs of individuals but also the norms of an entire community. Safer sex must be legitimized by the community. It has been reported that individuals, despite being knowledgeable about HIV transmission, have perceived that unsafe sexual practices were expected by potential sexual partners, believed their personal inclinations toward safer sex were not shared by others, and feared potential rejection by sex partners (Legion, et al., 1990).

HIV prevention programs for youth need to be aware that substance use may be an important indicator of risk for HIV infection and AIDS through its association with unsafe sexual behaviors. "Nearly 50% of HIV-infected adolescents seen at an outpatient clinic in New York City reported heavy crack use... The likelihood of... sexual risk behaviors (among high school students) increases as substance use progresses from alcohol and cigarettes to marijuana, cocaine and other illicit drugs" (Lowry, et al., 1994, pgs. 1118-1119).

Romer et al., (1994) has suggested two prevention strategies to use with youth. First, shared parental monitoring, when parents of children's friends join together to monitor the behavior of their children, which is similar to the traditional practice of shared caregiving among African-American families, may be an effective prevention method for children. Second, the promotion of delayed sexual activity (or continued condom use) to youth within their friendship networks may influence the social norms of peers to favor risk reduction instead of enhancement.

AIDS education programs for adolescents must address the effects of peer pressure and community norms, poor socio-economic conditions, and substance use and abuse. It has been suggested that comprehensive interventions that combine skill building youth education programs with individual counseling, parental involvement and training, and community involvement would ensure access to social, health, and mental health services and reduce substance use and sexual risk behaviors (Lowry, et al., 1994).

People living with AIDS (PLWAs) can be effective in providing AIDS education to adolescents. PLWAs may play an important role in altering attitudes and behaviors based on fear and denial through addressing the impact of HIV/AIDS from personal experience. Because youth are still developing cognitively and have open minds, they can listen to PWAs and give truthful feedback. Guest speakers can also help PWAs in the audience connect with available resources. If the families of PWAs are involved in education efforts, they may benefit as well because this allows them to channel their grief through helping to educate and protect other people's children (Legion, et al., 1990).

Since the mid-1980s, many schools throughout the United States have implemented HIV/AIDS education programs for adolescents but there is little information available regarding their effectiveness (Holtzman, et al., 1994). More research is needed to study the longitudinal behavior changes of adolescents, especially those who engage in high risk behaviors, the effects of prevention programs on HIV-related knowledge and attitudes of adolescents, and to what extent knowledge about HIV affects their behavior.

The Severely and Persistently Mentally Ill (SPMI)

The severely and persistently mentally ill (SPMI) population, including mentally ill chemical abusers (MICAs) may be at risk for HIV due to their high rates of substance abuse and unsafe sexual activity. These two risk behaviors are not necessarily mutually exclusive. Cournos (1993) reported that a number of sexually active patients exchanged sex to support substance abuse habits, and, the use of drugs was associated with unsafe sexual activity — having multiple partners.

Regarding the sexual behavior of people with severe mental illness, Cournos (1993) found that between 50-66% had been sexually active within the past year; one in five male and female SPMIs reported a lifetime history of homosexual behavior; and, 90.2% of sexually active patients did *not* consistently use condoms. Similarly, Kaplan, et al. (1993) found that, of the 201 patients studied, 50% had been sexually active in the past six months, and 89% used condoms inconsistently or not at all.

Furthermore, chronic psychiatric patients, including MICAs, did not eliminate risk behavior based on knowledge of risk factors (Fine, 1993). According to Kaplan, et al. (1993), the psychiatric patients studied, despite exhibiting knowledge of HIV modes of infection and the consequences of seropositivity, "reported low rates of condom use."

Since SPMI and MICA clients have limited knowledge and understanding of HIV disease, and usually do not apply this knowledge to changing behavior, more work needs to be done in developing risk reduction training programs specifically for this population. According to Fine (1993), there have been a few reported psycho-educational group programs for psychiatric patients and MICAs that have demonstrated improvements in attitudes and knowledge regarding transmission risk factors and a reduction in risk behaviors. Additionally, Kaplan, et al. (1993) recently developed an HIV risk reduction group intervention training module targeting people with severe mental illness. However, despite these gains, there is still a need for more data on modifying HIV risk behavior and attitudes in the severely and persistently mentally ill (Kelly, et al.; 1992, Fine, 1993).

Immigrants

AIDS prevention programs must be sensitive to the cultural beliefs and values of different ethnic groups. "Cultural diversity is evident in the different languages, cultural practices and beliefs regarding illness and health seeking behavior. Thus, it may be more effective to develop and implement health education programs that are adapted to a community's existing practices and beliefs, rather than trying to change them to fit the program" (Bayer, 1994, pg. 895).

AIDS programs that are *not* culturally sensitive and culturally appropriate will be ineffective "because they will not reach their intended audience, will not be understood by those who are reached, and will not be accepted by those who understand" (Bayer, 1994, pg. 895).

Unfortunately, both the widespread stigmatization of special population groups, including people of color, continues to create obstacles in fighting the AIDS pandemic. Discrimination and stigmatization may increase as there is more awareness of the disproportionate number of people of color who are infected with HIV (National Commission on AIDS, 1993). In addition to stigmatization, another barrier in combating this pandemic is the lack of information regarding the effects of HIV/AIDS on certain populations, particularly Asians and Pacific Islanders (see section below). The number of actual AIDS cases may be significantly under-counted for these communities because the actual ethnicity is sometimes misrepresented in AIDS service organization records and on death certificates (National Commission on AIDS, 1993). Therefore, it is essential that HIV/AIDS statistics be interpreted and used carefully.

Due to the limited information and inaccurate data available, aggressive outreach to immigrant and other special population groups is essential. Those individuals may not seek out services because they do not perceive themselves to be at risk. If targeted HIV prevention is postponed until there are large numbers of AIDS cases, then the opportunity will be missed to prevent those cases from occurring (National Commission on AIDS, 1993).

Asians and Pacific Islanders

The relatively small number of cases among Asian and Pacific Islander individuals, as compared to other racial groups, as well as the limited understanding of the epidemiology of HIV/AIDS among these populations have: 1) resulted in a complacency and a lack of attention by public health officials and community members to develop prevention efforts; 2) often been used to justify low levels of program funding for health, mental health and social services targeting these groups; and 3) sent an inaccurate message to these communities that they don't have to worry about AIDS.

Even though the number of AIDS cases among Asians and Pacific Islanders (A&PIs) currently appears to be relatively low, these communities are still in the early stages of a growing HIV pandemic. As previously mentioned, with South and Southeast Asia quickly becoming epicenters of the HIV/AIDS pandemic, with the heterosexual rate of transmission increasing, and with the increase of Asian immigrants (representing 25% of all immigrants) to New York City in the 1980s, Asian and Pacific Islanders are at high risk for HIV infection (*The Newest New Yorkers,* 1992).

Therefore, it is essential to target prevention efforts to the Asian and Pacific Islander community in general, and to immigrant women in particular. For example, the Asian and Pacific Islander Coalition on HIV and AIDS (APICHA) has a unique program where outreach workers distribute HIV/AIDS brochures, condoms and other materials in immigrant communities in Brooklyn, Manhattan, and Queens (Mangaliman, 1994). Unless additional HIV prevention strategies are implemented for the Asian and Pacific Islander populations and other populations currently under-represented statistically, the course of the pandemic in these relatively insular communities may resemble that of the African-American and Hispanic/Latino populations.

Latino Populations

In the Latino community, culturally prescribed gender roles and condom use is an important issue. In the traditional Latino culture, women are not expected to be knowledgeable about sexuality, nor to raise issues such as condom use. In contrast, Latino men are socialized to be informed about sexuality and may have sexual contacts outside of marriage. Condoms are viewed as birth control and for preventing infection from prostitutes by Latino men. Thus, with the emphasis on procreation in the Latino culture and the prohibition of contraception by the Catholic church, Latinos are less likely to use condoms (Maldonado, 1990).

There are many implications for prevention campaigns targeted to Latino men. Given the machismo element of the Latino culture with male dominance and women in subordinate relationships with their sexual partners, prevention campaigns may need to support the aspects of machismo which focus on the male's responsibility for protecting his family. Messages which emphasize AIDS as a threat to the family, promote condom use as a way of protecting the family, and encourage the empowerment of women may be more effective prevention approaches (Maldonado, 1990).

Caribbean Populations

The Caribbean has been described as an area of 'high risk' for AIDS. "Although the means of transmission may vary, it is the poorest sections of society and the poorer countries of the world that are most vulnerable to HIV/AIDS" (Livingston, 1992, pg. 3).

Presently, Caribbean populations constitute the largest number (15%) of immigrants entering the United States, and more than 1 million of them are Haitians (Rey, 1993). In addition, it is estimated that there are about 5 million undocumented immigrants in America. Given the high per capita rates of AIDS cases in the Caribbean, the increasing numbers of new Caribbean immigrants, as well as the incoming refugees from Guantanamo Bay, prevention, outreach and education to these populations are a high priority (Rey, 1993).

Prevention and health education strategies must take into account that 91% of the cumulative adult AIDS cases in the Caribbean are the result of sexual transmission (53% heterosexual, 38% homosexual and/or bisexual) (Livingston, 1992). Additionally, in developing countries, which may have low literacy rates, the reading of AIDS education materials is difficult for most people. Therefore, the government must find other ways to inform the public about the disease.

In the Haitian population, HIV is primarily spread through heterosexual transmission. While a small number of HIV infected Haitian males admitted to bisexuality, sex with different partners, or prostitutes, none, however, admitted to homosexuality or IV drug use. Haitian women with AIDS were often offered money for sex. Prevention programs targeting the Caribbean population must address how cultural and socio-economic factors, including beliefs about health care and cures, affect behavior. In addition, an understanding of the cultural attitudes toward gender, sex, sexuality, and sexual behavior is essential (Rey, 1993).

Health promoting behaviors vary among socio-economic classes. Due to the high rate of illiteracy in Haiti, there is limited access to printed educational materials. People who live in rural areas of Haiti have much less knowledge about using condoms to prevent HIV transmission than people living in urban areas. In the United States, there is a high rate of illiteracy among Haitian-American parents and the lack of participation in community and school activities limits their exposure to educational materials. While in the higher socio-economic strata, individuals visit physicians, those in the lower strata do not. Highly educated Haitians, despite having knowledge about HIV, continued to engage in high risk behavior including unprotected sex and multiple sex partners (Rey, 1993).

Many Haitians believe in prayers, voodoo practices, and folk and herb remedies as possible cures. Haitians, especially women, believe that HIV-infected persons are victims of a "Hex" by voodoo or witchcraft and since AIDS is caused by a spirit then only a magical intervention can be effective in prevention and healing. HIV positive Haitian males often feel that they can eliminate the virus (which they believe is the result of a spirit or curse) by having multiple sexual encounters, by expelling the "evil" sperm (Rey, 1993).

Haitian women have a dependent role and experience difficulty discussing sexual issues, and negotiating condom use. In contrast, as testimony of their "machismo," Haitian men often discuss with each other issues regarding sex and having multiple sexual partners, including prostitutes. Men, not women, often decide on having "protected sex" and take the responsibility of obtaining condoms (Rey, 1993).

Consequently, the development of HIV prevention, outreach and education programs must exist concomitantly with cultural realities and include knowledge about Haitian, and other cultural belief systems regarding issues such as health care, sexuality, and death. The most effective prevention approaches are comprehensive, culturally-relevant health promotion campaigns that carefully utilize both mass media strategies and face-to-face personal and community-based programs (Livingston, 1992; Business Publishers, 1994). Prevention strategies must target multiple systems including youth, families, schools, workplaces, communities, organizations, and the media. Additionally, professional folk healers need to be involved in outreach and prevention efforts because they are highly respected by their communities, can be teachers, give practical meanings to symbols, and provide guidance to both Caribbean people and prevention educators.

Middle-Aged and Older People

Due to the increasing availability of treatments for the many HIV-related illnesses, many people are living longer and growing older. Many HIV prevention and education programs have neglected to address the issues of older adults due to false assumptions that they are not at risk for HIV and are not sexually active (Grossman, 1994). Little attention has been focused on the epidemiology of AIDS in older persons who are at risk as much as the larger population. It is important for health and mental health providers who work with older persons to be aware that AIDS can affect geriatric patients of both sexes (Ship, et al., 1991). As aforementioned, among the 11% of cumulative adult cases age 50 and over in New York City, 51% were due to having unprotected (homosexual and heterosexual) sex, 34% were related to intravenous drug use, and 1.4% were from blood transfusions (DOH *AIDS Surveillance Update*, October, 1994).

Age does not decrease sexual desire or activity, and sexual activity may increase with age. It has been reported that two-thirds of males and one-third of females over the age of 60 are sexually active. Many adults over age 50 may not use condoms because there is little concern about pregnancy after menopause, and also the false perception that older people do not get AIDS. Men who are having (or who have had) unprotected sex with other men are at high risk for HIV infection. There are over 1 million gay men in the U.S. over the age of 65, and this does not include men who are sexually involved with men who do not identify themselves as being gay.

Older alcohol and drug users have been ignored by health professionals and the general public because of the false belief that older people seldom used or abused drugs. However, a number of middle-aged and older individuals have drug and alcohol abuse histories, which often leads to impairments in memory and decision making which can result in unsafe sexual and drug use behaviors. Therefore, it is essential to have thorough assessments to determine both drug and alcohol histories, and the cause of memory loss, if exhibited, which could be due to HIV infection, alcohol and other drug use, and/or old age.

A significant number of older adults have received one or more blood transfusions for illnesses or health complications. They, as well as other recipients of blood transfusions, are at high risk if they received a transfusion prior to March, 1993 when HIV screenings were initiated.

HIV/AIDS affects older people in a variety of other ways. Many middle-aged and older adults have become caregivers for their adult children and/or grandchildren who have AIDS. They must deal with grief, bereavement and loss issues on a regular basis. Often, older relatives become the legal guardians to children who have been orphaned by AIDS.

Furthermore, it has been reported that older individuals have less knowledge than younger people regarding HIV prevention, transmission, and antibody testing (Catania, et al., 1989). Consequently, there is a need for additional prevention programs specifically developed to address the needs and reduce the risks for middle-aged and elderly people.

It is essential to provide extensive outreach due to the difficulties in reaching the at-risk older population. Older gay men may be more secretive about their sexual orientation than younger gay men and thus isolated from the gay community and its resources. Additionally, it is difficult to identify and target older people who have had multiple sexual partners, or blood transfusions prior to 1985.

Prevention strategies with older people need to address the sex-related changes that come with age, along with cultural and historical differences in attitudes about sex, illness, and death. Previous research has indicated that brief interventions focusing on being supportive and providing specific information and suggestions can cause significant changes in sexual behavior and attitudes among older individuals (Catania, et al., 1989).

It has been suggested that interventions should involve mass media including television, the press, mailings and radio. Basic education is needed to eliminate the myth that older people do not get AIDS. Transmission modes, both past and present, that affect the elderly must be highlighted. Risk factors include prior blood transfusions, intravenous drug use, having multiple sexual partners, or having sex with someone who has had prior transfusions, uses or used intravenous drugs, or has had multiple sexual partners. Older individuals need to be encouraged to obtain HIV antibody testing if they are at risk and obtain information about the test, what it is, how to obtain it, the cost, etc (Catania, et al., 1989).

Prevention strategies must also be implemented at community-based or institutional programs. In groups and on the individual level, older individuals can discuss the use of condoms, learn communication skills to negotiate safer sex behaviors, and obtain cognitive-behavioral interventions to help them recognize and avoid situations that can lead to risk behaviors. All of the above methods must be tailored to address the needs of specific subcultures and ethnic groups. For instance, it may be effective to reach older gay men who are secretive about their sexual orientation through anonymous telephone hot lines such as those being used in Seattle (Catania, et al., 1989).

People With Disabilities

People with disabilities, particularly mental retardation and developmental disabilities (MR/DD), are at high risk for HIV/AIDS. These populations may have cognitive limitations and poor impulse control, as well as being easily manipulated into engaging in high risk behaviors (both sexually and/or using intravenous drugs) (Jacobs, et al., 1991).

Caretakers and agency staff often tend to think of MR/DD clients as asexual and thus may not provide appropriate information about how HIV is transmitted sexually. Peer education programs are considered to be an effective and desirable component of AIDS education. According to Jacobs, et al. (1989), the "Health Belief Model" of AIDS prevention has been adapted for developmentally disabled clients. This model emphasizes that people with disabilities: 1) must be taught to perceive HIV infection as a threat; 2) must be empowered to protect themselves and realize they can control whether or not they get the virus; 3) must be taught in a simple and concrete manner the necessary preventive health behaviors to allow them to make informed decisions; 4) must participate in peer support groups which function to reinforce AIDS educational messages through positive support or confrontation; and 5) must be reassured they can be sexually satisfied while using condoms.

For many individuals with disabilities who are now living in communities, it is important that both program staff and families, relatives and caretakers/caregivers be educated about HIV/AIDS risk reduction behavior for these populations. These risk reduction techniques must be reinforced not only by staff in the agencies, but also by caretakers in the home or residence of the disabled individual.

Conclusion

In summary, public health officials, researchers, health and mental health professionals, and community-based service providers must all work together in order to develop a better understanding of the role of cultural, behavioral, and socioeconomic factors in HIV transmission, the stages of the disease, and access to care. The information resulting from these efforts should be integrated into the design of HIV prevention and treatment services (National Commission on AIDS, 1993). Comprehensive HIV/AIDS services need to be targeted to all people, including those at risk, health care and social service personnel, indigenous healers, immediate and extended family members, workers, students, religious and spiritual leaders: basically, the entire community (Livingston, 1992).

ACKNOWLEDGEMENTS

I am indebted to Darryl L. Wong, M.P.H. and Angela Christofides, M.S.W. for their editorial contributions and support, as well as, Arnold Korotkin, A.C.S.W., M.B.A., Stacy Lamon, Ph.D., and to Ketty H. Rey, J.D., Ph.D., Director of the Office of Services to Special Populations of the N.Y.C. Department of Mental Health, whose expertise on these issues, particularly in the area of special populations and multi-cultural concerns proved invaluable.

REFERENCES

Alexander, V. (December, 1990). Black Women and HIV/AIDS. *SIECUS Report*, 19(2), 30-32.

Bayer, R. (1994). AIDS Prevention and Cultural Sensitivity: Are They Compatible? *American Journal of Public Health*, 84, 895-898.

Business Publishers, Inc. (1994, September 6). Service Coordination Key for People With AIDS. *Mental Health Report*, 18(18), 140.

Cantania, J.A., Stall, R., Coates, T.J., Pelham, A. O., & Sacks, C. (1989). Issues in AIDS Primary Prevention. *Generations, 8*(4), 50-54.

Cournos, F. (1993, June 25). *HIV Seroprevalence and Sexual Risk Behavior*. Paper presented at the HIV/AIDS and the Mentally Ill Conference (pp. 1-6). Columbia University College of Physicians & Surgeons, New York, N.Y.

Fine, J. (1993, June 25). *Substance Use and HIV Risk Behavior*. Paper presented at the HIV/AIDS and the Mentally Ill Conference (pp. 15-26). Columbia University College of Physicians & Surgeons, New York, N.Y.

Greenspan, A., & Castro, K.G. (1990). Heterosexual Transmission of HIV Infection. *SIECUS Report,* 19(1), 1-8.

Grossman, A. (Ed.) (1994). *Reaching Out to Middle Age and Older People: The Challenge of HIV/AIDS*. New York: New York University, AIDS/SIDA Mental Hygiene Project, pp. 9-22.

Holtzman, D., Lowry, R., Kann, L., Collins, J. L., & Kolbe, L.J. (1994). Changes In HIV-related Information Sources, Instruction, Knowledge, and Behaviors Among U.S. High School Students, 1989 and 1990. *American Journal of Public*

Health, 84(3), 388-393.

Jacobs, R., Samowitz, P., Levy, J.M., & Levy, P.H. (1989, August). Developing An AIDS Prevention Education Program for Persons with Developmental Disabilities. *Mental Retardation, 27*(4), 233-237.

Jacobs, R., Samowitz, P., Levy, J.M., Levy, P.H., & Cabrera, G. (1991). Young Adult Institute's Comprehensive AIDS Staff Training Program. In A. C. Crocker, H. J. Cohen, & T.A. Kastner (Eds.), *HIV Infection and Developmental Disabilities* (pp. 161-169). Baltimore, MD.: Paul H.Brooks Publishing Company.

Johnson, A.M. (1994). Condoms and HIV Transmission. *New England Journal of Medicine, 331*, 391-392.

Kaplan, M., Herman, R., & Bailum, S. (1993, June 25). *Training Professionals to Help Patients Stay Safe: Risk Interviewing and Risk Reduction Techniques*. Paper presented at the HIV/AIDS and the Mentally Ill Conference (pp. 33-37). Columbia University College of Physicians & Surgeons, New York, N.Y.

Kelly, J.A., Murphy, D.A., & Bahr, G.R. (1992). AIDS/HIV Risk Behavior Among the Chronically Mentally Ill. *American Journal of Psychiatry, 149*, 886-889.

Lerner, S. (1994, June). Microbicides: A Woman-controlled HIV Prevention Method In the Making. *SIECUS Report*, 10-13.

Lifshitz, A. (1990, December). Critical Cultural Barriers that Bar Meeting the Needs of Latinas. *SIECUS Report*, 19(2), 38-39.

Livingston, I.L. (1992, September). AIDS/HIV crisis in developing countries: The Need for Greater Understanding and Innovative Health Promotion Approaches. *Journal of the National Medical Association, 84*(9), 755-770.

Lowry, R., Holtzman, D., Truman, B. I., Kann, L., Collins, J. L., & Kolbe, L.J. (1994). Substance Use and HIV-related Sexual Behaviors Among U.S. High School Students: Are They Related? *American Journal of Public Health, 84*(7), 1116-1120.

Maldonado, M. (1990, December). Latinas and HIV/AIDS: Implications for the 90s. *SIECUS Report, 19*(2), 33-37.

National Commission on AIDS. (1993, March). The Challenge of HIV/AIDS in Communities of Color. *AIDS Reference Guide*. Washington, D.C.: Atlantic Information Services Inc., 1114, 1-16.

New York City Department of Health-Office of AIDS Surveillance. (1994, October). *AIDS Surveillance Update*.

Odets, W. (1994). AIDS Education and Harm Reduction for Gay Men: Psychological Approaches for the 21st century. *AIDS & Public Policy Journal, 9*(1), 3-15.

Osborn, J. (1990, December). Women and HIV/AIDS: The Silent Epidemic? *SIECUS Report, 19*(2), 23-26.

Perez, E. (1990, December). Why Women Wait to be Tested for HIV Infection. *SIECUS Report, 19*(2), 28-29.

Philipson, T.J., Posner, R.A., & Wright, J.H. (1994, Spring). Why AIDS Prevention Programs Don't Work. *Issues in Science and Technology*, 33-35.

Potts, M. (1994). The Urgent Need for a Vaginal Microbicide in the Prevention of HIV Transmission. *American Journal of Public Health, 84*, 890-891.

Rey, K. (1993, May 7). *Cultural Beliefs Affecting AIDS Education in the Haitian Community*. Paper presented at an Inter-Agency Meeting Regarding the Guantanamo Bay Haitian Refugees (pp. 1-31). New York City Department of Mental Health, Mental Retardation and Alcoholism Services, New York, N.Y.

Romer, D., Black, M., Ricardo, I., Feigelman, S., Kaljee, L., Galbraith, J., Nesbit, R., Hornik, R. C., & Stanton, B. (1994). Social Influences on the Sexual Behavior of

Youth at Risk for HIV Exposure. *American Journal of Public Health*, 84(6), 977-985.

Saag, M. (1994). Yokohama Update: Tenth International Conference on AIDS. *HIV Information Network*. New York, NY: World Health Communications Inc., 4.

Ship, J.A., Wolff, A., and Selik, R.M. (1991). Epidemiology of Acquired Immune Deficiency Syndrome in Persons Aged 50 Years or Older. *AIDS Reference Guide*. Washington, D.C.: Atlantic Information Services Inc.,114, 1-5.

Signorile, M. (1994, October). Unsafe Like Me. *Out Magazine*, pp. 22-24, 128-129.

Ungvarski, P.J. (1994, October 26). *Epidemiological Trends in HIV/AIDS*. Fact sheet distributed at the HIV Disease: Yesterday's Assumptions, Today's Realities Conference. New York University, New York, New York.

AIDS IN THE BLACK/AFRICAN-AMERICAN COMMUNITY: A CENTRAL HARLEM EXPERIENCE

Janet L. Mitchell, Rosalind Thompson, Betty W. Carrington,
Pearila B. Namerow, Lawrence Brown,
Patricia O. Loftman and Sterling B. Williams

When the National Commission on AIDS released the report of their three years of study on January 11, 1993 in Washington, D.C., the following statement was included:

> The continuing widespread stigmatization of people of color creates enormous difficulties for effectively combating the HIV/AIDS epidemic. Perhaps the greatest of these is that communities of color fear that stigmatization and discrimination are likely to increase as the public becomes more aware of the disproportionate number of people of color who are infected with HIV. For these communities, disproportionate representation raises the fear that they will be saddled with the disease — blamed for it, stigmatized by it, and left to deal with it on their own. As one witness stated: As the American public becomes increasingly aware of AIDS as a significant health problem in the black community, there will both be danger and opportunity. The opportunity is to deal comprehensively rather than haphazardly with the problem as a whole, to see it as a social catastrophe brought on by

> years of economic deprivation and to meet it as other disasters are met, with an adequacy of resources. The danger is that AIDS will be attributed to some innate weakness of black people and used to justify further neglect and to rationalize continued deprivation. (Thomas, 1992) pp.2,3.

No evidence exists that race is a biological risk factor for HIV infection. Rather, social explanations provide the most relevant reasons toward understanding the disproportionate racial impact of HIV on the black community and to understanding the length of time from diagnosis to death (National Commission, p7). We do know that poverty and illiteracy are correlated with increases in illness and decreased access to health education and health care. The question then has been and is how can we get health education messages out to the black community?

The health education message for the prevention of HIV and STD's is straightforward. The avoidance of sexual intercourse altogether or restricting sex to partners documented to be uninfected will prevent infection and is the most effective approach. If this strategy is not chosen, the next highly effective approach is the correct and consistent use of latex condoms (Roper, Peterson, Curran, 1993, pp. 501, 502).

While the health education message is straightforward, a positive cultural force and a strong barrier have existed. Positively, the use of word of mouth for transmitting messages of critical importance to the African American community has existed since the period of slavery from the 1600s through 1863 and the Emancipation Proclamation. Escapes and utilization of the Underground Railroad were orchestrated through verbal messages. These messages were also transmitted through music by way of the Negro Spirituals, "Steal Away, Steal Away Home" is an example. Therefore, if a health message is seen as positive and in the best interest of the black community, it is discussed by neighbors, in barber and beauty shops and in other social settings and family gatherings. It is posited that the message about condom usage would be passed along in the urban black community in the same manner. And, this verbal message would be validated by public health messages using video and print media and promotion by the black church.

The strong barrier against the acceptance of education about the high risk behaviors which foster HIV transmission exists if the black community feels that theirs is the only community targeted for the health message. For this reason, skepticism about family planning and the use of contraception has and continues to exist because of the fear of contrived plans of genocide of the African American community (Turner and Darity, 1973 and Gould, 1984). If the health threat is perceived to endanger an entire society, it is carefully weighed and evaluated within the social framework of the Black/African American community as to the legitimacy of the threat and the benefits for complying with the recommended interventions.

The Central Harlem Community[1]

The population of Central Harlem has become more ethnically diverse since 1980. The percentage of residents who were born outside the United States doubled between 1980 and 1990 and includes people from all parts of Africa, the Caribbean and Latin America. Along with this increased diversity, the overall population has decreased 37% from 159,267 in 1970 to 99,519 in 1990. However, available housing units have declined by 32% since 1970 but current rebuilding and recent renovation efforts have started to reverse this trend.

In 1990, Central Harlem had the highest infant mortality rate and incidence of low birth weight of all the health districts in New York City, more than twice that of New York City overall and substantially higher than other predominately African American communities in the city. These babies are not only more likely to die but are also more vulnerable. Compared to New York City as a whole, babies in Central Harlem are almost twice as likely to be born too soon and twice as likely to be born too small.

In terms of family life, over 30% of households with children were headed by women, more than twice the rate in New York City overall. Many Harlem women are juggling work and family. In 1990, more than half of the working women had children under 18 years old living at home. In 1990, almost 3,000 children were served by child development programs.

Regarding employment: in 1990, almost 20% of employed Central Harlem residents held professional or executive management positions; more than in 1980. More than 50% of people working were in clerical or service professions. However, the unemployment rate for men was more than twice as high in Harlem as in New York City overall.

Deaths from heart disease are still more than twice as frequent as in New York City overall. Heart disease is still the leading cause of death for both men and women in Central Harlem.

Harlem Hospital Medical Center (HHMC)

The Harlem Hospital Medical Center is a New York City municipal hospital and is an affiliate of the Columbia University College of Physicians and Surgeons. It is the largest health provider to the citizens of Central Harlem and neighboring communities. It has served the citizens of Harlem for over one hundred years. As such HHMC has a wealth of experience in the provision of health care to the urban poor. AIDS and HIV represent another major health disorder with a greater preponderance in this community as compared to most others in the United States.

In 1987 there were 154 new cases of AIDS diagnosed at Harlem Hospital Center. Sixteen per cent were women. Harlem Hospital sees one third of all cases of AIDS in Manhattan. At any one time one fourth of the hospital beds are filled with AIDS patients. Intravenous drug use is the risk behavior for 80% of the AIDS cases at Harlem Hospital Center.

The Department of Obstetrics and Gynecology (OBS/GYN) at the Harlem Hospital Center offers a full range of services to women, especially those in Central Harlem. The obstetrical service has averaged approximately 3000 deliveries per year. In 1989, the obstetrical clinics at Harlem Hospital serviced 2,347 women for a total of 15,773 patient visits. These women were seen in the regular OBS clinic, the High Risk Obstetrical clinic for women with medical or prenatal illnesses, and the Special Obstetrical Clinic for women with substance abuse problems. The racial distribution was 62% African American, 35% Hispanic/Latina and 3% other. The median age was 23 years.

The Special Prenatal Program for Chemically Dependent Women at Harlem Hospital, established in 1985, services pregnant women with a recent history of drug abuse. The patients are referred from within the hospital, neighborhood health centers; drug treatment programs throughout the city; and, other community based services and programs. The unit is staffed with a nurse clinician, a drug counselor, a social worker, a health educator/nutritionist, community liaison worker, attending level physicians, and two senior midwives. Psychiatric and other addiction services are immediately available since the clinic is located adjacent to Harlem Hospital Center's outpatient methadone detox and maintenance unit. The Chief of Perinatology (and first author) was Director of the Special Prenatal Clinic as well as the Obstetrical High Risk Clinic.

The Special Prenatal Clinic has four sessions weekly. Since 1985, over fourteen hundred women received prenatal and drug treatment services in this clinic. Approximately 80% of the patients receiving care list crack and/or cocaine as their first drug of choice. Fifteen percent have a history of injection drug use.

The Gynecology clinics at Harlem Hospital recorded 18,753 patient visits in 1989. These were the visits of women seen in the Family Planning Clinics (6,646), and the regular gynecology clinics (12,107). In 1989 and 1990, the unregistered delivery rate at Harlem Hospital averaged about 16%. Over 80% of this population had a urine toxicology positive for cocaine at delivery. Harlem Hospital has also seen an increase in neonatal syphilis. The majority of these babies were born to unregistered mothers. HIV/AIDS counseling and testing are being offered to all women who present for prenatal care or gynecological services at Harlem Hospital Center and the affiliated neighborhood health centers. Women are also offered counseling and testing through drug treatment programs and alternative testing sites. Women at high risk because of their own drug abuse or that of their sexual partners are encouraged to enroll in a comprehensive study funded by the Centers for Disease Control (CDC) on perinatal transmission coordinated by the City Health Department.

Based on New York City's record blood surveillance of Central Harlem, Harlem Hospital Medical Center can expect to deliver 90-120 HIV infected mothers (three to four percent of the 3,000 deliveries) annually. If the state estimate of 1,000 infected babies (calculated on a 40% transmission rated of a predicted 2500 infected women) is correct, this would mean between 60-72 infected babies delivered at Harlem (New York State Department of Health, 1988).

Because of the needs of the surrounding community, the Harlem Hospital Center has been a leader in providing care and developing prevention programs for HIV infection. It has worked in collaboration with other institutions while focusing on the needs of differing populations within this community. Another initiative, the Maternal Infant Transmission Study funded by the CDC in 1986 comprised the focus for providing HIV-infected and non-infected pregnant women with education and supportive services around HIV issues. This study was instrumental in assisting staff to design and modify strategies to enable women infected and at high risk for infection to decrease risk to themselves, to their partners, and subsequently to their children. Recruitment into this study focused on the Special Prenatal Program for Chemically Dependent Pregnant Women. Although prevention has never been the goal of this CDC-funded study, staff at HHMC recognized the need and seized the opportunity to provide the Harlem community with needed health information and medical services.

In 1989, the Departments of Obstetrics and Pediatrics were funded by the Human Resources and Services Administration (HRSA) to provide care and HIV education and prevention strategies to women delivering with little or no prenatal care — the Family Care Program. The crack cocaine epidemic introduced a new risk for HIV acquisition, especially for women. Early data on women who delivered at the HHMC with little or no prenatal care and with no history of injection drug use or sexual activity with an injection drug user (IDU) or HIV-infected partner showed an HIV seroprevalence rate of 9%. Of importance was the fact that all of these efforts were focused equally on those who were infected and those who were not, which is evidence of the philosophy and commitment of the institution toward prevention.

Unintended pregnancies and lack of family planning services go hand-in-hand. In a study of women delivering with limited prenatal care (N=249) at the HHMC, Department of Obstetrics and Gynecology, the same women who declared that for their most recent pregnancy they were not thinking about becoming pregnant, also said that either they did not want any more children or that they did not want them for another three years or more.

The Perinatal HIV and AIDS Reduction and Education Demonstration Activity (PHREDA) Project, 1989–1992 [2]

The Harlem Hospital Center/Columbia University Perinatal HIV and AIDS Reduction and Education Demonstration Activity (PHREDA) project implemented an enhanced service provision model targeting three groups of women:(1)women who delivered at the Harlem Hospital Center without prenatal care, considered to be four or less visits(NPC), N=249; (2) women attending Harlem Hospital's Special Prenatal Clinic (SPNC) N=83, a prenatal program for chemically dependent women; and (3) women, N=325, in four methadone treatment clinics at the Addiction Research and Treatment Corporation (ARTC).

Harlem Hospital Center's (HHMC) PHREDA project, in the Department of Obstetrics and Gynecology, attempted to impact upon the perinatal transmission of HIV through the increased use of effective family planning methods. Its major purpose was to change the knowledge, attitude, and behaviors relative to both HIV and family planning, through one-on-one risk-reduction counseling, among women who were either HIV infected or are at high risk of becoming infected. Heretofore, family planning was not a component of the postpartum visit. Secondarily, the project proposed to evaluate the role of provider (institutional) attitudes and knowledge about HIV and contraception in socially high risk women. The project used a certified nurse midwife (CNM) as the designated provider for postpartum and follow-up care including the provision of HIV education and family planning counseling. Additionally, at ARTC the researchers wanted to test the hypothesis that women at a methadone maintenance treatment program (MMTP) would access an on-site gynecologist if one was available.

Objectives of PHREDA

The education and prevention objectives of this HIV study were to encourage a reduction in high risk behaviors by:

(a) reducing the frequency of having unprotected sex with multiple partners,
(b) reducing the risk associated with having sex with past or current intravenous drug users,
(c) increasing the frequency of condom usage when having sex,
(d) improving the knowledge levels and attitudes about HIV.

The pregnancy planning objectives were:

(a) the reduction of unintended pregnancy,
(b) to increase the frequency with which contraception is used relative to the frequency of having sex and
(c) to increase the level of correct use of contraception.

Additional pregnancy planning behavioral objectives for the two groups of recent obstetric patients were:

(d) to increase the number of women returning for their postpartum examinations,
(e) to increase the number of women returning for their postpartum examinations who adopted a family planning method with emphasis on latex condoms and a spermicidal foam or cream.

The expected outcome hypothesized was a reduction in the incidence of pregnancy among three groups of women at high risk of perinatal transmission of HIV.

Another objective was the gathering of data on a population of women for which very little information exists. Although there are numerous data available about the effective use of contraceptive methods, there is very little information about the differences in perceptions and attitudes among ethnic and cultural groups. There is also little information available on the impact or the attitudes and perceptions of the sexual partner on the effective and continued use of contraception. There are minimal data on contraceptive use among female drug users. Much of this is probably due to a misconception that female IDU's are infertile.

Methodology

At both Harlem Hospital Medical Center (HHMC) and the Addiction Research and Treatment Corporation (ARTC) recruitment was conducted by the research assistants (RA) — one at HHC and one at ARTC. The recruitment process was conducted as described in the following narrative.

At HHMC 332 women were assessed initially by face-to face interviews conducted by the project's research assistant. The No Prenatal Care (NPC) women were interviewed and recruited postpartum while still on the hospital unit, approximately 24 to 48 hours after delivery, while the SPNC women were interviewed during their third trimester, in the Special Prenatal Clinic (SPNC).

Since unregistered patients are not candidates for early discharge and must be inpatients for a minimum of 48 hours, time was available for the research assistant to conduct an interview with each woman agreeing to participate in the study. Each morning the research assistant examined the obstetrical admissions log; delivery room log; recovery room log; and patient charts to determine the patient's clinic status. If the patient did not have more than four clinic visits she was eligible for participation in the cohort of women assigned to the unregistered delivery group. Interviews with this unregistered cohort occurred either at the woman's bedside or in the administrative inner office on the obstetrical unit. The woman determined where and when the interview was to occur. It was discovered by the research assistant that the women actually preferred to be interviewed at their bedsides with the bedside curtains drawn for privacy.

A potential problem was averted because the HRSA Family Care Program, which provided primary care, social service support, and HIV pretest counseling and testing using a case management approach since November, 1988, recruited patients from the same obstetrical admissions population as the PHREDA study. To minimize the number of times patients were approached and to maximize the recruitment process, the PHREDA project's RA and the HRSA staff member responsible for recruitment informed patients of the existence of both projects. Since both projects administer survey instruments to their patients, the demographic portions of both questionnaires were combined to form a generic questionnaire.

Once one project obtained the information it was shared with the other project. The remainder of the questionnaire containing project-specific questions was administered separately by each project. This process actually allowed two patients to be recruited at once, while minimizing the number of patient contacts. Patients received $10.00 for completion of the initial interview and $7.00 for the follow-up.

The NPC women were given two-week appointments, prior to discharge, with the project's designated health care provider, the certified nurse-midwife (CNM) who would provide care for the woman over an 18 month period. The SPNC women who attended the clinic on the other two session days returned to their prenatal care providers for their first postpartum appointment and were then scheduled for visits with the CNM six weeks later.

The research assistant (RA) who scheduled the two week postpartum appointment, did so within 48 hours of delivery, giving the woman an appointment slip which was noticeably different from the traditional one with the name and telephone number of the midwife and two full-time project staff to contact in case she could not keep her appointment; and the exact location, date and time of the appointment. The patient was told to ask for the midwife by name, rather than simply stating that she had an appointment in the clinic. These strategies — the special appointment slip and use of the midwife's name to gain entry — proved to be very successful tools; both provided tangible ways of assisting the patient to navigate the hospital system. These tools helped to empower the woman to deal effectively with the system. The patient also received a reminder in the mail, as a reinforcement and in case the original slip was misplaced, and a telephone call from the RA (all with the patient's prior consent).

Reinforcement to keep the appointment was ongoing. Ideally, all project participants were to meet the CNM before discharge from the OBS unit. However, due to the historical difficulty of recruiting midwives to a municipal hospital, the project was only able to hire a midwife at 20 percent effort; 23% of the women met with the midwife prior to the first appointment. At this meeting, the CNM greeted the woman; introduced herself, and described her role; and addressed any immediate concerns the woman had.

One week post delivery, prior to the initial postpartum visit, the CNM telephoned those patients she had not met, as well as those she had met, and asked about the woman's well-being; explained the postpartum visit, addressing any concerns the patient may have had about this visit; began a discussion of contraceptive usage and HIV education; and reinforced the appointment time, date and location. The CNM reinforced the project's woman-focused message, that the clinic was her time to discuss any concerns she may have had, whether they were physical or emotional. The patient was encouraged to bring her partner with her for her appointment.

At the postpartum visit, the CNM provided pregnancy planning and counseling, and HIV/AIDS education and counseling to the women, reviewing the women's responses to the initial questionnaire, using an encounter form which summarized the pertinent issues, designed by the CNM and the project coordinator/director. A six week visit and three-month interval visits were subsequently scheduled. Follow-up visits included discussion of contraceptive use; HIV counseling and education; physical exams; and referrals.

At ARTC, family planning and HIV counseling were provided by the on-site gynecologist. The RA at ARTC scheduled appointments for patients from three of the clinics: Kaleidoscope (KL), Starting Point (SP), and Third Horizon (TH) with the on-site gynecologist, for those who wished an appointment within two weeks of the interview. The patients at the fourth clinic, Bushwick (BK) were referred to family planning clinics.

ARTC was organized in 1969 to deal with the unique problems of the minority group drug addict. As a nonprofit, minority operated organization, ARTC has provided a wide range of comprehensive health care and treatment services to well over 20,000 patients since its founding. It provides treatment to 2,100 opiate addicted patients enrolled in the six outpatient clinics referred to previously, located in Central Harlem, East Harlem, and the Fort Greene, Bushwick and Brownsville sections of Brooklyn. The mean age of these patients was 32.9 years. Thirty-five percent of the patients are female. The racial distribution is 50% African American, 40% Hispanic/Latina and 10% other.

The services provided by ARTC include chemotherapy for opiate addiction, counseling for individuals, groups, and alcoholics, self-help groups such as Narcotics Anonymous, vocational evaluation and placement, educational evaluation and placement, medical care services, life skills training, women's groups, mental health services and AIDS education. For 1990, the overall seroprevalence rate of HIV in the population seen at ARTC was 59%. For women that rate was 61%.

A total of 325 women were recruited by the RA from the following ARTC clinics: KL and STP in Central Harlem; TH, in East Harlem and BC in Brooklyn. The ARTC system of "pulling cards" to ensure patient compliance with appointments was utilized. Under this system the RA presented a daily list of patients to be seen to the security desk guard. The security guard pulled the clinic card according to this list. The RA held these cards until the patient arrived and was instructed by the security guard to see the RA. Since patients could not be treated without a clinic card, the patient would of necessity go to the RA. This method insured compliance.

Since the ARTC clinics were open from 8:00 a.m. until 1:00 p.m., approximately four patients could be reasonably interviewed per day. However, at least 15 cards were pulled each day to take into account no shows. The RA had the assistance of the clinic counselors in reinforcing compliance with no-shows. All participants were reimbursed $10 for completion of the initial questionnaire and $7 each for the follow-up survey.

At three of the ARTC clinics — KL, SP and TH the patient was offered an appointment with the project's on-site gynecologist. If the patient elected to see the gynecologist, an appointment was made within a two week period, with any patient who required an emergency visit receiving an immediate appointment. At the Bushwick Clinic, patients were referred off-site for family planning services.

Staff Training

Although staff at both sites: HHMC and ARTC were experienced in the delivery of care to the defined population it was mandatory to increase the knowledge level about HIV transmission and family planning issues and appropriate ways to convey those messages. Cultural differences in attitudes toward reproductive health and the delivery of the message in culturally sensitive modes were emphasized. The project's consultant, chosen to design and conduct a portion of the staff training, was an expert in ethnic/cultural issues, especially as it related to women and reproductive issues. Since 34% of HHC's population and 41% of ARTC's population were of Hispanic origin, presentations were needed to familiarize the staff with traditional Hispanic cultural values and the impact of these values on: patient attitudes, beliefs and behaviors related to sexuality, reproduction, family planning, drug use, and, HIV/AIDS. A provider needs assessment had been developed earlier by the consultant which evidenced misinformation about HIV and specific cultural practices.

Obstacles

At the beginning of the project, recruitment was slow and it was discovered by the RA that many of the women thought the project was solely for people with AIDS. Once the introduction of the project was clarified to emphasize the health care aspects and dubbed the "Health Mother's Project" by the RA, recruitment increased. In addition, the results of a random telephone survey highlighted the need to explain the two week postpartum appointment in greater detail, for some women had anticipated and feared an internal exam would be done at that time.

Upon speaking with women who had not returned for postpartum care we found that it was important to demonstrate flexibility in the rescheduling of appointments for this population of women; and that since the appointment slip was frequently lost, the appointment needed to be placed on the back of the general clinic card.

Confidentiality

All patients were given an informed consent to read and sign prior to the administration of the questionnaire. The form was also explained to the patient by the RA. This informed consent received approval from the hospital's Institutional Review Board. The informed consent form included a telephone number for the patient to call if she had any further questions or concerns about the study. Questionnaires were maintained in a locked cabinet and the patient's locator form with her name and address were maintained separately. Chart numbers and research numbers were maintained separately as well. The survey instruments were hand-carried to the evaluation unit.

DATA MANAGEMENT

Coding and Data Entry

The intake and follow-up questionnaires used in conjunction with this project contained primarily closed-ended questions assessing women's sociodemographic backgrounds, and a wide range of knowledge, attitudes and behavior related to the prevention of the perinatal transmission of HIV. Because of the closed-ended nature of the questions, virtually all were pre-coded, thereby facilitating the process of data entry. In this project, the SPSS-PC data entry package was used. Prior to the onset of data entry, several data entry files were constructed. Several distinct files were needed because the data collection instruments were quite lengthy, and differed somewhat for the women enrolled at the Harlem and ARTC sites. Separate data entry files for the intake versus the follow-up interviews were also constructed. Data review for completeness and internal consistency as well as data cleaning were performed by Columbia University staff.

MAJOR FINDINGS AND IMPLICATIONS REGARDING HIV EDUCATION

Knowledge Measures

Improving women's knowledge about HIV was an important objective of this project. Therefore, in both the intake and follow-up interviews, we incorporated one of the National Center for Health Statistics (NCHS) knowledge scales. This scale contains nine items measuring such issues as ways to prevent HIV, modes of transmission, and symptoms characteristic of people who are HIV positive. Each of the items in this scale has response categories of "Definitely True," "Probably True," "Probably False," and "Definitely False" which were assigned scores between one and four, depending upon the correct response for the item. Thus, an individual's total scores could potentially fall between nine and 36. These total scores were then adjusted for the number of items each respondent answered, and therefore ranged between one and four, representing the average score on each item answered. Respondents who did not answer at least 70% of the items, were considered missing on this scale.

The change in HIV knowledge score was arrived at by subtracting the final score at intake from the final score at follow-up. T-tests were used to assess differences between the comparison groups. As Table 3 indicates, women who did see the certified nurse-midwife during the postpartum visit had significantly higher change scores than women who did not see the midwife. The difference between women who had received prenatal care in the SPNC program versus the NPC group was not statistically significant.

Given this important finding regarding the effectiveness of the nurse-midwife in improving women's knowledge about HIV, information is presented about the individual items on the scale. For each item in the scale, the percentage of women who knew the correct answer was reported. The percentages reported as correct include only those women who said the item was definitely true if it was true and false for those items that were definitely false.

Of the items considered, it was noted that women were least knowledgeable about the use of bleach to clean needles and drug paraphernalia, and most knowledgeable about heterosexual and perinatal transmission of HIV. Women who had seen the nurse-midwife differed significantly from women who had not on several of the specific items. These included knowledge that an HIV infected man could transmit the virus to a woman during penile vaginal intercourse; that the virus which causes AIDS could be present in a man's body fluids such as his semen; that a man could infect a woman with HIV and that a woman could infect a man; and that withdrawal was not as effective as condoms in preventing HIV transmission.

In addition to this general knowledge scale, a more specific two item measure focused on the transmission of HIV. The two items, one regarding the role of casual contact in HIV transmission and the other addressing sharing needles or drug use, were combined into one measure. As noted in Table 3, there was very little change between intake and follow-up in women's knowledge on this measure, and women in the two sets of comparison groups did not differ with respect to the amount of change observed.

The final knowledge measure that was investigated related to women's familiarity with the time during the menstrual cycle that they were most likely to be able to get pregnant. At follow-up, 17% of the women correctly answered this item. Although the findings did not attain statistical significance, compared to the women who did not see the CNM, twice as many women who did see her during the postpartum appointment, moved from incorrect to correct responses between intake and follow-up on this item.

Of the 332 women enrolled in the study, 76 were successfully followed and completed at least one follow-up interview. The social and demographic characteristics of these women are presented in Table 1, along with the characteristics of all of the women enrolled in the study, those who participated in the SPNC Program, and those who received little or no prenatal care prior to delivery. As can be seen in Table 1, the women who were followed had a mean age of 28 and nearly all were African American. More than half of these women received public assistance while growing up, and on average, had completed 11 years of education. Approximately four-fifths had never been married, and at enrollment into the project, 81% were not working. Nearly three out of five of these women were receiving public assistance; and more than half reported public assistance as their main source of support. Most women said that they had a permanent place to live, but 3 percent reported that they lived in temporary housing.

In Table 2, it is noted that the women who were followed did not differ from the women who were lost to follow-up on any of the key sociodemographic variables. Similarly, among the 76 women who were followed, there were no differences on any of these characteristics between those who received the intervention of seeing the CNM during the postpartum visit, and those who did not see the CNM. In comparing the women who were enrolled in the special prenatal program versus those who received little or no prenatal care, again focusing on those who were followed, only one difference occurred between the two groups. A greater proportion of the women in the SPNC group than of the other women were receiving welfare at the time of enrollment into the project. Thus, although the size of the follow-up sample was small, relative to the sample originally enrolled, few differences were found between the women who were followed and those lost to follow-up. The remaining tables assessed the effects of the intervention upon a diverse set of outcomes. A limitation of the project was the small number of cases in the follow-up group.

The tables present information related to HIV testing and the status of women recruited from both the Harlem Hospital and ARTC sites. In each of the tables, there are three columns of information. The first column was based on data obtained during the intake interviews from all women enrolled at the specific site. The second column was also based on intake data, but reflects information obtained from those women who were followed up at least once. The third column presents follow-up data, and is therefore of course limited to those women who completed follow-up interviews.

Among the women recruited from Harlem Hospital approximately three-fifths, at intake, had been tested for HIV, but by follow-up this figure had risen to 80%. Of those tested, slightly more than two-thirds reported knowing the results of their tests at intake, while at follow-up, this figure had risen to 79%. Of those tested and knowledgeable of their results, at intake 10% reported positive results, while by follow-up that figure had risen to 14.6%. In absolute numbers, of all of the Harlem Hospital women enrolled in the study, nine women reported that they were HIV positive at intake; three of these women were in the group who were followed at least once. At the time of follow-up, a total of seven women were HIV positive.

Of the women recruited from the ARTC sites, slightly more than three-quarters said they had been tested for HIV at the intake interview. The comparable figure at follow-up was 91%, which reflected an increase between intake and follow-up. About four-fifths of the women who had been tested at intake said that they knew the results of the test and this figure had risen slightly to 89% by follow-up. Of those who knew the results of their tests, slightly more than three-quarters were negative, while 16% of all women enrolled in the study, and 19% of those who would eventually be followed, were positive at intake. By the time of follow-up, 23 reported positive results, 76% had negative results and the percent refusing to report results was negligible. In terms of absolute numbers, there were 34 ARTC women who were positive at intake, 23 of whom were eventually followed up. By the time of the follow-up interview, however, there were a total of 36 women who had had positive HIV test results.

Discussion and Implications

It was found that women were more receptive to HIV/AIDS information when that information was integrated into the regular clinic activities and when their general health care needs were met. Although there may be objections to a traditional clinic setting based upon previous negative encounters a woman may have had with this system, when a designated health care provider was assigned to the woman and the care was individualized, the receptivity to the educational and skills building messages increased.

One-on-one risk reduction counseling may actually work most effectively with this population of high risk women who have been outside of the mainstream of health care and experience competing priorities, as opposed to multi-session group activities.

Additionally, those women who have been outside of the health care system were at highest risk. While 80% of the women in ARTC's drug treatment programs, and 69% of the women in the SPNC had been tested for HIV, only 34% of those women delivering with little or no prenatal care had been tested. Programs which are tailored to this group of women are most needed.

Another approach, used by this project, with important implications for counseling high risk women was the use of multiple reinforcements of the patients' appointments as well as reinforcement of the risk reduction message by all who encountered the patient. The team approach to counseling as well as the provision of a designated health care provider increased the frequency of delivery of the AIDS prevention and pregnancy planning messages.

This project's findings point to staff sensitivity as a key factor in encouraging women to return for care. Seventy-four percent of the women in the SPNC, the program that provided prenatal care and drug treatment options to women with a history of chemical dependency within a year of pregnancy, returned for postpartum/family planning care, as opposed to 12% of the NPC women. Many of the women had negative perceptions of physicians, a factor which kept them from returning for their postpartum appointment. The CNM, the project's designated health care provider was highly rated by all who returned to her for care. Data highlight the need for increased provision of information about the availability and accessibility of free counseling and testing for HIV. Only 51% of the women in the HHC project, who had not been tested, knew where they could receive free testing.

The project's data demonstrated that knowledge of one's HIV status impacts upon condom use, with 85% of the HIV infected women reporting consistent use of a contraceptive message, while 60% of the HIV negative women reported using no method. This finding has far-reaching implications for increasing the availability of testing and counseling.

In a sample of 572 women (NPC, SPNC, and ARTC), initially surveyed, 83% had previously used one or more established methods of birth control. While the most frequently used method was birth control pills, which 61% had used at some time in the past, the next most commonly used method was condoms, with their use at 58%. Although nearly half of this population brought with them no prior condom use experience and the prevalence of use within the four weeks prior to their participation in the study was quite low, 55% of the women who returned to the midwife for postpartum care (N=45) selected condoms as their primary method of choice. When asked about changes in sexual behavior because of AIDS, the majority of women in all three groups responded that they had increased or begun condom use. While the women's desire to use condoms does exist, their behavior often contradicts this intent. A prime opportunity exists to reduce this dissonance through appropriate counseling.

While virtually all of these women said it was important that a birth control method prevent venereal disease and HIV, be safe, and that it effectively prevent pregnancy, when questioned about why they would not want to use condoms to keep from getting pregnant, many felt that condoms were not effective because they frequently break. To these women the condom appears to be an ineffective method of choice. These responses highlight the value of structuring counseling sessions with the patient's health care provider to allow time for misinformation to be corrected.

At ARTC, despite the short period of time that the gynecologist was on staff, 38 women kept their appointments with him. Ninety-four percent of those given an appointment with the project's on-site gynecologist kept their appointments as compared to 80 percent of those who were referred to off-site family planning clinics (assessed through self-report). This demonstrates the importance of providing on-site health care to women at drug treatment facilities. Additionally, many of the women who refused care with the gynecologist, and some of those who did not, expressed a desire for a female gynecologist.

The primary method of choice for both the HHC women who saw the CNM and the ARTC women who saw the on-site gynecologist was the condom, while the contraceptive method chosen by those receiving care off-site at a traditional family planning clinic was an oral contraceptive. These data demonstrate that when care is provided in an environment which is public health oriented, supportive or accessible, women may choose a method which lowers their risk of HIV infection as well as unintended pregnancy. At that time traditional family planning clinics had not been providing HIV counseling.

Impact

This study concluded in 1991 but there is some evidence that condom usage has increased nationally and locally. As of June 8th, 1993, a New York Times/CBS poll showed Americans had an improved knowledge about AIDS. In the poll, respondents were asked what had they done to avoid being infected by HIV. Three answers were dominant: limiting the number of sexual partners, having safer sex and abstaining from sex.

Advance Data, a publication of the Centers for Disease Control and Prevention/Nation Center for Health Statistics, from Vital and Health Statistics (Number 260, February 14, 1995) reported that between 1988 and 1990, the proportion of women 15-44 years of age in the United States whose partners were using the condom for their current method of birth control increased from 9 to 11 percent, which continued the trend observed between 1982 and 1988.

However, since HIV infection rates have been increasing steadily in women (Centers for Disease Control, 1982, 1983, 1984, 1985, 1986, 1987a, 1989, 1990a, 1991, 1992), the proven interventions around supportive care and education are suggested for general use. Difficulties persist, however, if most men avoid birth control responsibility and HIV prevention information is not accessible. According to a Harris Poll released on May 22, 1995 and cited in The New York Times (Section B, p. 10) on May 23, 1995, the lack of male involvement contributes to unplanned pregnancies (estimated at 40% of births) and also accounts for men failing to support a partner who is informed about birth control. The poll also shows that men are less likely to use a condom when asked to do so.

However, according to the New York City Department of Health Bureau of Maternity Services and Family Planning, in the years 1991-1993 condom usage had increased for women (n= an average of 7500) presenting to a community-based walk-in pregnancy testing program from 10% to 16%. (Ashton, 1994) Condoms used alone without a spermicide may lead to unplanned pregnancies. So, whether by word of mouth or by public health messages in the media, condom use has increased because of concern about HIV and STD's, but more information needs to be shared with men and women about increasing the effectiveness of condom usage to prevent unintended pregnancies.

A final recommendation of the National Commission on AIDS in Part 1 of its chapter, "The Challenge of HIV/AIDS in Communities of Color" states: "Public health officials should work with researchers, health professionals, and community-based service providers to gain a better understanding of the role of cultural and socioeconomic factors in the transmission of HIV, the disease process, and access to care. Information gleaned from these efforts should be taken into account in designing HIV prevention messages, services, and programs, and in providing expanded treatment opportunities." The Harlem PHREDA has contributed to the fulfillment of this recommendation.

References

Ashton, D., Graham, E. H. (1994). *Community-based Walk-in pregnancy Testing: A Strategy for Engaging High Risk Women Into Care Early.* Paper presented at the 122nd Annual Meeting of the American Public Health Association, Washington, DC, 1994.

Centers for Disease Control. (1982). *AIDS Weekly Surveillance Report*, United States, Dec. 22, 1-2.

Centers for Disease Control. (1983). *AIDS Weekly Surveillance Report*, United States, Dec. 22, 1-3.

Centers for Disease Control. (1984). *AIDS Weekly Surveillance Report*, United States, Dec. 31, 1-3.

Centers for Disease Control. (1985). *AIDS Weekly Surveillance Report*, United States, Dec. 30, 1-3.

Centers for Disease Control. (1986). *AIDS Weekly Surveillance Report*, United States, Dec. 29-1-4.

Centers for Disease Control. (1987a). *AIDS Weekly Surveillance Report*, United States, Dec. 28, 1-5.

Centers for Disease Control. (1987b). Public Health Service Guidelines for Counseling and Antibody Testing to Prevent HIV Infection and AIDS. *Morbidity and Mortality Weekly Report*, 36, 509-514.

Centers for Disease Control. (1989). *HIV/AIDS Surveillance*, U.S. Department of Health and Human Services, 1-14.

Centers for Disease Control. (1990). *National HIV Seroprevalence Surveys*. U.S. Department of Health and Human Services, 1-26.

Centers for Disease Control. (1991). *HIV/AIDS Surveillance*, U.S. Department of Health and Human Services, 1-22.

Centers for Disease Control. (1992). *HIV/AIDS Surveillance*, U.S. Department of Health and Human Services, 1-22.

Centers for Disease Control. (Feb. 14, 1995). *Advance Data from Vital and Health Statistics*, 1-14.

Centers for Disease Control. (May 25, 1995). *Monthly Vital Statistics Report, Final Data*, 43(11)(S), 1-24.

Centers for Disease Control. (June 13, 1995). *Monthly Vital Statistics Report, Provisional Data*, 43(12), 1-24.

Gould, Ketayun H. (1984). *Black Women in Double Jeopardy: A Perspective on Birth Control.* NY: National Association of Social Workers Inc., 96-104.

Kagay, Michael R. (June 8,1993). Poll Finds Knowledge About AIDS Increasing. *The New York Times*, p. C5.

National Commission on AIDS. (1992). *The Challenge of HIV/AIDS in Communities of Color.* Washington DC: US Government Printing Press, 1 -76.

Roper, W., Peterson, H. B., & Curran, J. W. (April, 1993). Commentary: Condoms and HIV/STD Prevention - Clarifying the Message. *American Journal of Public Health*, 83(4), 501-503.

Steinhauer, J. (May 23, 1995). Most Men Avoid Birth Control Responsibility, Poll Finds. *The New York Times*, B10.

Turner, C. and Darity, W. (1973). Fears of Genocide Among Black Americans as Related to Age, Sex and Region. *American Journal of Public Health* , 63(12), 1029-1034.

TABLE 1
SOCIAL AND DEMOGRAPHIC CHARACTERISTICS

	All WOMEN ENROLLED AT HARLEM HOSPITAL (N=332)	SPECIAL PRENATAL (N=83)	NO PRENATAL (N=249)	WOMEN WHO WERE FOLLOWED (N=76)
AGE		PERCENT		
≤ 19	6.1	3.6	12.9	10
20—24	13.8	15.7	25.7	18.6
25—29	28	44.6	29.7	35.7
30—34	25	19.3	22.9	20
35+	27.1	16.9	8.8	15.7
Mean	30	28.6	26.1	27.7
RACE/ETHNICITY				
African—American	71.8	85.4	89.6	95.7
Hispanic	25.2	14.6	9.6	4.3
Other	3	0	0.8	0
RELIGIOUS AFFILIATION				
Protestant	48.3	56.6	57.3	65.7
Catholic	34.7	27.7	20.2	15.7
None/Other	17	15.7	22.6	18.6
RECEIVED PUBLIC ASSISTANCE WHILE GROWING UP				
Yes	54.3	46.2	63.4	55.4
No	45.7	53.8	36.6	44.6

EDUCATIONAL ATTAINMENT				
No High School Diploma	60.2	67.1	55.6	60.9
High School Diploma (GED)	30.4	29.3	30.2	30.4
More Than High School	9.4	3.7	14.1	8.7
Mean	11.12	10.87	11.2	11.1
MARITAL STATUS				
Never Married	65.6	71.1	80.7	81.4
Currently Married	15.6	12	10	10
Separated, Divorced, Other	18.9	16.9	9.2	8.6
EMPLOYMENT STATUS				
Working	11.8	32.5	10.4	18.6
Not Working	88.2	67.5	89.6	81.4
CURRENTLY RECEIVING PUBLIC ASSISTANCE				
Yes	68.7	69.9	48.2	57.1
No	31.3	30.1	51.8	42.9
SOURCE OF MOST INCOME DURING PAST YEAR				
Public Assistance	62.5	53.1	44.6	52.3
Job	12.1	21	14.5	13
Friends/Family	18.8	13.6	34.9	30.4
Other	6.7	12.3	6	4.3
CURRENT PLACE OF RESIDENCE				
Permanent Housing	93.3	85	94.3	97.1
Temporary Housing	6.7	15	5.7	2.9

TABLE 2

COMPARING WOMEN WHO WERE AND WERE NOT FOLLOWED AT HARLEM HOSPITAL CENTER, AND OF THOSE FOLLOWED, WOMEN WHO HAD A POSTPARTUM APPOINTMENT WITH THE NURSE MIDWIFE VERSUS NOT, AND WOMEN WHO WERE ENROLLED IN THE SPECIAL PRENATAL CLINIC VERSUS THOSE WHO RECEIVED LITTLE OR NO PRENATAL CARE

	WOMEN FOLLOWED VS. NOT FOLLOWED	OF THOSE FOLLOWED, SAW NURSE MIDWIFE AT POSTPARTUM APPOINTMENT VS. NOT	OF THOSE FOLLOWED, SPECIAL PRENATAL VS. NO PRENATAL
Age	NS	NS	NS
Race	NS	NS	NS
Past Welfare	NS	NS	NS
Educational Attainment	NS	NS	NS
Marital Status	NS	NS	NS
Employment	NS	NS	NS
Current Public Assistance	NS	NS	p<.01
Place of Residence	NS	NS	NS

TABLE 3
KNOWLEDGE MEASURES (HARLEM HOSPITAL CENTER COHORT)

	PERCENT CORRECT OR MEAN FOR WOMEN FOLLOWED	SIGNIFIGANT DIFFERENCE BETWEEN THOSE WHO SAW NURSE MIDWIFE AT POSTPARTUM APPOINTMENT AND THOSE WHO DID NOT	SIGNIFICANT DIFFERENCE BETWEEN THOSE IN SPECIAL VS. NO PRENATAL
General HIV Knowledge Scale[b]	0.097	Yes	No
A person who has the AIDS virus can look and feel healthy and well.[a]	57%	No	No
A man with the AIDS virus can pass it on to a woman during sexual intercourse (vaginal sex).[a]	92%	Yes	No
A pregnant woman who has the AIDS virus can give the AIDS virus to her baby.[a]	93%	No	No
Cleaning needles for drug use with bleach is a good way of killing the AIDS virus.[a]	33%	No	No
The virus which causes AIDS may be present in a man's body fluids, such as his semen.[a]	80%	Yes	No
It is possible to become infected with the AIDS virus after having sex just once.[a]	86%	No	No
A man can give AIDS to a woman, but a woman cannot give AIDS to a man.[a]	83%	Yes	No

In terms of preventing AIDS, withdrawing the penis before ejaculation (before "coming") is just as safe as using a condom.[a]	72%	Yes	No
The virus which causes AIDS may be present in a woman's body fluids, such as her menstrual blood.[a]	59%	No	No
HIV Transmission Scale[b]	-0.088	No	No
Period of Fecundity During the Menstrual Cycle[a]	17%	No*	No*

*Substantive results suggest that statistical significance would be attained if sample size were larger.

[a] This is a follow-up measure.

[b] This measure reflects the difference between the score at follow-up and the score at intake.

TABLE 4
ATTITUDINAL AND BEHAVIORAL INTENTION MEASURES (HARLEM HOSPITAL CENTER COHORT)

TOPIC	PERCENT OR MEAN FOR WOMEN FOLLOWED	SIGNIFICANT DIFFERENCE BETWEEN THOSE WHO SAW NURSE MIDWIFE AT POST-PARTUM APPOINTMENT AND THOSE WHO DID NOT	SIGNIFICANT DIFFERENCE BETWEEN THOSE IN SPECIAL VS. NO PRENATAL
fertility AND BIRTH CONTROL			
General birth control attitudes[b]	-0.05	No	No
Condom attitudes[b]	0.05	No	No
Perception of ability to avoid pregnancy[a]	3.8	No	No
Chances of getting pregnant next year[a]	1.8	No	No
HIV			
Perception of ability to prevent HIV[a]	3.8	No*	No
Chances of getting HIV within next year[a]	1.4	No	No
Risk Scale[b]	0.026	No	No

TABLE 4 (CONTINUED)

TOPIC	PERCENT OR MEAN FOR WOMEN FOLLOWED	SIGNIFICANT DIFFERENCE BETWEEN THOSE WHO SAW NURSE MIDWIFE AT POST-PARTUM APPOINTMENT AND THOSE WHO DID NOT	SIGNIFICANT DIFFERENCE BETWEEN THOSE IN SPECIAL VS. NO PRENATAL
Intends to discuss HIV with new partners[a]	93%	No	No
Intends to ask new partners about their sexual histories[a]	90%	No	No
PSYCHOLOGICAL MEASURES			
Locus of control[b]	-0.01	No	No

*SUBSTANTIVE RESULTS SUGGEST THAT STATISTICAL SIGNIFICANCE WOULD BE ATTAINED IF SAMPLE SIZE WERE LARGER.

[a] THIS IS A FOLLOW-UP MEASURE.

[b] THIS MEASURE REFLECTS THE DIFFERENCE BETWEEN THE SCORE AT FOLLOW-UP AND THE SCORE AT INTAKE.

TABLE 5
BEHAVIORAL OUTCOMES (HARLEM HOSPITAL CENTER COHORT)

OUTCOME[a]	PERCENT OR MEAN FOR WOMEN FOLLOWED	SIGNIFICANT DIFFERENCE BETWEEN THOSE WHO SAW NURSE MIDWIFE AT POST-PARTUM APPOINTMENT AND THOSE WHO DID NOT	SIGNIFICANT DIFFERENCE BETWEEN THOSE IN SPECIAL VS. NO PRENATAL
FERTILITY AND BIRTH CONTROL			
Returned for a post-partum appointment	80%	Not Applicable	No*
Pregnant since last birth	28%	No*	No*
Used a birth control method at last intercourse	56%	No	No
Frequency of birth control use within past month	2.4	No	No
Used condoms within past month	2.1	No	No
HIV RISK BEHAVIORS			
Sex for money	7%	No	No
Sex for drugs	1%	No	No

TABLE 5 (CONTINUED)

OUTCOME[a]	PERCENT OR MEAN FOR WOMEN FOLLOWED	SIGNIFICANT DIFFERENCE BETWEEN THOSE WHO SAW NURSE MIDWIFE AT POST-PARTUM APPOINTMENT AND THOSE WHO DID NOT	SIGNIFICANT DIFFERENCE BETWEEN THOSE IN SPECIAL VS. NO PRENATAL
Sex with anyone besides main partner within past month	11%	No*	No
MAIN PARTNER:			
Is/was an IV drug user	14%	No	No
Had sex with other men	2%	No	No
Has been imprisoned	37%	No	No
Has been tested for HIV	70%	No	No
Is HIV positive	3%	No	No

*Substantive results suggest that statistical significance would be attained if sample size were larger.

[a] All outcomes in this table are measured at follow-up.

TABLE 6
SOCIAL AND DEMOGRAPHIC CHARACTERISTICS

	ALL WOMEN ENROLLED AT ARTC (N=325)	WOMEN WHO WERE FOLLOWED (N=177)
	PERCENT	
AGE		
≤ 19	0	0
20—24	1.8	0.6
25—29	20.6	23.8
30—34	28.2	26.2
35+	49.4	49.4
MEAN	34.3	34.4
RACE/ETHNICITY		
African-American	50.9	51.7
Hispanic	42.6	41.9
Other	6.5	6.4
RELIGIOUS AFFILIATION		
Protestant	38.2	39
Catholic	50.5	48.8
None/Other	11.3	12.2
RECEIVED PUBLIC ASSISTANCE WHILE GROWING UP		
Yes	47.1	44.4
No	52.9	55.6
EDUCATIONAL ATTAINMENT		
No High School Diploma	63.6	64.7
High School Diploma (GED)	29.9	30.6
More Than High School	6.5	4.7
Mean	10.6	10.5

TABLE 6: (CONTINUED)

	ALL WOMEN ENROLLED AT ARTC (N=325)	WOMEN WHO WERE FOLLOWED (N=177)
	PERCENT	
MARITAL STATUS		
Never Married	46.9	43.6
Currently Married	22.7	26.7
Separated, Divorced, Other	30.4	29.7
EMPLOYMENT STATUS		
Working	6.8	6.5
Not Working	93.2	93.5
CURRENTLY RECEIVING PUBLIC ASSISTANCE		
Yes	89.2	90.7
No	10.8	9.3
SOURCE OF MOST INCOME DURING PAST YEAR		
Public Assistance	83.7	85.5
Job	6.5	8.1
Friends/Family	4.3	3.5
Other	5.5	2.9
CURRENT PLACE OF RESIDENCE		
Permanent Housing	93.8	91.9
Temporary Housing	6.2	8.1

TABLE 7

SELECTED FAMILY PLANNING OUTCOMES AMONG ARTC WOMEN

FREQUENCY OF BIRTH CONTROL	
Use During Past Month (1 = Never; 5 = Every Time)	2.3
FREQUENCY OF CONDOM USE	
With Main Partner During Past Month (1 = Never; 5 = Every Time)	2.9
PERCENT (%) USING A METHOD	
at Last Intercourse	57
CHANCES OF GETTING PREGNANT IN NEXT YEAR	
(1 = Very Unlikely; 4 = Very Likely)	1.4
HOW MUCH CAN DO TO PREVENT PREGNANCY IN NEXT YEAR	
(1 = Nothing; 4 = A Lot)	3.7
KNOWS WHEN DURING MENSTRUAL CYCLE	
Pregnancy is Most Likely	14

TABLE 8
PATTERNS OF FAMILY PLANNING SERVICE UTILIZATION AND SATISFACTION AMONG ARTC PATIENTS

		ARTC-ON-SITE *GYNECOLOGIST*	OTHER FAMILY PLANNING *CLINICS*
Given an appointment for a family planning visit?			
	Yes	58%	11%
Of those given an appointment, was the appointment kept?			
	Yes	94%	80%
Ever visited the ARTC gynecologist?			
	Yes	54%	NA
Was a method of birth control received at the family planning visit?			
	Yes	33%	75%
Of those receiving a method, type received?			
	Pills	17%	67%
	IUD	4%	0%
	Diaphragm	9%	33%
	Condoms	65%	0%
	Foam	4%	0%
Level of satisfaction with receptionist and clerical staff at the family planning clinic?			
	Mean	3.1	3.5

TABLE 8 (CONTINUEDO

	ARTC-ON-SITE *GYNECOLOGIST*	OTHER FAMILY PLANNING *CLINICS*
Level of Satisfaction with the gynecologist at the family planning clinic?		
Mean	3.0	3.0
Feeling regarding waiting time to see the gynecologist?		
Much too long	14%	67%
A bit too long	17%	33%
Not long at all	61%	0%
Length of time actually waited to see the gynecologist?	28 Min.	55 Min.
Length of time of the visit with the gynecologist?	22 Min.	30 Min
Feelings regarding the amount of time spent with the gynecologist?		
Much too short	14%	67%
A bit too short	48%	0%
A bit too long	32%	33%
Much too long	6%	0%
Were the day and time of the family planning visit convenient?		
Yes	87%	75%

TABLE 9
HIV STATUS OF THE ARTC WOMEN

	INTAKE		FOLLOW-UP
	ALL WOMEN	WOMEN WHO WERE FOLLOWED	WOMEN WHO WERE FOLLOWED
EVER TESTED			
Yes	78.8	78.6	90.7
No	21.2	21.4	9.3
KNOWS RESULTS OF TEST			
Yes	82.5	83.7	89.1
No	17.5	16.3	10.9
RESULTS OF TEST			
Negative	79.7	77.2	76.0
Positive	16.0	18.7	23.4
Refused	4.3	4.1	0.6

TABLE 10
HIV STATUS OF THE HARLEM WOMEN

	INTAKE		FOLLOW-UP
	ALL WOMEN	WOMEN WHO WERE FOLLOWED	WOMEN WHO WERE FOLLOWED
EVER TESTED			
Yes	57.2	58.8	80.3
No	42.8	41.2	19.7
KNOWS RESULTS OF TEST			
Yes	67.9	72.5	78.7
No	32.1	27.5	21.3
RESULTS OF TEST			
Negative	89.5	86.2	85.4
Positive	9.5	10.3	14.6
Refused	1.0	3.5	0.0

[1]THE FOLLOWING DESCRIPTION OF THE POPULATION WAS SUPPLIED BY THE HARLEM BIRTH RIGHT COMMUNITY HEALTH DIALOGUES AND INITIATIVES PROJECT, A PROJECT OF THE NEW YORK URBAN LEAGUE (CDC FUNDED) AND BASED ON 1990 CENSUS DATA.

2 The research was supported by the Centers for Disease Control, Grant No. 13-118

Relevant Measurement of HIV/AIDS Prevention Beliefs for African American Youth

Helen M. Rupp and Howard C. Stevenson

With the rise of HIV/AIDS cases in this country, investigators have worked to find interventions to effectively change the sexual risk taking behaviors of certain populations. According to Wyatt (1994) these interventions have been created without a broad understanding of both sexuality itself and environmental factors in a person's life which may encourage risk taking behaviors. She suggests three phases in research on human sexuality issues. The first phase is an examination of sexuality in general which helps one to understand normative practices and differences which emerge. "Sexual practices should be described within the context of age, income, gender, sexual orientation, religious beliefs, and cultural values (Wyatt, 1994, 751)." Phase two should focus on environmental factors which may lead to risk taking. Phase three is the development of interventions (informed by the first two phases) and their evaluation. Measurement is an underlying theme in all three of Wyatt's phases. Psychometrically sound measures are needed in order to measure differences between and within groups, to develop appropriate educational programs and in the evaluation of the effectiveness of these programs (Catania,

Gibson, Chitwood & Coates, 1990; DiClemente, Boyer & Mills, 1987; Kelly, St. Lawrence, Hood & Brasfield, 1989; Koopman, Rotheram-Borus, Henderson, Bradley & Hunter, 1990; Perkel, 1992). When conducting research or developing an educational intervention, the importance of reliable and valid measures cannot be ignored. This study will explore the measurement of African American adolescent's beliefs about preventing AIDS in light of Wyatt's call for informed research and intervention. This paper will review the prevalence of HIV/AIDS in adolescence, explore the relevance of the theory of reasoned action as a guiding theoretical framework, and discuss the Beliefs About Preventing AIDS scale developed by Koopman, Rotheram-Borus, Henderson, Bradley and Hunter in 1990.

HIV/AIDS in Adolescents

The number of HIV/AIDS cases involving adolescents is on the rise. Although the exact number of individuals infected with HIV/AIDS is unknown (Hein, 1992), some informative statistics are available. As of January 1989, 336 cases of AIDS were reported to the Centers for Disease Control for people aged 13-19 years (Rotheram-Borus & Koopman, 1991). By 1993, that number had risen to 1,412 cases in adolescents aged 13-19 years (accounting for one percent of reported cases; Centers for Disease Control [CDC], 1993). People ranging in age from 20 to 29 made up 21% of the reported AIDS cases in 1988 (Hein, 1989), this suggests that many people are being exposed to HIV during their teenage years, as the latency period for the disease is seven to 10 years (Flora & Thoresen, 1989; Rotheram-Borus & Koopman, 1992).

There are a number of differences in the pattern of AIDS cases between adolescents and adults. According to Hein (1989), these differences include a greater number of asymptomatic adolescents; a greater proportion of females when compared with all adults (14% versus seven percent), and higher percentages of minority individuals (53% versus 38%). Transmission rates also differ across these two age groups with a higher percentage of teen cases being acquired by heterosexual transmission (nine percent versus four percent). In 1993, the CDC reported 977 cases of AIDS in males aged 13-19 (less than one percent of the total cases reported for males). Three percent of these cases were infected through heterosexual contact. Of the 435 infected females aged 13-19 (one percent of total cases for females) 54% resulted from heterosexual contact (CDC, 1993). Adolescents in general face a number of risks due to behaviors common for their age group. Engaging in impulsive behaviors, feeling invulnerable to disaster (Quadrel, Fischhoff & Davis, 1993; Weinstein, 1989), sexual exploration and experimentation (Rotheram-Borus & Koopman, 1991), peer pressure in the areas of sexuality and drug use, and reliance upon peers as sources of information (Peterson & Hamburg, 1986) can all lead to greater risk of infection.

By the end of 1989, 35.8% of those diagnosed with AIDS between the ages of 13 and 19 were African American, even though they comprised only 15% of the population. African Americans aged 20 to 24 represent 31.6% of those diagnosed with AIDS and 28.6% of those aged 25 to 29 (Hein, 1992). African American adolescents may also have some special risk factors. These include a general distrust by the African American community toward public health efforts (Stevenson, 1994), a belief that AIDS was not a problem that African Americans in general needed to worry about, and the continued belief in traditional sex roles, including machismo beliefs and behaviors (Jenkins, Lamar & Thompson-Crumble, 1993). African American youth living in urban environments may also be faced with more immediate life threatening events (such as a higher threat of crime or violence and higher rates of poverty and un/underemployment) which can take precedence over the threat of a disease which may take years to surface (Jenkins, Lamar & Thompson-Crumble, 1993; Stevenson, Davis, Weber, Weiman & Abdul-Kabir, in press).

Behavior change is the only way to prevent or decrease the spread of AIDS. In order to encourage or change a behavior one must understand the determinants of that behavior (Fishbein & Middlestadt, 1989). The theory of reasoned action, put forth by Fishbein and Ajzen in the 1970s, and Ajzen's extension theory of planned behavior (Ajzen & Madden, 1986) can provide a helpful framework for looking at the beliefs and attitudes held by adolescents in regards to the prevention of HIV/AIDS.

The Theories of Reasoned Action and Planned Behavior

The theory of reasoned action holds that behavior is the result of specific intentions. These intentions are a function of the balance between the individual's attitudes toward the behavior and the subjective norms surrounding that behavior. Attitudes toward a behavior reflect the person's estimate that a given behavior will lead to a specific consequence (outcome expectancies) and evaluations of these consequences. Subjective norms are a function of the person's perceptions of what others think should be done and the person's motivation to comply with these referents ("What do others think?" and "Are their opinions important to me?"; Jemmott and Jemmott, 1991, 1992). The theory of planned behavior encompasses reasoned action. This theory holds that in some cases an individual's behavior might not be under their volitional control, but depend upon the presence of appropriate skills or opportunities, upon another's actions, or take place within the context of strong emotions. At these times, any prediction of intentions should consider not only attitudes and subjective norms, but perceived behavioral control as well. This is the perceived ease or difficulty of performing the behavior, and reflects past experiences, anticipated obstacles, resources, and opportunities. In essence, this theory places Bandura's research on self-efficacy (described below) within a larger framework of behavior, intentions, beliefs, and attitudes (Ajzen & Madden, 1986; Jemmott & Jones, 1993).

Bandura (1989) states that people need to feel that they are capable of exercising personal control. Perceived self-efficacy is a person's belief that they *can* exert control over their motivation and behavior and over their social environment. Self-efficacy affects what people choose to do, how much effort they put forth, how long they persevere in the face of adversity, whether they engage in negative self-talk, and the amount of stress and depression they experience during taxing situations. In regards to AIDS prevention, self protecting behaviors can conflict with interpersonal pressures and sentiments. The influences of social acceptance, social pressures, situational constraints, and fear of rejection or embarrassment can override the influence of the best informed judgement, and the lower the person's perceived self-efficacy the more easily swayed they will be in the face of these pressures.

These theories of reasoned action and planned behavior also hold that the interactions between and relative importance of each area of influence on behavior (self-efficacy, subjective norms, attitudes, etc.) may vary from behavior to behavior and across different populations (Fishbein & Middlestadt, 1989; Jemmott & Jones, 1993) thus allowing the flexibility needed to investigate gender and cultural differences. These theories have been utilized by previous researchers and are relevant in the measurement of attitudes and beliefs about HIV/AIDS prevention (Jemmott & Jemmott, 1992; Pendergrast, DuRant & Gaillard, 1992; and Stevenson, et al., in press).

Psycho-Social Variables that Influence At-Risk Behaviors

All of the aforementioned issues have an impact on a person's willingness and ability to engage in self protecting behaviors. The rules and mores regarding sexuality in a teen's peer group and community also affect the use of self protective behavior (Stevenson, et al., in press). Stevenson, et al (in press), also state that beliefs about self-control and self-efficacy have a major impact on whether or not teens engage in or endorse risky behaviors.

Another important aspect of adolescents' lives which may influence their abilities to protect themselves from HIV/AIDS is religion and religious affiliations (Mays, 1989). Religiosity's importance in terms of predicting "at-risk" behaviors has been documented (Benson & Donahue, 1989; Hadaway, Elifson & Petersen, 1984). Benson and Donahue (1989) found, using multiple regression, that religiousness was one of the three (out of 10 possible) strongest negative predictors of behaviors such as cigarette smoking, binge drinking and drug use among both white and African American youths. This means that the more religious the teens were, the less likely they were to engage in these risky behaviors. Hadaway, Elifson and Petersen (1984) studied the effects of religiousness on attitudes toward drug use and actual drug and alcohol use among white, Catholic and Protestant high school students. They found that "religion has an independent constraining effect" above and beyond other sources of social control and moral influence, such as parents

(p. 125). The influence of religion was found to have a larger effect on behaviors with few other constraining influences, such as alcohol use. When a behavior was more universally condemned, such as use of drugs other than marijuana, religion played less of a restraining role in relation to other societal constraints. Religion must also be considered when preparing HIV/AIDS interventions and evaluations as it may influence many aspects of a person's sexuality, such as ideas regarding intercourse, sexual practices, contraceptives and premarital relationships (Mays, 1989). Religion can also be important as an avenue for intervention or to provide a view of support systems and social networks in African American communities (Mays, 1989).

Beliefs About Preventing HIV/AIDS

In order to change behavior one must change the underlying attitudes or subjective norms which influence the behavior (Fishbein & Middlestadt, 1989). Before one can change attitudes and beliefs, one must be able to measure them. One scale available within the belief domain is the Beliefs About Preventing AIDS scale developed by Koopman, et al., (1990) for use with adolescent homosexual males and runaways of both genders. Koopman, et al., used focus groups to review and reword questions from already existing scales of AIDS knowledge and beliefs and to develop additional items for their scale. New focus groups were then formed to review the revised scale. The scale was pilot tested with adolescent runaways, sex offenders and gay males in order to revise the instrument and instructions based on feedback from those sampled and to ensure the feasibility of administration to their target population of gay and runaway youth. Two advisory councils were then created to review the measure and to "ensure accuracy, clarity and comprehension at the sixth-grade reading level" (Koopman, et al., 1990, p 61). Based upon their review of earlier prevention research, Koopman, et al., defined five domains of AIDS prevention beliefs. The first domain is that of self efficacy, or the belief that one is capable of avoiding the contraction of AIDS. Domain two, perceived threat, is the belief that AIDS actually poses a personal danger. Self control in high risk situations, one's perception of being in control of one's sexual behavior, is the third domain. The fourth area queries about peer support for safe acts and the last domain asks about the individual's expectation to act to prevent pregnancy.

Current Measurement of HIV/AIDS Variables

Despite the increasing AIDS rate among adolescents and an increase in attempts at intervention, there remains an important need for a measurement technology which is statistically sound, developmentally appropriate and theoretically driven. Currently, continuity of measures across investigators is minimal and many investigators create scales for their own purposes, usually comprised of only a few items, raising questions about the issues of reliability and validity (e.g., Belgrave, Randolph, Carter, Braithwaite & Arrington, 1993; Dusenbury, Botvin, Baker & Laurence, 1991; Goodman, & Cohall, 1989; and Jemmott, Jemmott & Fong, 1992). While many investigators are driven by a theoretical orientation, measurement theory is often not considered. Exceptions do exist, but they are few (e.g., a Condom Attitude Scale by Sacco, Levine, Reed & Thompson, 1991). The above problems lead to a lack of generalizability across studies, and possibly to conflicting results. A psychometrically sound measure of HIV/AIDS beliefs which can be used across populations is needed.

It was the intent of the authors of the current study to expand and validate a measure that already existed in the literature on adolescents. Measures that are currently known are more likely to be used if revised. Therefore, the purpose of the current study was to explore the measurement of beliefs about preventing AIDS within the context of Wyatt's (1994) call for informed interventions and to theoretically connect the findings to the theory of reasoned action. In the first study, factor analytic work with the Beliefs About Preventing AIDS scale was conducted to determine if the domain areas developed by Koopman, et al. (1990) hold up to statistical analysis for an African American adolescent population. In the second study, this revised scale was used to investigate the relationship of prevention beliefs to selected psychosocial variables that influence safe-sex behaviors for African American adolescent girls and boys.

Experiment 1

Method

Participants

The 350[1] African American adolescents in this study were enrolled in a summer career development program across three years in a large Northeastern city. These students were participants in a larger study of AIDS education to be described below. The adolescents who fully completed the study ranged in age from 14 to 18, with a mean age of 14.49 years, 108 (30.9%) were male and 242 (69.1%) were female. Classes were held in community centers in different areas of the city. Class membership was determined by geography, as students were assigned to classes based on the proximity of the center to their home. Each class contained 15 to 20 students.

The current assessment study was nested within a larger intervention research program, the AIDS, Culture and Education Project, across three years. In Year One the effectiveness of a culturally similar AIDS education video to improve AIDS/HIV knowledge was evaluated (Stevenson & Davis, 1994). Year Two studied the differences in learning between groups of students viewing a culturally similar video that was produced, directed and acted by teenagers and students viewing a professional video — both of which followed the same script (Stevenson, Gay & Josar, 1994). In Year Three the effectiveness of a culturally relevant AIDS education intervention was examined. The intervention included role plays and discussions around the issues of sexuality and culture. Measures of beliefs and attitudes that were administered during the pre-test phase of the project across all three years were analyzed.

Measures

Beliefs About Preventing AIDS.

The Beliefs About Preventing AIDS scale was found to be internally consistent overall (alpha = .81). Within the domains reliability ranged from moderately high to fair (alpha = .78 for self-efficacy to alpha = .52 for perceived threat). Validity for this scale was based on the procedures used in its development.

General AIDS Knowledge

The AIDS Knowledge Test, also developed by Koopman, et al. (1990), consists of 52 true-false items. It was found to exhibit good internal consistency (alpha = .82, p.0001) and test-retest reliability (1 week, r = .82).

Mediating Variables

A number of questions were included to evaluate their potential relationship with AIDS knowledge and beliefs. These included questions about previous AIDS education, intuitive perception of one's AIDS knowledge ("Compared to most people, how much would you say you know about AIDS?"), fear of contracting AIDS in the future, and religiosity (a factor comprised of the two questions: "How often do you attend religious services?" and "How religious are you?"). Demographic data were also collected, including gender, parental education, level of sexual activity, condom usage, etc.

Procedure

All classes completed the full set of measures over the course of one to three one-hour sessions. The questions were read aloud to the students in order to counteract any possible problems due to varied reading abilities. The measures were immediately followed by the intervention in years one and two, with the post session two weeks later. For year three, the intervention was presented during its own session about one week after the measurement sessions, with the post administered, on average, the week following.

Results

Ward's procedure was used to check for multidimensionality and Bartlett's Chi-Square was found to be significant (2 = 3409.38, p.001). Ward's procedure resulted in the possibility of two to 10 factors. The 39 items of the Beliefs About Preventing AIDS scale were then subjected to common factor analysis. Factor solutions were evaluated against the following criteria: 1) the solution should meet the constraints of Cattell's scree test; 2) each unrotated factor should account for greater than five percent of the total variance; 3) rotated factors should retain at least five appreciable loadings of >.30; 4) rotated factors should yield reasonable internal consistency for salient items; and 5) the resulting factor solution should make psychological sense, both in terms of psychological meaningfulness and item retention (McDermott, 1993).

Exploratory analyses using common factor analysis were performed. Cattell's scree allowed for a maximum of six factors. Two- through four-factor solutions were attempted using varimax and equamax rotations. A three-factor solution, similar across both rotations, seemed to best represent the data. A promaxian rotation (with k=2) was attempted with this solution. The resulting structure added two items to the first factor with the other factors remaining stable. Factor one (Self-Efficacy, SE) and factor two (Self-Control, SC) were found to be reliable (SE, alpha = .72; SC, alpha = .71). The SE factor had an eigenvalue of 5.1463 and accounted for 35.09% of the total variance. It included 13 items, with possible scores ranging from 13 to 52. The SC factor had an eigenvalue of 1.6363 and accounted for 32.83% of the total variance. It included six items, resulting in a possible range of six to 24. For factor three, a possible condom efficacy factor containing seven items, reliability was found to be low (alpha = .58). This factor had an eigenvalue of 1.3349 and accounted for 17.30% of the total variance (see Table 1 for items loading on each factor). The intercorrelation between SE and SC was found to be reasonable, r = .38, and the factor solution remained stable after partialling out the effects of gender. Test-retest reliability for the factors was found to be fair after one week, alpha = .33, p=.03 for SE and alpha = .59, p.0001 for SC.[2] Confirmatory, Oblique Principal Components Cluster Analysis was performed and showed that the promaxian solution was indeed a viable solution.

Experiment 2

Method

Participants

Subjects in Experiment 2 were comprised of the 138[3] students involved in the third year of the study. The 50 males (36.2%) and 88 females (63.8%) ranged in age from 14 to 16 with a mean age of 14.34.

Procedure

Analyses of variance were performed using the two reliable factors found in Experiment 1 as dependent variables. Demographic data and psychosocial variables of interest were used as the independent variables. These included 1) gender, 2) self reported level of sexual activity, 3) self appraised AIDS knowledge, determined by the question "Compared to most people, how much would you say you know about AIDS? A Lot, Some, Little or Nothing" (no student reported knowing nothing about AIDS), 4) actual AIDS knowledge, measured by the AIDS Knowledge Test (Koopman, et al., 1990), 5) self reported condom use, measured by the question "How often have you used a condom during the past year? Never, Rarely, Occasionally, Usually or Always," and 6) religiosity, measured by the sum of two questions, "How often do you attend religious services? Never, A Little, Some, Often, or Very Often" and "How religious are you? Not Much, A Little, Sometimes, Most of the Time, or All of the Time."

Results

Descriptive Information

Forty-five students (32.6%) reported no sexual activity and 25 (18.1%) reported engaging in intercourse only once for a total of 70 students (50.7%) having sex once or less in the six months prior to completing the questionnaires. Sixty-eight students (49.3%) reported engaging in sexual intercourse more than once within the six months prior to completing their questionnaires. "A lot" was the response of 57 (42.2%) students when asked how much they thought they knew about AIDS. Fifty-six (41.5%) said "some" and 22 (16.3%) felt they knew "little." No student felt they knew "nothing" about AIDS. Of those who engaged in intercourse, 55 (59.1%) used condoms always or usually, 13 (14.0%) used them occasionally and 25 (26.9%) used them rarely or never. In terms of religiosity, 50 students (36.2%) were not religious,

52 (37.7%) were moderately religious and 36 (26.1%) were very religious.

Correlational Analysis

All three of the factors found in study one were significantly correlated with the total scores on the AIDS Knowledge Test; $r = .21$, p=.01 for SE, $r = .31$, p.001 for SC, $r = .39$, p.001 for Condom Efficacy. The higher one's score on any of the three factors, the higher one's score on the AIDS Knowledge Test. SE was positively correlated to self reported AIDS knowledge ($r = .18$, p.05). This means that the more these teens thought they knew about AIDS, the higher their SE scores. SE was negatively correlated to self reported sexual activity, $r = -.17$, p.05, meaning that the more often the teens engaged in sexual intercourse the less they endorsed SE beliefs. SC was positively correlated to gender ($r = .24$, p.01) and negatively related to sexual activity ($r = -.37$, p.001). Females and those who were less sexually active scored higher on SC. Females were also less likely to be sexually active ($r = -.39$, p.001). Factor three, a condom efficacy factor, was positively correlated with self reported condom use, $r = .34$, p.001. Those with higher condom efficacy scores were more likely to say they used condoms regularly. Also those who engaged in sex more often were more likely to report regular condom usage ($r = .40$, p.001).

Analyses of Variance

Self-Efficacy

A one-way ANOVA showed a significant main effect for level of religiosity, where $F(2,135) = 4.57$, p=.01. Tukey's HSD revealed that those who were least religious scored significantly lower on SE ($M = 45.16$, $SD = 6.85$) than those who were moderately religious ($M = 48.44$, $SD = 3.43$). Those who were very religious ($M = 45.69$, $SD = 6.90$) tended to score lower than moderates, as the mean difference approached significance.

An analysis of covariance revealed an effect for self reported condom use when sexual activity was controlled ($F(3,134) = 4.84$, p.01). The adjusted mean for those who never or rarely used condoms (44.57) was significantly lower than the adjusted mean for those who usually or always used condoms (48.26). Those who occasionally used condoms (adjusted mean = 47.25) did not differ significantly from either group. No other effects were found for the Self-Efficacy factor.

Self-Control

Three one-way ANOVAs showed the main effects for Self-Control. For SC, the mean score for females (20.38, $SD = 3.73$) was significantly higher than for males (18.38, *SD* = 4.37), *F*(1,136) = 8.05, *p*.01. Those who were sexually active (*M* = 18.26, *SD* = 4.55) scored lower on SC than those who engaged in intercourse once or less in the prior six months (*M* = 21.00, *SD* = 3.01), *F*(1,136) = 17.43, *p*.001. Finally, those receiving low scores on the AIDS Knowledge Test scored significantly lower (*M* = 18.71, *SD* = 4.62) on SC than those receiving higher AKT scores (*M* = 20.44, *SD* = 3.38), *F*(1,136) = 6.39, p=.01. No other main effects were found to be significant.

In regards to condom use, an ANOVA revealed findings similar to those for Self-Efficacy. When controlling for sexual activity, those who stated they never or rarely used condoms and those who only occasionally used condoms scored significantly lower on SC than those who regularly used condoms (adjusted means are 18.32, 18.13 and 21.23 respectively), F(3,134) = 9.73, p.001.

A three-way ANOVA revealed an interaction between gender, sexual activity and actual AIDS knowledge, where F(1,130) = 3.91, p=.05. Figure 1 shows that SC scores for females remained stable across low and high actual AIDS knowledge whether they were sexually active or not, although scores tended to be lower for those females engaging in sexual activity (see Table 2 for means and standard deviations). For the males this was not the case. Non-active males scored higher than active males on SC if their actual AIDS knowledge was low. The reverse was true for those whose AIDS knowledge was high, with the active males scoring higher on SC than non-active males.

A two-way ANOVA revealed an interaction between self appraised AIDS knowledge and religiosity, where F(4,126) = 2.77, p.05. Those who were moderately religious and very religious maintained relatively stable SC scores across levels of self appraised AIDS knowledge (see Table 3 for means and standard deviations). For those who were not religious this was not the case. Subjects who were not religious and who held moderate appraisals of their knowledge scored significantly lower than those who were moderately religious (see Figure 2).

Discussion

The purpose of the present study was to help in the development of a psychometrically sound measurement technology for the assessment of HIV/AIDS prevention attitudes and beliefs. The Beliefs About Preventing AIDS scale (Koopman, et al., 1990) was subjected to factor analysis. The resulting three-factor solution, while not confirming Koopman, et al._s (1990) structure, does fit within the theories of reasoned action and planned behavior (Ajzen & Madden, 1986; and Jemmott & Jemmott, 1991, 1992). Self-Efficacy as comprised here, seems to measure one's thoughts regarding one's ability to act to prevent HIV infection. It pulls for cognitive beliefs regarding theoretical questions about intercourse and HIV/AIDS and also somewhat taps outcome expectancies. Self-Control pulls more for situation specific behaviors, how capable one feels in handling sexual situations (which corresponds with the theory of planned behavior). The third factor, while not highly reliable, seems to be a condom efficacy factor. It measures one's comfort with and knowledge of condom use.

Self-Efficacy and Self-Control measure different constructs as determined by the low inter-correlations and their differential relationships to relevant psychosocial variables. For example, Self-Efficacy scores varied depending upon levels of religiosity, with those reporting moderate religiousness scoring higher than those who were least religious. For Self-Control, this relationship only held for those who reported a moderate appraisal of knowledge about AIDS. Self-Control was also related to other psychosocial variables which Self-Efficacy was not, i.e., gender, actual AIDS knowledge and sexual activity. These results add support to the differential validity of the two reliable factors.

Convergent validity is supported by the similar findings for condom use when sexual activity is controlled. Those who did not regularly use condoms scored lower than regular users on both Self-Efficacy and Self-Control. The only difference between the factors was the scores for those using condoms only occasionally. For Self-Efficacy these participants tended to differ from those not using condoms, for Self-Control they scored significantly lower than those using condoms regularly. It is possible that these teens feel capable of preventing AIDS in the abstract (Self-Efficacy), but know that they may have difficulties following through in real life situations (Self-Control). It makes sense that to engage in regular condom use, one must have significant self-control over one's sexual behavior or in the least one is expending cognitive energy thinking about the consequences of one's actions.

A number of implications for prevention efforts arise from the current analysis. Results suggest that educators should devise HIV/AIDS intervention strategies aimed at homogeneous groups, based upon the differences found across both gender and levels of sexual activity. For example, the results illustrated in Figure 1 show this need. For those males who were not sexually active, having low AIDS knowledge did not hurt their untested sense of Self-Control. For sexually active males, having more knowledge contributed to their sense of Self-Control. If a teen is active it is better for them to be knowledgeable about HIV/AIDS, especially if that teen is male. This suggests that active versus not active groups may represent two different types of teenagers who have different sociocultural experiences as a function of their choices. Stevenson, et al. (in press) also support the idea that teens may need different interventions based upon their culture, community and/or gender. Future research needs to investigate the differential outcomes in homogeneous versus heterogeneous groups, possibly through the use of randomized field tests in schools or other groups with large numbers of adolescents.

Future studies need to examine the relationship between religiosity and Self-Efficacy and Self-Control. It remains to be seen if Self-Efficacy can be increased for people at the extremes in terms of religiosity. Can those who are not religious get the support given by religion through a different avenue, and can those who are very religious learn how to think about intercourse and HIV/AIDS without going against their religious beliefs?

A number of possible limitations exist within this study. First, the data collected were all based upon self report. This possible limitation can be discounted by the fact that the relationships found make psychological sense and follow what one could deduce logically. Second, this research focused solely on young, urban, African American adolescents. More research is needed with other and/or older African American adolescents to see if these factors hold in rural and suburban areas and in different geographic regions. Assessment is also needed with other racial and ethnic groups to see if the Beliefs About Preventing AIDS scale is valid for use with these groups. One note of concern in terms of the factor analysis is that all items in the Self-Control and Condom-Efficacy factors are reversed. This suggests the possibility of a difficulty factor (i.e., the items grouped together based upon the negatively phrased questions rather than because they measured the same construct). This possibility was balanced by the fact that the items in these factors did have psychological meaning. Further research with these factors, such as positively phrasing some items or work with other subjects, could help to clarify this possible difficulty. Future work should also focus on bolstering the Condom Efficacy factor with items which might help to increase its reliability. In conclusion, this study investigated the reliability and validity of the Beliefs About Preventing AIDS scale, as well as its ability to differentiate among subgroups of African American youth. Results indicate the necessity for homogeneous groups when providing HIV/AIDS education.

References

Ajzen, I. & Madden, T. J. (1986). Prediction of Goal-directed Behavior: Attitudes, Intentions, and Perceived Behavioral Control. *Journal of Experimental Social Psychology,* 22, 453-474.

Bandura, A. (1989). Perceived Self-efficacy. In V. M. Mays, G. W. Albee, & S. F. Schneider (Eds.), *Primary Prevention of Psychopathology, Vol XIII: Primary Prevention of AIDS: Psychological Approaches* (pp. 129-141). Newbury Park, CA: Sage.

Belgrave, F. Z., Randolph, S. M., Carter, C., Braithwaite, N. & Arrington, T. (1993). The Impact of Knowledge, Norms, and Self-efficacy on Intentions to Engage in AIDS-preventive Behaviors Among Young Incarcerated African American Males. *Journal of Black Psychology,* 19, 155-168.

Benson, P. L. & Donahue, M. J. (1989). Ten-year Trends in At-risk Behaviors: A National Study of Black Adolescents. *Journal of Adolescent Research,* 4, 125-139.

Catania, J. A., Gibson, D. R., Chitwood, D. D. & Coates, T. J. (1990). Methodological Problems in AIDS Behavioral Research: Influences on Measurement Error and Participation Bias in Studies of Sexual Behavior. *Psychological Bulletin,* 108, 339-362.

Centers for Disease Control and Prevention. (1993). *HIV/AIDS Surveillance Report,*

5(3).

DiClemente, R. J., Boyer, C. B. & Mills, S. J. (1987). Prevention of AIDS Among Adolescents: Strategies for the Development of Comprehensive Risk-reduction Health Education Programs. *Health Education Research: Theory and Practice,* 2, 287-291.

Dusenbury, L., Botvin, G. J., Baker, E., & Laurence, J. (1991). AIDS Risk Knowledge, Attitudes, and Behavioral Intentions Among Multi-ethnic Adolescents. *AIDS Education and Prevention,* 3, 367-375.

Fishbein, M. & Middlestadt, S. E. (1989). Using the Theory of Reasoned Action as a Framework for Understanding and Changing AIDS-Related Behaviors. In V. M. Mays, G. W. Albee, & S. F. Schneider (Eds.), *Primary Prevention of Psychopathology, Vol XIII: Primary Prevention of AIDS: Psychological Approaches* (pp. 93-110). Newbury Park, CA: Sage.

Flora, J. A. & Thoresen, C. E. (1989). Components of a Comprehensive Strategy for Reducing the Risk of AIDS in Adolescents. In V. M. Mays, G. W. Albee, & S. F. Schneider (Eds.), *Primary Prevention of Psychopathology, Vol XIII: Primary Prevention of AIDS: Psychological Approaches* (pp. 374-389). Newbury Park, CA: Sage.

Goodman, E. & Cohall, A. T. (1989). Acquired Immunodeficiency Syndrome and Adolescents: Knowledge, Attitudes, Beliefs, and Behaviors in a New York City Adolescent Minority Population. *Pediatrics,* 84, 36-42.

Hadaway, C. K., Elifson, K. W. & Petersen, D. M. (1984). Religious Involvement and Drug Use Among Urban Adolescents. *Journal for the Scientific Study of Religion,* 23, 109-128.

Hein, K. (1989). AIDS in Adolescence: Exploring the Challenge. *Journal of Adolescent Health Care,* 10 (Supplement), 10S-35S.

Hein, K. (1992). Adolescents at Risk for HIV Infection. In R. J. DiClemente (Ed.), *Adolescence and AIDS: A Generation in Jeopardy* (pp. 3-17). Newbury Park, CA: Sage.

Jemmott, L. S. & Jemmott, J. B. (1991). Applying the Theory of Reasoned Action to AIDS Risk Behavior: Condom Use Among Black Women. *Nursing Research,* 40, 228-234.

Jemmott, L. S. & Jemmott, J. B. (1992). Increasing Condom Use Intentions Among Sexually Active Inner-city Black Adolescent Women. *Nursing Research,* 41, 273-278.

Jemmott, J. B, Jemmott, L. S. & Fong, G. T. (1992). Reductions in HIV Risk-associated Sexual Behaviors Among Black Male Adolescents: Effects of an AIDS Prevention Intervention. *American Journal of Public Health,* 82, 372-377.

Jemmott, J. B. & Jones, J. M. (1993). Social Psychology and AIDS Among Ethnic Minorities: Risk Behaviors and Strategies for Changing Them. In J. Pryor & G. Reeder (Eds.), *The Social Psychology of HIV Infection* (pp. 183-224). Hillsdale, NJ: Lawrence Erlbaum Associates.

Jenkins, B., Lamar, V. L., & Thompson-Crumble, J. (1993). AIDS Among African Americans: A Social Epidemic. *Journal of Black Psychology,* 19, 108-122.

Kelly, J. A., St. Lawrence, J. S., Hood, H. V. & Brasfield, T. L. (1989). An Objective Test of AIDS Risk Behavior Knowledge: Scale Development, Validation, and Norms. *Journal of Behavior Therapy* and *Experimental Psychiatry,* 20, 227-234.

Koopman, C., Rotheram-Borus, M. J., Henderson, R., Bradley, J. S., & Hunter, J. (1990). Assessment of Knowledge of AIDS and Beliefs About AIDS Prevention Among Adolescents. *AIDS Education and Prevention,* 2, 58-70.

Mays, V. M. (1989). AIDS Prevention in Black Populations: Methods of a Safer Kind. In V. M. Mays, G. W. Albee, & S. F. Schneider (Eds.), *Primary Prevention of Psychopathology, Vol XIII: Primary Prevention of AIDS: Psychological Approaches* (pp. 246-279). Newbury Park, CA: Sage.

McDermott, P. A. (1993). National Standardization of Uniform Multisituational Measures of Child and Adolescent Behavior Pathology. *Psychological Assessment,* 5, 413-424.

Pendergrast, R. A., DuRant, R. H. & Gaillard, G. L. (1992). Attitudinal and Behavioral Correlates of Condom Use in Urban Adolescent Males. *Journal of Adolescent Health,* 13, 133-139.

Perkel, A. D. (1992). Development and Testing of the AIDS Psychosocial Scale. *Psychological Reports,* 71, 767-778.

Peterson, A. C. & Hamburg, B. A. (1986). Adolescence: A Developmental Approach to Problems and Psychopathology. *Behavior Therapy,* 17, 480-499.

Quadrel, M. J., Fischhoff, B. & Davis, W. (1993). Adolescent (in) Vulnerability. *American Psychologist,* 48, 102-116.

Rotheram-Borus, M. J. & Koopman, C. (1991). AIDS and Adolescents. In R. M. Lerner, A. C. Petersen, & J. Brooks-Gunn (Eds.), *Encyclopedia of Adolescence, Vol 1: A-L* (pp. 29-36). New York, N.Y.: Garland Publishing, Inc.

Rotheram-Borus, M. J. & Koopman, C. (1992). Adolescents. In M. L. Stuber (Ed.), *Children and AIDS* (pp. 45-67). Washington, DC: American Psychiatric Press, Inc.

Sacco, W. P., Levine, B., Reed, D. L. & Thompson, K. (1991). Attitudes About Condom Use as a AIDS-relevant Behavior: Their Factor Structure and Relation to Condom Use. *Psychological Assessment: A Journal of Consulting and Clinical Psychology,* 3, 265-272.

Stevenson, H. C. (1994). The Psychology of Sexual Racism and AIDS: An Ongoing Saga of Distrust and the "Sexual Other." *Journal of Black Studies,* 25, 62-80.

Stevenson, H. C. & Davis, G. (1994). Impact of Culturally Sensitive AIDS Video Education on the AIDS Risk Knowledge of African-American Adolescents. *AIDS Education and Prevention,* 6, 40-52.

Stevenson, H. C., Davis, G., Weber, E., Weiman, D. & Abdul-Kabir, S. (in press). Gender Differences in Beliefs About AIDS Prevention Among Urban African American Youth. *Journal of Adolescent Research.*

Stevenson, H. C., Gay, K. M., & Josar, L. (1994). Culturally Sensitive AIDS Education and Perceived AIDS Risk Knowledge: Reaching the "Know-it-all" Teenager. *AIDS Education and Prevention,* 7, 134-144.

Weinstein, N. D. (1989). Perceptions of Personal Susceptibility to Harm. In V. M. Mays, G. W. Albee, & S. F. Schneider (Eds.), *Primary Prevention of Psychopathology, Vol XIII: Primary Prevention of AIDS: Psychological Approaches* (pp. 142-167). Newbury Park, CA: Sage.

Wyatt, G. E. (1994). The Sociocultural Relevance of Sex Research: Challenges for the 1990s and Beyond. *American Psychologist,* 49, 748-754.

Acknowledgement

The authors gratefully acknowledge the assistance of Paul A. McDermott, Ph.D. for his statistical input and Margaret Beale Spencer, Ph.D. for her comments on an early draft of this article.

Notes

1. 281 additional subjects were not included in the analyses because of failure to completely answer all of the items on the measures. A total of 350 subjects completed all data.
2. Alpha coefficients are based upon the scores of the 42 control subjects who completed all relevant measures in year three.
3. 149 additional subjects were not included in the analyses due to incomplete measures.

TABLE 1
FACTOR STRUCTURE OF THE BELIEFS ABOUT PREVENTING AIDS SCALE

ITEM	FACTOR LOADING
SELF-EFFICACY (ALPHA = .72)	
I know how to have safe sex.	.54
I plan on being very careful about who I have sex with.	.54
I will have safe sex even if people make fun of me for it.	.48
It doesn't bother me if others make fun of me because I believe in having safe sex.	.46
In the future I will always be able to practice safe sex.	.44
AIDS is a health scare that I will take very seriously.	.42
My partner will know I really care about him/her if I ask to use condoms.	.41
There is still time for me to protect myself against AIDS.	.39
In the future, whenever I have sexual intercourse with a member of the opposite sex, I plan to make sure we are using birth control.	.37
Not getting pregnant (or not getting a girl or woman pregnant) is very important to me.	.36
AIDS is the scariest disease I know.	.33
A person who gets AIDS has a good chance of being cured.[a]	.30
I feel almost sure that I will get AIDS.[a]	.30
SELF-CONTROL[b] (ALPHA = .71)	
If I wanted to have sex with a member of the opposite sex, and did not have protection,I would go ahead and have intercourse anyway.	.61
Once I get sexually excited, I lose all control over what happens.	.59
Trying to have safe sex gets in the way of having fun.	.58
Using condoms would be a sexual "turn off" for me.	.43
I have no control over my sexual urges.	.40

If I was going to have sex with someone and they made fun of me for wanting to have safe sex, I would probably give in.	.36
CONDOM EFFICACY (ALPHA = .58)	
If I ask to use condoms, it might make my partner not want to have sex with me.	.49
I would be too embarrassed to carry a condom around with me, even If I kept it hidden.	.48
I don't know how to use a condom.	.41
I would feel uncomfortable about buying condoms.	.39
People will think I am afraid of having sex if I bring up the subject of AIDS.	.37
There is a good chance I will get AIDS during the next 5 years.	.34
I have a high chance of getting AIDS because of my past history.	33

[a]ITEM WHOSE SCORE MUST BE REVERSED.
[b]ALL OF THE ITEMS IN FACTORS TWO AND THREE WERE REVERSED.

TABLE 2
MEAN SELF-CONTROL SCORES AS A FUNCTION OF GENDER, LEVEL OF SEXUAL ACTIVITY AND ACTUAL AIDS KNOWLEDGE

		ACTUAL AIDS KNOWLEDGE	
LEVEL OF SEXUAL ACTIVITY		LOW	HIGH
MALES			
	Not Active	21.43 (2.82)	19.17 (3.25)
	Active	15.81 (4.57)	20.13 (3.28)
FEMALES			
	Not Active	20.83 (3.56)	21.35 (2.57)
	Active	18.17 (4.71)	19.47 (4.45)

NOTE. NUMBERS IN PARENTHESES ARE STANDARD DEVIATIONS.

TABLE 3
MEAN SELF-CONTROL SCORES AS A FUNCTION OF RELIGIOSITY AND SELF APPRAISED AIDS KNOWLEDGE

SELF APPRAISED AIDS KNOWLEDGE			
RELIGIOSITY	LITTLE	SOME	A LOT
Not Religious	19.78 (3.73)	16.13 (4.15)	19.30 (3.85)
Moderately Religious	20.25 (4.71)	21.45 (2.92)	19.27 (4.46)
Very Religious	20.20 (4.92)	20.50 (3.03)	20.67 (3.89)

NOTE. NUMBERS IN PARENTHESES ARE STANDARD DEVIATIONS.

Figure Captions

Figure 1. Self-Control as a function of gender, sexual activity and actual AIDS knowledge.

Figure 2. Self-Control as a function of religiosity and self appraised AIDS knowledge.

Sexual Abstinence: A Viable Option for Young Adolescents in HIV/AIDS Prevention

Ifeanyi Emenike

What is Sexual Abstinence?

Sexual abstinence is the voluntary avoidance of sexual intercourse. It is the safest kind of sex because there is no exchange of semen, vaginal secretions, saliva, or blood. Abstinence can be taken to mean anything from avoiding all forms of sexual activity to avoiding only those, such as intercourse or oral sex, in which fluids are exchanged in a way that can transmit disease (Williams and Knight, 1994). There is no doubt that sexual expression is a natural form of animal behavior; indeed for the human species, sexual feelings can be a relatively constant experience. But people can choose to abstain from sexual activity. Certain people for religious reasons practice lifelong sexual abstinence (sometimes called celibacy, which literally means remaining unmarried). Some individuals refrain from sexual interaction, particularly sexual intercourse, until they marry. Still others refrain from sexual interaction because they fear the closeness and intimacy implied by sex or they have strong negative feelings regarding sex (Edlin and Golanty, 1992).

Sexual abstinence can also provide an opportunity to develop a new set of personal and relational experiences. It provides a way to discover new dimensions in interpersonal relationships. Without the distractions of sexual activities an individual can focus on self-development, career, or school, and put energy into long-time relationships. New relationships can also develop without the pressure for sex early in the relationship, thus permitting the partners to develop trust and caring before becoming sexual (Edlin and Golanty, 1992).

According to Cox, (1993), everyone has sexual feelings. Yet, before we express these feelings, we need to think about our own value system, our potential partner, and his or her feelings. We need to ask ourselves questions such as:

1. Will having sex with this person add to the relationship?

2. Am I (and is my partner) approaching sex freely or because of being talked into it or being made to feel guilty if sex is refused?

3. Is having sex in agreement with my own value system? My partner's?

4. Am I willing to risk a sexually transmitted disease, especially something as deadly as AIDS?

5. Will my decision hurt others? My partner? My friends? My parents?

Sexual Behavior of Teenagers

Trends concerning sexual behavior in the United States show that the percentage of adolescents reporting sexual intercourse is increasing, and that the age at which intercourse is first experienced is decreasing (Finkle and Finkle, 1983). The dramatic increase in the number of active teenagers represents an escalation in unwed teenage pregnancy and a magnification in the risk of sexually transmitted diseases (STDs including HIV/AIDS) (Jacobson, Aldana and Beaty, 1994).

An estimated 78 percent of adolescent girls and 86 percent of adolescent boys have engaged in sexual intercourse by age 20 (National Research Council, 1987, Sonnenstein, 1989). Clearly for young adolescents the most effective means of preventing possible physical and psychological problems related to sexual intercourse is total abstinence or perhaps a postponement of sexual activity. However, teenage sexual activity is a complex issue, embedded in family, social and economic factors. Intervention to prevent associated negative health outcomes must address those factors if they are to succeed.

Initiation of sexual intercourse by teenagers is associated with a number of factors, including academic achievement, religiousness, relationships between parents and their children, puberty, and other developmental characteristics, race and socioeconomic status. Sexual activity at young ages is more common among young adolescents from low socioeconomic status families, and among adolescents who smoke, use alcohol or other drugs, or have evidence of delinquency (Hogan, 1983, Jessor, et al., 1983, National Center for Health Statistics, 1985).

The increase in teenage sexual activity since 1970 has contributed to increases in STDs (including HIV/AIDS) (CDC, 1992). Many adolescents are at risk for exposure to the human immunodeficiency virus (HIV) because they experiment with high-risk behaviors, such as intravenous (IV) drug use and unprotected sexual intercourse (Haffner, 1988). Currently, approximately 21% of all acquired immunodeficiency syndrome (AIDS) cases are diagnosed in persons between 20 and 29 years of age, (CDC, 1987) and many of these cases resulted from HIV infection during adolescence. Furthermore, of 167,803 reported AIDS cases through February 1991, 659 cases involved 13 to 19-year olds, an increase of 173 cases from the number reported in 1990 (CDC, 1991).

Factors Influencing Sexual Behavior

It has been suggested that the primary reasons why many teenagers engage in sexual intercourse are peer or social pressure, curiosity, and sexual feelings/desires (Harris and Associates, 1986; Neuman and Beard, 1989). Developing sexually responsible attitudes and behaviors while fulfilling intimacy needs is part of the normal developmental process, beginning with adolescence. Attitudes and abilities to withstand peer and social pressure toward sex can be developed in three areas:

(a) the educational structure:

> Making intelligent choices based on fact requires sequential and accurate information with appropriate timing. It has been suggested that 51.4% of most sexual information is learned during the ages of 12 and 13 (Thornburg, 1981). However, schools only account for about 15% of information related to sex education (Thornburg, 1981), and less than 10% of adolescent children are exposed to anything approaching a meaningful sexuality education program (Gordon, 1986).

(b) the parent(s):

> Undeniably, familial environment influences teen sexual behavior. Indeed, teens who communicated with parents about sex were less likely to have sex than teens who had not communicated with

parents about sex (Moore, Simms, and Betsey, 1986). Early sexual experience can be linked to one or both parents': (1) early sexual experience (Newcomer and Udry, 1984), (2) low educational goals and poor education (Miller and Sneesby, 1988), (3) single status (Miller and Bingham, 1989), and (4) level of strictness and child supervision (Newcomer and Udry, 1984).

(c) and, a religious affiliation:

Religion has been related to teen sexual activity. Adolescents who reported attending church more frequently, and stated that religion was an important part of their lives, were less likely to have had sexual intercourse. Those with the highest level of sexual activity were more likely to have less religious affiliation (Thornton and Camburn, 1989).

Teenage Risk-Taking Behavior

Recent studies have found that most young people are knowledgeable about HIV/AIDS and safer-sex practices, yet many continue to practice high-risk sexual behavior (King and Anderson, 1994). Health risks are a significant issue for young adolescents. The Carnegie Council on Adolescent Development's report *Turning Points* (1989) estimated that seven million young people between the ages of 10 and 17 are highly vulnerable to high risk behaviors while another seven million are at moderate risk. These risky behaviors may result in health concerns that include sexually transmitted diseases, drug usage, and pregnancy. More recently, Scales (1991) concluded that if recent trends regarding young adolescents' health continue, these young people will have problems caused by early sexual activity and poor emotional health.

Current increase in sexually transmitted diseases makes it dangerous for anyone, especially young people to engage in casual sex. Initiation of sexual activity at a young age is a primary risk factor for unintended pregnancy. By age 21, approximately one in five young people have acquired a sexually transmitted disease. Because only some teenagers are sexually active, this amounts to a rate of at least 25% among those who are (CDC, 1989).

Sexual relationships among teenagers are often characterized by impermanence. The National Committee for Adoption (1985), indicated that as a result, 58% of sexually active young women aged 15 through 19 have had two or more sexual partners and seven percent have had 10 or more partners. The most recent data from the National Survey of Family Growth indicate that three quarters of young women have had sexual intercourse by their twentieth birthday.

Young's secondary analysis of a 1986 Harris Poll commissioned by Planned Parenthood showed that neither sex education nor knowledge are related to postponement of sexual intercourse or use of contraceptives among adolescents younger than 17: A knowledgeable 13-year-old is no more likely to use contraceptives than an uninformed 13-year-old. Young came to the conclusion that developmentally, younger teenagers are not able to effectively apply the knowledge that they have (Young, 1988). Thus educational programs must be age specific, promoting attitudes and skills that young adolescents can use until they gain more mature skills in managing their sexuality (Howard and McCabe, 1990).

Peers of the same gender are a major influence on adolescent attitudes about sexual activity. The proportion of their same-sex peers that teenagers believe are sexually active and how sexually active they believe them to be are powerful predictors of sexual experience among adolescent boys and girls (National Research Council, 1987). However, individual behavior and attitudes are more closely related to what adolescents think their friends are doing than what they are actually doing.

The Failure of Condom Education

America now has a track record of approximately 20 years of contraceptive-based sex education, where the emphasis has been on knowledge about sexuality, contraceptive methods and STDs (including HIV). However, during the period in which this knowledge has been disseminated, sexual activity has increased dramatically and, with it pregnancy rates and STDs (Bergman, 1993). Pediatrics (May, 1992) noted that "Knowledge about AIDS or HIV infection and its prevention was not associated with any change in risk behavior, nor were the number of sources of information about the epidemic, acquaintance with those who were infected, estimates of personal risk, or exposure to HIV counseling."

The April 1988 American Journal of Public Health reported that a study of condom education and distribution in San Francisco schools showed that a year-long effort resulted in only eight percent of males and two percent of females using condoms every time they had sex.

Condoms of American manufacture appear to have lower failure rates than those of foreign origin. It should be noted that condoms occasionally fail (approximately a 10% failure rate) due to manufacturing defects but more often due to human failure to use them properly. Thus, condoms are not a foolproof guarantee of avoiding HIV/AIDS infection.

The AIDS and HIV crisis of the mid-1980s caused an increase in the efforts to teach "safe" and then "safer" sex. Condoms were advocated as the solution (Bergman, 1993). What then is the better approach? The unequivocal answer is promoting abstinence as a viable option to young people all over the United States of America.

Abstinence is the Better Choice, Healthy People 2000: Risk Reduction Objectives

National health objectives for the year 2000 include efforts to reduce the number of adolescents who engage in sexual intercourse. These risk reduction objectives are:

> * Reduce the proportion of adolescents who have engaged in sexual intercourse to no more than 15% by age 15 and no more than 40% by age 17. (Baseline: 27% of girls and 33% of boys by age 15; 50% of girls and 66% of boys by age 17; reported in 1988) (CDC).
>
> * Increase to at least 40% the proportion of every sexually active adolescents aged 17 and younger who have abstained from sexual activity for the previous 3 months. (Baseline: 26% of sexually active girls aged 15 through 17 in 1988) (CDC).

According to a recent study of adolescents in Utah, half of the adolescents who reported that they were sexually active stated that they desired not to be (Governors Task Force on Teenage Pregnancy Prevention: 1988). Programs that address these feelings of ambivalence about sexual activity present these feelings as normal and encourage teens to postpone further sexual activity in order to avoid further risks to their health (U.S. Department of Health and Human Services, 1995).

Abstinence (avoidance) from both drugs and sex is the safest way to prevent HIV infection at the present time. Yet in our free and easy society, it is especially hard to say "NO" to sex. The advent of the birth control pill, bringing with it a revolution in sexual culture, has made it as difficult to say "NO" to sex as it used to be to say "Yes." The young person who says "No" to sex may be criticized by friends as being "uncool," "old-fashioned," "square," "a nerd," etc. Lines such as "Everyone does it," "If it feels good, do it," "If you loved me you would," are very hard to resist. Yet to say "Yes" these days puts one at a great risk of being exposed to HIV infection as well as other sexually transmitted diseases (Cox, 1993).

Many young people do not deliberately plan to have sex with their date, but end up saying "It just happened." Today, sex is too risky an activity to let it "just happen." There are too many serious consequences that can completely alter one's life to just let sex happen without thought and the exercise of personal responsibility (Cox, 1993).

According to Bergman (1993), an approach to sex education based on promoting abstinence from premarital sexual activity (that is, from behavior that causes teen pregnancy and spreads HIV and other STDs) must be instituted. This approach can encourage attitudes that lead to marriage and the formation of stable families.

About 50% of unmarried girls and 40% of unmarried boys aged 15 through 19 have not yet had intercourse. These people are practicing abstinence. Also 83% of Japanese teenage girls are virgins, and 73% of America's highest achieving high school students have never had sexual intercourse (Bergman, 1993).

Bergman (1993) noted that secondary abstinence is based on the idea that teens who have been sexually active can choose to stop. They can start all over. That is a sure way to protect not only their health but their lives.

Successful Programs Designed to Help Teenagers Postpone Sexual Intercourse

HIV/AIDS education has in the main emphasized the protective use of condoms with the assumption that young people are going to engage in sexual intercourse no matter what. This assumption is based on the failure of normal sex education to significantly reduce the number of young people engaging in sexual activities.

A study of adolescent development shows that cognitive growth lags behind physical maturation. Until about the age of 16 adolescents are still using concrete thinking skills. As a result, young teenagers have limited ability to recognize the potential impact of their choices; they are less likely than older teenagers to think about the future and consider the consequences of their actions (Howard and McCabe, 1990). These are well known scientific facts, but young people ought to be given the opportunity to make their choices based on all possible options, not on limited intellectual assumptions. By this, it is suggested that teenagers should be exposed to the concept of abstention or postponing sexual intercourse as a viable option.

There are currently a number of potentially promising behavioral intervention models designed to reduce the rate of onset of behaviors such as smoking in adolescents. These include: (a) interventions using a social influence model that aim to "inoculate" adolescents against negative social influences. This model is based on the concept that young people engage in such behaviors, including early sexual activity, partly because of societal influences, both in general and more specifically, from their peers. The model uses the public health concept of immunization as a strategy for combating social and peer pressures that encourage negative health behaviors. By exposing young people to these "noxious" social influences in small doses, while at the same time enabling them to examine such influences and develop skills to deal with them, this strategy helps young people eventually build up an "immunity" to them. Programs based on this model rely on specific activities that help students identify the origins of pressures to use drugs, drink or have sex, to examine the motivations behind those pressures and to develop skills to respond effectively; and, (b) interventions that aim to reduce adolescents' motivation to engage in specific negative behaviors by providing them with the life skills they will need to support their positive decisions. These interventions focus on increasing adolescents' competence in decision-making, building social skills and social supports, and enhancing self-esteem (Millstein, 1989).

Based on the knowledge that young teenagers do not respond to lectures, Emory University School of Medicine/Grady Memorial Hospital Teen Services Program developed a "Social Influence Model," an outreach program called Postponing Sexual Involvement. According to Howard and McCabe (1990), young people respond most favorably to programs promoting postponement of sexual intercourse when the information about how and why to say "no" comes from peers slightly older than themselves. The curriculum was presented to all eighth grade students (13-14 year-olds) in a local school system. The materials depicting "Postponing Sexual Involvement" were presented in a five session series by older, socially successful student leaders who were recruited, trained and supervised on-site. The program primarily focuses on the social and peer pressures that lead young people into early sexual involvement and on ways to resist such pressures. The emphasis is on why young people are having sex and how they might avoid it, rather than on the consequences of such behavior. Examples of pressures from the media as well as scenes depicting problems young people face in relating to peers are presented on video tape or slides in five classroom periods. Each session concentrates on variations of a single message — how and why to postpone sexual involvement.

The major goal of the Grady Memorial Hospital's Postponing Sexual involvement program given in eighth grade was to assist young people in postponing sexual intercourse. Overall, nearly three-quarters of the students in the program group had not had sexual intercourse before participating in the program. Based on the reports of these students, the study found that almost all (95%) who had not had sexual intercourse and who participated in the hospital's program felt the information personally would be helpful in saying no to sexual involvement. In fact, those who took part in the program did delay sexual involvement. By the end of eighth grade, students who had not participated in the program were as much as five times more likely to have begun having sex than were those who had taken part in the program. Program students were also more likely to continue to postpone sexual involvement. By the end of ninth grade, 24% of the students who were participants in the program had begun having sex, compared with 39% of those who were not. The program appeared to help both boys and girls to postpone sexual activity.

Other programs that have been successful in promoting abstinence among teenagers include the San Marcos, Texas, unified school district Teen AID abstinence program. Reported pregnancies dropped from 147 to 20, an 88% reduction. Similar programs (Sex Respect, Best Friends, Free Teens) have shown very promising results. For example, students who received the Sex Respect curriculum show significant changes in attitude over the course of their participation. There are consistent increases in the extent to which students (grades seven through nine) feel that sex among unmarried teens is wrong and that teens who have sex outside of marriage would benefit by deciding to stop and wait for marriage.

Research supports widely held beliefs that adolescents can also respond positively to directive counseling from adults about sexuality. One such research supports the creation of environments within communities that support teen decisions to postpone sexual activity. Some successful programs have taken a community approach involving the media, the school and the clergy in preventing teenage pregnancy. Barrier methods, particularly the condom, provide substantial protection against sexually transmitted diseases, but are most likely to be used ineffectively by adolescents because they are not generally effective users of any protective measures. Thus, decreasing the level of sexual activity should significantly improve adolescent health by decreasing unintended pregnancies and sexually transmitted diseases, particularly HIV infection (Bergman, 1993).

The philosophy of Postponing Sexual Involvement by Howard and McCabe, (1990) is that:

> * Persons younger than 16 are not able to fully understand the implications of their actions.
>
> * Persons younger than 16 generally are not mature enough to deal with the consequences of their sexual actions. Furthermore, the needs that young people are trying to meet through sexual intercourse could be met in other ways.
>
> * Young people under 16 are often pressured into doing things they really do not want to do. Teenagers report that social pressure is the chief reason why their peers do not wait until they are older to have sexual intercourse. Pressure to have sexual intercourse comes from peers and also from images presented by the media.

Truly 100% safe sex means abstinence. Particularly for young people, abstinence may be a very wise choice; it protects them from the dangers of situations in which they may lose sexual control, and it guarantees that they will indeed have many years in the future for safe and fulfilling sex (Hales, 1991). The once popular view of adolescence as a period of inevitable storm and stress has been replaced by one that emphasizes the potential of this developmental stage for constructive adaptation and maturation (Millstein, 1989).

The April 1993 American Journal of Public Health states that we should be able to agree that premature initiation of sexual activity carries health risks. Therefore, we must exercise leadership in encouraging young people to postpone sexual activity. Adolescents are bombarded with messages encouraging them to "do it." We need to strive for a climate supportive of young people who are not having sex and so help to create a new health-oriented social norm for adolescents and teenagers against premature sexual activities.

References

Bergman, W. L.(1993). It's Not Just AIDS: Uninformed and Misinformed, Teens Face an Epidemic of Sexually Transmitted Diseases. *The World and I.* The Washington Times Corporation.

Carnegie Council on Adolsescent Development. (1989). *Turning Points: Preparing American Youth for the 21st Century.* New York: Carnegie Corporation.

Centers for Disease Control. (1991). *Division of STD/HIV Prevention Annual Report, 1990.* Atlanta: U.S. Department of Health and Human Services, Public Health Service.

Centers for Disease Control. (1990). *Sexually Transmitted Disease Surveillance, 1989.* Atlanta, GA.

Cox, F. D.(1993). *The AIDS Booklet.* Dubuque, IA: Wm. C. Brown Publishers.

Discussion Guide on Human Sexuality. (1987). Atlanta: Emory/Grady Memorial Hospital.

Edlin, G., and Golanty, E. (1992). *Health and Wellness: A Holistic Approach.* Boston: Jones and Bartlet Publisher.

Emory/Grady Teen Services Program. (1987). *Making Responsible Decisions.* Atlanta: Grady Memorial Hospital.

Finkle, M. C., and Finkle, D. J. (1983). Male Adolescent Sexual Behavior, the Forgotten Partner: A Review. *Journal of School Health,* 53(9), 544-547.

Gorden, S. (1986). What Kids Need to Know. *Psychology Today,* 20(10), 22-24.

Harris, L., et al. (1986). *American Teens Speak: Sex Myths, TV, and Birth Control.* The Planned Parenthood Poll (Project No. 864012). New York: Planned Parenthood Federation of America.

Haffner, D. W. (1988). AIDS and the Adolescent: Education Must Begin Now. *Journal of School Health.* 58, 154-155.

Hein, K. (1993). "Getting Real" About HIV in Adolescents. *American Journal of Public Health.* 83(4), 492-494.

Hales, D. (1991). *Your Health.* Redwood City, CA: The Benjamin/Cummings Publishing Company Inc.

Howard, M. and McCabe, J. B. (1990). Helping Teenagers Postpone Sexual Involvement. *Family Planning Perspectives,* 22(1), 21-26.

Jacobson, H. R., Aldana, S. G., and Beaty, T. (1994). Adolescent Sexual Behavior and Associated Variables. *Journal of Health Education* 25(1), 10-12.

Kegeles, S. M. et al. (1988). Sexually Active Adolescents and Condoms: Changes Over One Year in Knowledge, Attitude and Use. *American Journal of Public Health,* 78(4), 460-461

King, B. M. and Anderson, P. B. (1994). A Failure of HIV Education: Sex Can Be More Important Than a Long Life. *Journal of Health Education.* 25(1), 13-18.

Ku, L., Sonnenstein, F. L., and Pleck, J. H. (1993). Factors Influencing First Intercourse for Teenage Men. *Public Health Reports,* 106(6), 680-694.

Miller, B. C. and Bingham, C. R. (1989). Family Configuration in Relation to Sexual Behavior of Female Adolescents. *Journal of Marriage and the Family,* 51, 499-506.

Miller, B. C. and Sneesby, K. R. (1988). Education Correlates of Adolescents' Sexual Attitudes and Behavior. *Journal of Youth and Adolescence,* 17, 521-530.

Millstein, S. G.(May, 1989). Adolescent Health: Challenges for Behavioral Scientists. *American Psychologist,* 44(5), 837-842.

National Committee for Adoption. (1985). *Adoption Factbook: United States Data,*

Issues, Regulations, and Resources. Washington DC: The Committee.

National Research Council. (1987). *Risking the Future: Adolescent Sexuality, Pregnancy and Childbearing.* Washington DC: National Academic Press.

Neuman, B. and Beard, B. J. (1989). Teen Sexuality in a Rural Community. *Journal of Community Health Nursing,* 6(4), 245-253.

Newcomer, S., and Udry, R. (1988). Adolescent Honesty in a Survey of Sexual Behavior. *Journal of Adolescent Research,* 3, 419.

Public Health Service (1995). *Healthy People 2000: National Health Promotion and Disease Prevention Objectives-full Report, with Commentary.* Washington DC: U.S. Department of Health and Human Services, Public Health Service, DHHS Publication No. (PHS) 91-50212.

Scales, P. C. (1991). *A Portrait of Young Adolelscents in the 1990s: Implications for Promoting Healthy Growth and Development.* Chapel Hill, NC: Centers for Early Adolescence.

Sonnenstein, F. L. and Pittman, K. (1984). The Availability of Sex Education in Large City School Districts. *Family Planning Perspective,* 16, 19-25.

Thornburg, M. D. (1981). Adolescent Sources of Information on Sex. *Journal of School Health,* 51, 274-277.

Thornton, A. D. and Camburn, D. (1988). Religious Participation and Adolescent Sexual Behavior. *Journal of Marriage and Family,* 51, 641-653.

Udry, J. R. and Billy, J. (1987). Initiation of Coitus in Early Adolescence. *American Social Review,* 52, 841-855.

Williams, B. K., and Knight, S. M. (1994). *Healthy for Life: Wellness and the Art of Living.* Pacific Grove, CA: Brooks/Cole Publishing Company.

Young, M. (1988). *The Planned Parenthood Poll: A Secondary Analysis of National Data.* Paper presented before the American Alliance for Health, Physical Education, Recreation and Dance, Kansas City, Mo., April 6-10.

Selected Bibliography

Airhihenbuwa, C. O. (1995). *Health and Culture: Beyond the Western Paradigm.* Thousand Oaks, CA: Sage Publications.

Airhihenbuwa, C. O. (1989b). Perspectives on AIDS in Africa: Strategies for Prevention and Control. *AIDS Education and Prevention,* 1, 57-69.

Airhihenbuwa, C. O., DiClemente, R. J., Wingood, G. M. & Lowe, A(1992). AIDS Education and Prevention Among African-Americans: A Focus on Culture. *AIDS Education and Prevention,* 4, 267-276.

Bell, N. K. (1989). AIDS and Women: Remaining Ethical Issues. *AIDS Education and Prevention,* 1, 22-30.

Cochran, S. D. (1990). Women and HIV Infection: Issues in Prevention and Behavior Change. In V. M. Mays, G.W. Albee, & S.F. Schneider (Eds.),*Primary Prevention of AIDS:Psychological Approaches.* Newbury Park, CA: Sage Publications.

Dawit, S. (1993). Women and AIDS. In G. Young, V. Samarasinghe & K. Kusterer (Eds.), *Women at the Center.* West Hartford, Connecticut: Kumarian Press.

Fisher, J. D. (1988). Possible Effect of Reference Group-based Social Influence on AIDS-risk Behavior and AIDS Prevention. *American Psychologist,* 43, 914-920.

Fullilove, M., Fullilove, R. E., Haynes, K. K. and Gross, S. (1990). Black Women and AIDS Prevention: A View Toward Understanding the Gender Rules. *Journal of Sex Research,* 27(1), 47-64.

Gwede, C. & McDermott, R. J.(1992). AIDS in Sub-saharan Africa: Implications for Health Education. *AIDS Education and Prevention,* 4(4), 350-361.

Hankins, C. A. (1990). Issues Involving Women, Children, and AIDS Primarily in the Developed World. *Journal of Acquired Immune Deficiency Syndrome,* 3, 443-448.

Low, N., Egger, M., Gorter, A., Sandiford, P., Gonzalez, A., Pauw, J., Ferrie, J. & Smith, G. D.(1993). AIDS in Nicaragua: Epidemiological, Political and Socio-cultural Perspectives. *International Journal of Health Services.* 23(4), 685-702.

Mays, V. M. & Cochran, S. D. (1988). Issues in the Perception of AIDS Risk and Risk Reduction Activities by Black and Latino Women. *American Psychologist,* 43, 949-957.

Mitchell, J. L.(1988). Women, AIDS and Public Policy. *AIDS and Public Policy Journal,* 3(2), 50-52.

Morales, E. S.(1987). AIDS and Ethnic Minority Research. *Multicultural Inquiry and Research on AIDS,* 1, 2.

Nichols, M. (1990). Women and Acquired Immunodeficiency Syndrome: Issues for Prevention. In B. Voeller, J. M. Reinisch, & M. Gottlieb (Eds.), *AIDS and Sex:*

An Integrated biomedical and Biobehavioral Approach. New York: Oxford University Press.

Obbo, C. (1993). HIV transmission: Men are the Solution. In S. M.James & A. P. A. Busia (Eds.), *Theorizing Black Feminisms: The Visionary Pragmatism of Black Women.* New York: Routledge.

Overall, C. & Zion, W. P. (Eds.)(1991). *Perspectives on AIDS: Ethical and Social Issues.* New York: Oxford University Press.

Peterson, J. L. & Bakerman, R. (1989). AIDS and IV Drug Use Among Ethnic Minorities. *Journal of Drug Issues,* 19(1), 27-37.

Pyne, H. H. (1995). AIDS and Gender Violence: The Enslavement of Burmese women in the Thai Sex Industry. In J. Peters & A. Wolper (Eds.), *Women's Rights human rights.* New York: Routledge.

Schinke, S. P., Botvin, G. J., Orlandi, M. A., Schilling, R. F. & Gordon, A. N. (1990). African-American and Hispanic-American Adolescents, HIV Infection, and Preventive Intervention. AIDS Education and Prevention, 2(4), 305-312.

Scott, S. J. & Mercer, A. M. (1994). Understanding Cultural Obstacles to HIV/AIDS Prevention in Africa. *AIDS Education and Prevention,* 6(1), 81-89.

Sepulveda J., Fineberg, H. & Mann J. (1992). *AIDS, Prevention Through Education: A World View.* New York: Oxford University Press.

Seidel, G. (1993). The Competing Discourses of HIV/AIDS in Sub-Saharan Africa: Discourses of Rights and Empowerment vs. Discourses of Control and Exclusion. *Social Science and Medicine,* 36, 175-194.

Stevenson, H. C., Gay, K. M. & Josar, L. (1995). Culturally Sensitive AIDS Education and Perceived AIDS Risk Knowledge: Reaching the "Know-it-all" Teenager. *AIDS Education and Prevention,* 7(2), 134-144.

Stevenson, H. C. & White, J. J. (1994). AIDS Prevention Struggles in Ethnocultural Neighborhoods: Why Research Partnerships With Community Based Organizations Can't Wait. *AIDS Education and Prevention,* 6(2), 126-139.

Stevenson, H. C. & Davis, G. (1994). Impact of Culturally Sensitive AIDS Video Education on the AIDS Risk Knowledge of African-American Adolescents. *AIDS Education and Prevention,* 6(1), 40-52.

Sullivan, C. (1991). Pathways to Infection: AIDS Vulnerability Among the Navajo. *AIDS Education and Prevention,* 3(3), 241-257.

Walters, J. L., Canady, R. & Stein, T. (1994). Evaluating Multicultural Approaches in HIV/AIDS Educational Materials. *AIDS Education and Prevention,* 6(5), 446-453.

Weiss, E. & Gupta, G. R. (1993). Women Facing the Challenge of AIDS: Prevention and Policy Concerns. In G. Young, V. Samarasinghe & K Kusterer (Eds.), *Women at the Center.* West Hartford, CT: Kumarian Press.

Contributors

Caroline Blair is Project Officer, AIDS at the Kenya Country Office of the United Nations's Fund (UNICEF).

Nora K. Bell (Argyle/Denton) is currently the Dean of Arts and Sciences at the University of North Texas and Professor of Philosophy/Bioethics. She was formerly the Director of the Center for Bioethics at the University of South Carolina. She is a member of the Board of Directors of the National Leadership Coalition on AIDS. She received the South Carolina Women of Achievement Award in 1992, was a Commissioner on the South Carolina Commission on Aging from 1989—1993 and is listed in Who's Who Among University Teachers.

Lawrence Brown is affiliated with the Addiction Research and Treatment Center (ARTC). He is Assistant Clinical Professor of Medicine at Columbia University College of Physicians and Surgeons and an Attending Physician in the Department of Medicine at Harlem Hospital Center.

Betty W. Carrington is currently a CNM Research Associate in the Department of Obstetrics and Gynecology at the Harlem Hospital Center and is a Fellow of the American College of Nurse-Midwives.

John B. F. De Wit is Assistant Professor in the Department of Social and Organizational Psychology, University of Utrecht, the Netherlands.

Ifeanyi N. Emenike is Assistant Professor of Health Education at Benedict College, Columbia, South Carolina.

Sepali Guruge is involved in numerous community and volunteer activities with a special interest in the Tamil community in Toronto. Presently, she is conducting a joint project with Lynn Morrison and Kym Snarr to identify social/cultural and behavioral factors that may put the Tamil-speaking Sri-Lankan population of Toronto at risk for HIV/AIDS.

Dishon Gogi is the District Health Education Officer in Homa Bay District, Kenya.

Edward J. Hart is a Professor of Health Promotion at Bridgewater State College, Bridgewater, Massachusetts. He was formerly the Chairperson, Department of Health Education, State University of New York, Cortland, New York. He has published three books and several articles in professional journals. He is a consultant to many professional organizations.

Harm J. Hospers is Assistant Professor in the Department of Health Education and the Research Institute Health, Maastricht HEALTH University, the Netherlands.

Deborah J. Isenberg is the Training Coordinator for the Emory HIV/AIDS Mental Health Training Project and a Masters candidate in the Rollins School of Public Health of Emory University, Atlanta, Georgia.

Gerjo Kok is Professor and Scientific Director in the Department of Health Education and the Research Institute Health, Maastricht HEALTH University, the Netherlands.

Marietta Federici-Lafarge is a graduate student in Forensic Psychology. She is a volunteer of the Manhattan Plaza AIDS Project for the past nine years. She teaches cancer and AIDS patients the use of yoga skills to reduce stress and pain.

Patricia O. Loftman is the Director of Midwifery Services at the Harlem Hospital in New York City and a CNM authority in HIV education and health care of HIV infected women.

J. Stephen McDaniel is the Principal Investigator for the Emory HIV/AIDS Mental Health Training Project; Medical Director of Mental Health Services at Grady Health System Infectious Disease Program; Instructor of Family and Preventive Medicine and Assistant Professor of Psychiatry and Behavioral Sciences, Emory University School of Medicine, Atlanta, Georgia. His work on the paper in this volume was supported by Grant #1T15MH19894 from the Substance Abuse and Mental Health Services Administration, Center for Mental Health Services.

Debra G. Morris is the Training Director for the Emory HIV/AIDS Mental Health Training Project; Training Coordinator for the Southeast AIDS Training and Education Center, and Senior Associate, Department of Family and Preventive Medicine, Emory University School of Medicine, Atlanta, Georgia.

Lynn Morrison is currently a doctoral student in the Department of Anthropology at the University of Toronto. She is the Principal Investigator of a study on health and social issues including risk factors for HIV/AIDS in the Tamil-speaking Sri Lankan community of Toronto. Her past research experience in Romania focused on pediatric AIDS in the orphanages. She is the AIDS Education Coordinator of a project funded by the city of Toronto, at Ryerson Polytechnic University.

Frank Machlica is currently the HIV/AIDS Program Coordinator/Senior Consultant for the New York City Department of Mental Health, Mental Retardation and Alcoholism Services. His career includes eight years of experience in agency-based practice providing individual, family and group psychotherapy to children and adults. He is the HIV/AIDS program coordinator in charge of community based organizations and mental health services. He has written several documents including *HIV/AIDS Mental Hygiene Services in New York City.*

Janet L. Mitchell is chief of Perinatology at the Harlem Hospital Center in New York City and was the Principal Investigator for PHREDA.

Kabahenda-Nyakabwa earned a Masters Degree in Family Sociology from the University of Manitoba, Canada. She is a member of the Canadian Institute for Research on the Advancement of Women, The Women's Project AIDS Committee of Ottawa, the Canadian Association of African Studies and the Ottawa Chapter of UNIFEM.

Pearila B. Namerow is Associate Professor of Clinical Public Health in the Center for Population and Family Planning of Columbia University School of Public Health. During the PHREDA study (1989), she coordinated data management and analysis.

Uchenna C. Nwosu is Professor in the Department of Obstetrics and Gynecology, James H. Quillen College of Medicine, East Tennessee State University, Johnson City, Tennessee. He is widely published in several professional journals and serves as a consultant to various organizations.

Jerome O. Okafor is a Senior Lecturer in the Department of Health and Physical Education at Nnamdi Azikiwe University, Awka, Nigeria. He has published several textbooks on Health Education and articles in professional journals.

David Ojakaa is an independent consultant on family planning and AIDS.

S. A. Ochola is the Medical Officer of Health in Homa Bay District, Kenya.

Tim Rodgers was a doctoral candidate in Health Education at Southern Illinois University until his death in October, 1994. During the last few years of his life, he worked and studied extensively on the impact of HIV/AIDS on public health and society in general. He was actively involved in developing the groundwork for the Southern Illinois Regional Effort for AIDS (SIREA). The results of his commitment to maintain and improve the health and well-being of individuals who are infected with HIV continue to have long-lasting effects. This article was submitted on his behalf by Mark J. Kittleson, Department of Health Education, Southern Illinois University at Carbondale.

Helen M. Rupp is a doctoral student in the Psychology in Education Division, Graduate School of Education at the University of Pennsylvania.

Howard C. Stevenson is an Assistant Professor in the Psychology in Education Division, Graduate School of Education at the University of Pennsylvania. His work in this volume was supported in part by a W. T. Grant Foundation.

Robin Y. Swift is a Faculty Training Consultant for the Emory HIV/AIDS Mental Health Training Project and the Southeast AIDS Training and Education Center, and Senior Associate, Department of Family and Preventive Medicine, Emory University School of Medicine, Atlanta, Georgia.

Rosalind Thompson was the Project Coordinator of PHREDA study from 1989—1992. She is presently the Project Director of the Harlem Birth Right Community Health Dialogues and Initiatives Project which is funded by the Centers for Disease Control.

Minakshi Tikoo is an Assistant Professor in the College of Human Ecology, Kansas State University. She has published articles on Human Sexuality in professional journals.

Davidson C. Umeh is an Associate Professor in the Department of Physical Education and Athletics, John Jay College of Criminal Justice, The City University of New York. He has published articles in edited books and professional journals.

Charles B. U. Uwakwe is a Senior Lecturer in the Department of Guidance and Counselling at the University of Ibadan, Ibadan, Nigeria. He has published several articles on HIV/AIDS in professional journals and presented papers in conferences.

Claudia L. Windal is the HIV/AIDS Case Manager in the Indian Health Board of Minneapolis, Inc. Minneapolis, Minnesota.

Sterling B. Williams was the Chief of the Department of Obstetrics and Gynecology at the time of the PHREDA study at Harlem Hospital Center. He is a member of faculty of Columbia University College of Physicians and Surgeons. He is currently Associate Director of the Department of Obstetrics and Gynecology of the Columbia Presbyterian Hospital of New York City.

Gust A. Yep is a Professor in the Department of Speech and Communication Studies at San Francisco State University. He has contributed chapters in several books and published many articles in professional journals. He has received several research grants, teaching and service awards. He is a member of the Editorial Board for the *Journal of Social Behavior and Personality*.

INDEX

Sexuality, 9, 18, 30, 35-36, 49-51, 55, 62, 64, 66, 79, 81-83, 85-91, 99, 174, 178, 198-200, 204, 208-210, 212, 214, 221-222, 228-229, 244, 258-260, 276, 299-300, 302-303, 305, 319, 321, 325-327